ETHNOVETERINARY RESEARCH
AND DEVELOPMENT

ETHNOVETERINARY RESEARCH & DEVELOPMENT

Edited by
CONSTANCE M. McCORKLE, EVELYN MATHIAS
and
TJAART W. SCHILLHORN VAN VEEN

INTERMEDIATE TECHNOLOGY PUBLICATIONS 1996

Intermediate Technology Publications
103/105 Southampton Row, London WC1B 4HH, UK

© This selection: Constance M. McCorkle, Evelyn Mathias
and Tjaart W. Schillhorn van Veen

A CIP catalogue record of this book is available from the British Lit

ISBN 1 85339 326 6

Typeset by J&L Composition Ltd, Filey, North Yorkshire
Printed in UK by SRP Exeter

Contents

1. Introduction: ethnoveterinary research and development[1]

EVELYN MATHIAS, CONSTANCE M. McCORKLE
and TJAART W. SCHILLHORN VAN VEEN

THE TWENTIETH CENTURY has witnessed spectacular advances in both human and animal medicine and in both plant and animal agriculture. As a result, human lifespans and global food production have increased dramatically. These advances have, however, been accompanied by staggering population growth and by widespread environmental degradation in the form of biodiversity loss, water pollution, soil erosion and infertility, and much more. Moreover, while many people have benefited from these advances, many have not. In human healthcare, for example, 80 to 90 per cent of the planet's inhabitants still rely mainly on traditional treatments and practitioners, that is, on ethnomedicine (Duke 1992:59, WHO, cited in Plotkin 1988:260). Similar figures appear to hold for livestock and ethnoveterinary care. Yet prospects for the universal extension of 'high-tech' or high-input Western-style medical and agricultural technologies are dim when viewed in the context of such technologies' soaring prices, the shaky economies and politics of many nations, and burgeoning human and livestock populations. Nor is this to mention other considerations such as the escalating costs of generating new technological breakthroughs, consumer demand for more wholesome 'natural' products, or the growing threat of chemoresistance. Thus, whether in poor, Third World countries or in the relatively rich countries of the First World, the economic, environmental and biomedical sustainability of many modern technologies has been called into serious question.

Consequently, scientists and developers are increasingly searching for alternative paradigms—social as well as technical—to achieve continued progress in medicine and agriculture. This search is on-going in both human and veterinary medicine, plant and animal agriculture, First and Third Worlds, and at grassroots as well as government levels. It focuses on concerns such as affordability, environmental friendliness, socio-organizational and institutional manageability or 'implementability', and hence sustainability.

In biomedicine, these concerns have led to greater interest in and acceptance of disciplines previously relegated to the fringes of Western medical/veterinary practice: osteopathy, homoeopathy, acupuncture, chiropractic and herbal and holistic medicine. These are now seen as valid alternatives or complements to conventional approaches. (For discussions or examples of such trends in human medicine see Bannerman *et al.* 1983, Chesworth, in press, Eisenberg *et al.* 1993, Jacobs 1993, NIH 1994, WHO 1991a, 1991b; for veterinary medicine, Baïracli Levy 1991, deMaar 1992, Schoen 1994 and in progress.) Particularly noteworthy for veterinary medicine is the emergence of recognized professional societies such as the American Holistic Veterinary Medical Association, the American Veterinary Chiropractic Association and the International Veterinary Acupuncture Society.

In both First and Third World countries, the search for alternatives has also triggered a re-evaluation and appreciation of 'ethnoscience': local or indigenous knowledge and methods of cropping, stockraising, healing, managing natural resources, and so forth (Brokensha *et al.* 1980, McCorkle 1989a, Warren 1991a, 1991b, Warren *et al.* 1995). This sort of empirical agro-ecological and medical know-how has been elaborated down through generations; and it continues to be developed or modified by local groups as their ecological, economic, social, demographic and other circumstances change. Often, it is unique to a given culture or society and historically well-adapted to its biophysical and human ecologies. Usually it is transmitted orally rather than in writing. And it forms the basis for much of local-level decision-making and action in many facets of daily life.

Ethnoveterinary medicine constitutes one branch of ethnoscience. As the present volume suggests, ethnoveterinary research, development and extension (hereafter, ER&D) have emerged as a fertile field for the generation or regeneration and transfer of appropriate and sustainable medical/veterinary alternatives to people everywhere, but especially to Third World stockraisers. Briefly, ER&D can be defined as:

> . . . the holistic, interdisciplinary study of local knowledge and its associated skills, practices, beliefs, practitioners, and social structures pertaining to the healthcare and healthful husbandry of food-, work-, and other income-producing animals, always with an eye to practical development applications within livestock production and livelihood systems, and with the ultimate goal of increasing human well-being via increased benefits from stockraising
>
> (McCorkle 1995:53).

The paramount goal of ER&D is to further the search for development alternatives at the intersection of medicine and agriculture—that is, livestock healthcare—by building upon local veterinary and husbandry knowledge, practice and *materia medica* plus their associated human and socio-structural resources so as to increase the number of reliable animal healthcare options that are readily, comprehensibly, cost-effectively and sustainably available to producers generally. ER&D can also contribute to environmental health and conservation by identifying environmentally sound stockraising practices. It achieves these goals mainly through rescuing, testing, applying and disseminating little-known or disappearing local healthcare and husbandry knowledge and practice. Typically, traditional healers and stockraisers are themselves enlisted as partners in this effort. Often ER&D also leads to the enrichment of ethnoveterinary practice through inputs of formal scientific knowledge (and vice versa), a process referred to as techno-grafting or, more commonly, techno-blending.

The principal beneficiaries of (and participants in) ER&D are livestock producers. In this regard, it should be noted that virtually all rural peoples raise some species of livestock, from which they derive a galaxy of agricultural, ecological, nutritional, economic, social, cultural/religious and even psychological benefits (Fox and McCorkle 1995, McCorkle 1994c, 1994d or in press-b, and the references cited therein). Suffice it to say here that livestock indisputably constitute 'a driving force for food security and sustainable development' (Sansoucy 1994) as well as for human well-being generally.

ER&D seeks especially to serve smallholder stockraisers—including many peri-urban farmers (Mathias-Mundy *et al.* 1992) and women—and poor or remote rural groups who cannot afford or lack access to conventional veterinary services. Of course, having medical alternatives is important to *all* stockraisers whenever an emergency arises requiring immediate action to ameliorate a health problem, slow disease progression, or at least ease the patient's pain long enough for more specialized help to be called in.

While interest in ethnoveterinary medicine has grown dramatically over the last two decades (next section), a critico-analytic volume presenting the many facets, efforts and outcomes in this field has been lacking. The present anthology seeks to fill this gap. The chapters that follow offer reviews and case studies of ethnoveterinary knowledge and practice from different continents and societies, along with historical perspectives, theoretical discussions and methodologies of ER&D. The book seeks mainly to provide researchers, developers, and policy-makers working in agricultural and rural development with insights, ideas and approaches to the conduct of ER&D, plus ways to apply its results. At a broader level, however, the volume's overview of work in ER&D suggests a useful model for the study and application of local knowledge generally (McCorkle 1995). In this regard, the findings and experiences reported here will be of interest to professionals in other development sectors, as well as to academics interested in the applied health, agricultural, environmental and social sciences.

Ethnoveterinary R&D

Background and rationale
Since the domestication of animals some 10 000 years ago, stockraisers and handlers have naturally been concerned about livestock health (Bierer 1955). Probably for just as long, keepers of animals have been experimenting with and developing their own veterinary theories and techniques. Schwabe's chapter comparing ancient Egyptian veterinary knowledge and skills with the beliefs and practices of present-day Nilotic herders signals the depth of some ethno-veterinary traditions, along with the antiquity of such techniques as basic surgery and herbal veterinary medicine. The chapter by Anjaria notes a similarly long tradition of culturally unique veterinary medicine in India, documented as early as 269 BC (see also Shirlaw 1940). Indeed, the oldest known veterinary texts originate from Egypt, India and China (for example, Lin and Panzer 1994). The latter nation is particularly renowned for its early elaboration and use of acupuncture in animal healthcare, which is still based on the same principles and essentially the same techniques and equipment today.[2]

In fact, until the early 1900s most veterinary practices could be considered 'traditional' in the sense that they derived from long experience and underwent little fundamental change in many of their tools and techniques. For their *materia medica*, historically both human and animal medicine have relied heavily on plant materials. Indeed, most of today's major pharmaceutical companies started, a century ago, by selling plant extracts (Mez-Mengold 1971); and approximately a quarter of all prescription drugs currently sold in the Western world still use active ingredients derived from plants (Cox and Balick 1994). With the discovery of modern chemotherapeutics in the twentieth century, however, the First World began to abandon much of its own medical/veterinary tradition in favour of what is now viewed as conventional medicine.

This conventional paradigm is the one that—along with its costly bureaucratic institutions and infrastructure requirements—development projects have endea-voured to transfer to the Third World, typically in a heavy-handed top–down mode. However, certainly in veterinary medicine, these attempts have encoun-tered repeated and growing difficulties, for a host of reasons (for example,

Cheneau 1985, CTA/GTZ/IEMVT 1985, Daniels *et al*. 1993, de Haan and
Bekure 1991, de Haan and Nissen 1985, Leonard 1987, 1993, Schillhorn van
Veen 1993, 1994, Schillhorn van Veen and de Haan 1994, Umali *et al*. 1992,
Ward *et al*. 1993). It has become evident that, as in high-tech human medicine,
conventional veterinary medicine and formal-sector resources alone are inadequate for meeting the basic animal healthcare needs of a great many of the
world's stockraisers in any sustainable way. Thus, as Stem's chapter describes
for a number of livestock projects, in the mid-1970s scientists and developers
began to look increasingly to local healthcare knowledge, praxis and practitioners for fresh ideas that were more 'practical, low tech, and cost-effective'
(FAO 1991).

The origin and evolution of ethnoveterinary medicine as a recognized field of
R&D have been detailed elsewhere (McCorkle 1986). Here, only some of the
more integrative or sustained efforts in ER&D are referenced, for the convenience of readers interested in further case examples or additional continent-,
country- or species-specific information beyond that presented in this volume.

In these regards, an illustrative but critico-analytic annotated bibliography of
261 sources on ethnoveterinary medicine is available (Mathias-Mundy and
McCorkle 1989), as is a descriptive and largely non-duplicative data base of
300 items dealing mainly with ethnoveterinary botanicals (Zeutzius 1990). Other
significant bodies of work include: the pioneering studies in seven Asian nations
supported by the Food and Agriculture Organization of the UN (FAO–RAPA
1980 to 1992); also for Asia, an information kit on traditional animal healthcare
practices (IIRR 1994); the collective *oeuvre* of Tufts University's international
programmes in veterinary medicine (see Stem's chapter) and of the Small
Ruminant Collaborative Research Support Program (for example, Bazalar and
McCorkle 1989, Mathias-Mundy and Murdiati 1991 and 1992, McCorkle 1982
and 1989b, and other Mathias or McCorkle references cited below; Wahyuni *et
al*. 1991), including an analytic overview of ER&D in Africa (McCorkle and
Mathias-Mundy 1992); also for Africa, a compendium of ethnoveterinary treatments (Bizimana 1994) and the proceedings of a forward-looking conference on
ER&D continent-wide (Kasonia and Ansay 1994); and worldwide, a compilation
of ethnoveterinary ectoparasiticides in the tropics (Matzigkeit 1990) plus a
recent issue of the *Revue Scientifique et Technique de l'Office International
des Épizooties* (OIE 1994) devoted to traditional veterinary practices.

Principles and approaches
A paramount principle of ER&D is recognition of the complexity of variables
that impinge upon animal health and husbandry. These include both endogenous
and exogenous factors, defined respectively as internal and external to etiological agents and their hosts. Endogenous factors are essentially the purview of
veterinary science *per se*, at least etically. Exogenous factors span the biophysical, socio-cultural and religious, economic, educational, even legislative and
political systems in which animals and their keepers are embedded. Exogenous
factors naturally also embrace all husbandry and herding operations with implications for animal health.

As the professional diversity of the contributors to this volume testifies, the
interplay of so many variables defies the reach of any one scientific or development discipline. It also lies beyond the ken of scientists and development
experts alone. The perspectives and knowledge of the various social groups

involved in stockraising and in any associated operations that have implications for animal or human health (for example, produce harvesting, handling, processing, marketing, consumption) are equally imperative. This imperative reflects one of the fundamental tenets of ER&D: its equal attention to local actors' own (emic) knowledge and experience in all relevant realms, as well as to outsiders' Western-scientific (etic) understandings.

A corollary of the foregoing principles is that of holism: that is, in order to achieve any significant and sustainable net improvements in human well-being via stockraising, healthcare problems must be defined and tackled within the totality of endogenous and exogenous, emic and etic factors and insights. Otherwise, ER&D could 'succeed' at increasing livestock health and productivity but perhaps only by compromising environmental health or by stealing resources from other development sectors, such as cropping, crafting or social investments, for example, in family health or children's education (see McCorkle 1992 and 1994a and by Stem, this volume).

Methodological approaches to ER&D are many and eclectic, mirroring and often cross-cutting the diversity of factors and disciplines outlined above. Although the field as a whole is perforce multidisciplinary, there is need for unidisiciplinary library, laboratory and field investigations in order to provide important data-specific, contextual and comparative pieces of ER&D information that ultimately contribute to the holistic understanding of the animal healthcare puzzle. Such investigations might include: ethnosemantic, ethnobotanical, socio-economic, epidemiological and other surveys; obviously, review of the pertinent literature in human as well as veterinary medicine plus a search of historical, ethnographic and other records; bioassays, pharmacological tests *in vitro* and on lab animals *in vivo*; standard clinical, diagnostic, or other analyses of healthcare conditions; on-station and on-farm experiments with the livestock species of interest; gap-filling field or 'point' studies on virtually any health-related aspect of the livestock system under study; and more. This array of methods is illustrated or referenced throughout the present volume, and is also implied in the multiplicity of topics treated in ER&D (next section).

In its fullest and most dynamic form, however, ER&D emphasizes firsthand fieldwork undertaken ideally by an interdisciplinary team that includes not only scientists and developers but also men and women producers themselves, all working together under the real-world conditions to which the target beneficiaries and their animals are subject. In varying forms and degrees, such participatory approaches have come to characterize much of agricultural R&D (Okali *et al.* 1994). Acting as co-researchers and -developers, producers have immediate input into the definition of R&D problems. They then take active roles in the design, implementation and monitoring of on-farm trials to address the problems thus flagged.[3] Of course, as the final authority on end-user satisfaction, producers serve as the expert evaluators of ER&D outcomes. The chapters by Grandin and Young, McCorkle and Bazalar, Roepke and Stem all illustrate participatory aspects of ER&D.

When it comes to diffusing the information, practices or technologies thus validated or generated, then interested stockraisers, traditional healers, or veterinary input suppliers like traders and community storekeepers may also assume extension roles (Grandin and Young, Stem, McCorkle and Mathias, in progress). Thus, an R&D team is created that embraces not only scientists and the usual government or NGO (non-governmental organization) extensionists but also producers *cum* 'ethnoscientists', plus local volunteers, healthcare practitioners or businesspeople—with each of these groups contributing from their respective funds of knowledge, skills and collegial or community networks.

Topics in ER&D

With the history, evolution and general methodological approaches of ER&D already sketched above, below we turn to the multiplicity of other topics treated in ER&D (Table 1). Reference is made throughout to chapters in this volume that touch upon each issue, although not all topics can be fully represented between the covers of a single book. For greater detail on the subject matter outlined in this and the concluding section, readers are referred especially to Mathias-Mundy and McCorkle 1989 or 1995, Mathias and McCorkle, in press, McCorkle 1995.

Table 1. Topics in ethnoveterinary research and development

ER&D as a Field of Study
o History and evolution
o Methods

Ethnoveterinary Knowledge
o Semantic and taxonomic systems
o Etiology and diagnostics
o Epidemiology

Ethnoveterinary Practice
o Pharmacology and toxicology
o Immunization
o Surgery
o Manipulative and mechanical techniques
o Housing, feeding and watering
o Herding strategies
o Reproduction and genetics
o Pest, parasite and predator control
o Product harvest and by-product management
o Medico-religious practices

Applied/Develpment Topics
o Technology development
o Enterprise development
o Environmental topics
o Healthcare delivery
o Public health
o Education
o Socio-cultural and socio-economic topics
o Planning, policies and institutions

For analytic purposes, the following overview distinguishes ethnoveterinary knowledge from practice. The former informs, guides, and is expressed through the latter. Here, 'knowledge' should be understood as referring to cognitive phenomena; that is, how people classify livestock diseases; how they conceptualize the interrelationships, functions, and malfunctions of different organs and physiological systems; how they theorize about disease causation, progression, and modes of transmission, and thus settle upon one or another diagnostic hypothesis. These cognitive processes in turn guide selection of therapeutic (curative), prophylactic (preventive), or other (sale, slaughter) practices in response to disease. Both knowledge and practice figure in a third topical category in ER&D: their application in development contexts.

Ethnoveterinary knowledge

Semantic and taxonomic systems Ethnoscientific vocabularies and taxonomies for types of forages, varieties and classes of animals, the pests and, above all, the diseases that afflict livestock can be detailed and elaborate. Diseases are most often classified according to clinical signs (see within, Delehanty, Hefferman *et al.*) or perceived causes, whether natural or supernatural (see, Brisebarre, Lawrence, Perezgrovas, Shanklin). Epidemiological observations may also play a role (Heffernan et al., Köhler-Rollefson). The nature and the biosocial, geographic or demographic distribution of local terms and taxonomies for animal disease are often recorded as a first step in ER&D, with the aim of matching these to their approximate Western equivalents. As many of the foregoing authors demonstrate, rarely is there a one-to-one fit between ethnoveterinary semantic systems and Western-scientific ones, however.

Etiology and diagnostics A great deal of ethnoveterinary research—and nearly every chapter in this volume—has explored the causes local people assign to livestock disease and their corresponding ethnodiagnostic approaches. Even within a single culture, ethnoetiologies and -diagnoses may span both indigenous and introduced (Delehanty), traditional and modern (Brisebarre) ones. Besides post-mortem observations arising out of stockraisers' natural interest in elucidating disease causes and effects (Heffernan *et al.*), as Schwabe points out, necropsies and surgical procedures performed for religious or magical reasons have also long been a source of etiological and diagnostic (as well as physiological and anatomical) information in ethnoveterinary medicine. *Ceteris paribus*, however, ethno-diagnoses rely mainly on visible clinical symptoms, although some pastoralists have developed surprisingly accurate diagnostic tests (Köhler-Rollefson).

In addition to naturalistic observations, supernatural considerations also appear to figure in nearly all ethnoveterinary systems. These are not necessarily conflicting (see Medico-religious practices, below). Overall, however, research suggests that supernatural etiologies and diagnoses are most common for diseases that cause sudden death, are newly introduced, or have no easily detectable etiological agents or any clinical or post-mortem signs that are visible to the naked eye (Bonfiglioli *et al.*, Delehanty, Heffernan *et al.*).

Epidemiology In the course of examining local disease etiologies and prophylactic measures, most ER&D studies conducted at field level deal at least implicitly with ethno-epidemiological knowledge (for example, Heffernan *et al.*, Perezgrovas, Vondal). However, Grandin and Young make explicit provision for systematic investigation of this topic in their methodology for the collection and use of ethnoveterinary data. To date, ethno-epidemiology appears to have received the most explicit attention in connection with pastoral movements to avoid disease or manage its incidence. This is especially true for Africa (for example, Bonfiglioli *et al.*, Köhler-Rollefson, Schillhorn van Veen), where pastoralists control a great deal of often very subtle epidemiological knowledge (also see Immunization, below). A number of these and other studies (Shanklin, for example) also mention stockraiser awareness of epidemiological threats attendant upon the acquisition of new stock. And in her discussion of Saami reindeer raising, Anderson introduces an entirely new epidemiological concern: nuclear fall-out.

Ethnoveterinary practice
Pharmacology and toxicology Pharmacology is probably the most extensively studied domain of ethnoveterinary medicine. Almost no publication in ER&D— or any chapter in this volume—fails at least to mention the medicinal plants and other materials used to treat animals. Many also provide considerable historical and/or scientific information on the materials in question as well as pertinent findings from the literature in human pharmacology, pharmacognosy and phyto-chemistry (for example, Anjaria, Brisebarre, Malik *et al.*, Roepke). Ethnoveter-inary studies also often include details on specific local drugs and their modes of preparation, routes of administration, posology and reported or observed effects—nearly all of which mirror those of conventional pharmaco-therapeutics and -prophylaxis. However, Brisebarre reports on one, less familiar, technique: French shepherds' use of medicinal bouquets.

Compared to the wealth of literature on ethnoveterinary pharmacology, ethno-toxicology has received scant attention, despite the facts that poisonous plants figure prominently in all pharmacopoeia and that most stockraising peoples (especially pastoralists) possess considerable knowledge of the toxic plants in their environment. Ibrahim's chapter on ethnotoxicology among Nigerian agro-pastoralists thus constitutes an especially welcome contribution.

Immunization Descriptions of indigenous vaccinations mainly centre on those for poxes, contagious bovine pleuropneumonia, ecthyma and rinderpest (Bon-figlioli *et al.*, Köhler-Rollefson, Schillhorn van Veen), although many more are attested to in the wider literature. African pastoralists (ibid.), Indian poultry raisers, and other groups also have a number of indirect immunization techni-ques that, instead of vaccination, rely on the controlled exposure of animals to contagious disease.

Surgery Traditional surgical procedures found the world over and most frequently described in the literature span wound care, castration, venipuncture and other forms of bleeding, and branding/cauterization. Also commonly men-tioned are bone-setting, excision of tumours, lancing of abcesses, rumen trocar-ization and a panoply of obstetric procedures. (See Bonfiglioli *et al.*, Ghirotti and Woudyalew, Heffernan *et al.*, Lawrence, and Schwabe.) The larger literature also records a wide variety of surgical operations carried out for husbandry, hygiene, safety, identification or aesthetic purposes. These include hoof-trimming, nose-ringing, dental surgery, docking, dehorning, ear-cropping or -notching and horn-training.

Manipulative and mechanical techniques Massage, acupressure, hydrother-apy and exercise all fall into this category. Beside their therapeutic uses, many such procedures are aimed at 'seasoning' or 'conditioning' animals to the rigours of their environment and the duties required of them. Lawrence describes several such techniques employed by North American Indians to strengthen their horses; others are mentioned in Köhler-Rollefson's chapter on camel care in North Africa and India, and in Vondal's discussion of duck raising in Indonesian Borneo.

Housing, feeding and watering Most long-time stockraising peoples are aware of the relationship between adequate housing, feeding and watering on the one hand, and good animal health on the other (Ibrahim and Abdu, Perezgrovas, Shanklin, Vondal). Traditionally, such husbandry practices are usually closely adapted to a wide range of localized variables: climate, available construction and feed materials, predators, household socio-economic situation, and of course the ethology, sex, age, strength and reproductive status of the animals in question.

Herding strategies Under rangestock or pastoral conditions, herding strategies are a vital aspect of animal healthcare. Via herd or flock movement, mixed grazing, herd dispersal, quarantine/isolation, delayed turnout and still other strategies like social strictures on seasonal use of rangelands, traditional herding systems typically embody astute measures for avoidance of disease-bearing pests and climatic stresses, control of contagion and provision of key vitamins and minerals that promote animal health and productivity (Anderson, Bonfiglioli *et al.*, Köhler-Rollefson, Perezgrovas, Schillhorn van Veen). Although herding is most often thought of in regard to ruminants and sometimes pigs, poultry may also be herded. According to Indonesian duck farmers, for example, herding is crucial to their birds' fitness and disease resistance (Vondal).

Reproduction and genetics Like other aspects of animal husbandry, practices related to breeding can have direct implications for livestock health. Such practices may include controlling mating times, taking special precautions in the hygiene and feeding of breed stock, and of course selecting for tolerance or resistance to disease. The latter may be a conscious, intentional act—as when immigrant Fulani enhance their herds' adaptation to the diseases of a new area by breeding their cows with local bulls (Schillhorn van Veen). But genetic traits that make for better adaptation to local environments and husbandry regimes can also be favoured by management practices and beliefs that are performed for other reasons, including magical or religious ones (Ibrahim and Abdu).

Pest, parasite and predator control Indigenous control methods for pests, parasites and predators are many and diverse. Besides those already alluded to above, they can include: erecting fences and other kinds of barriers around livestock quarters, manually removing ectoparasites, lighting smudge fires near animal quarters, keeping companion species that kill and eat offending or disease-bearing rodents and insects or that guard against predators, seeing that stock regularly wallow or bathe, burning over or fencing off areas where diseased animals have died so as to prevent reinfestation, modifying habitat in various ways (burning, brush clearing) to make it less hospitable to dangerous species, co-ordinating grazing and watering hours with times of low pest activity, and many more. Bonfiglioli *et al.*, Ibrahim and Abdu, Köhler-Rollerfson, Perezgrovas and Schillhorn van Veen refer to several of such strategies.

Product harvest and by-product management Topics in this category span such activities as culling/slaughtering, dairying, and carcass, offal and product use—all in relation to how local practices may forestall or favour disease transmission among livestock or between livestock and humans. For example, people may bury or burn the carcasses of animals with diseases believed to be highly contagious or contaminating; or they may boil the meat extra-long before consuming it. Ferlo herders make sure to wash their hands after touching the flesh of an animal dead of certain diseases before they handle a healthy beast (Bonfiglioli *et al.*); but Samburu pastoralists almost invariably consume blood drawn from sick animals, no matter what the disease (Heffernan *et al.*); and Saami reindeer raisers are uncertain as to how best to cleanse their meat products of radioactive contamination (Anderson).

Medico-religious practices Almost innumerable studies attest that magic and religion form an integral part of ethnoveterinary practice. Schwabe's research on this topic has already been mentioned. Ghirotti and Woudyalew's, Perezgrovas', and Lawrence's descriptions of, respectively, bull castration in Ethiopia, equine healthcare among North American Indians, and Tzotzil Maya sheep management are representative of many more such cases of the interweaving of sacred and secular in animal healthcare and husbandry. Brisebarre and Shanklin also find hints of this interplay in both France and Ireland.

Indeed, people often surround their practical animal healthcare and husbandry measures with magical and religious ones such as prayers to saints and other supernatural beings, amulets and fetish bundles, chants and ceremonies, ritual feedings, or other kinds of special, apparently extra-medical attention[4] (much as Westerners may offer up prayers, send flowers or hold masses for a hospitalized friend or family member). But this does not necessarily mean that the associated veterinary or husbandry responses are irrelevant to the etically identified health problem. On the contrary, considerable epidemiological knowledge and practical veterinary acumen may be encoded in local cosmology and theology—as Ibrahim and Abdu discover in their study of Nigerian poultry raising.

In like vein, although ethnoetiologies and diagnoses are sometimes cast in a supernatural idiom, they can nevertheless lead to appropriate healthcare measures. For example, many stockraising peoples attribute some livestock diseases to supernatural phenomena like evil spirits and winds that haunt certain locales or that manifest at certain times of the day or night. Frequently, these explanations closely correlate with naturalistic phenomena such as: times and places where parasites, their hosts, or vectors abound; micro-climatic conditions that stress animals or foster the proliferation of poisonous plants, harmful bacteria, fungal mycotoxins, etc.; or sites where infectious spores lie long dormant in the soil, awaiting their next victims. One common ethnoveterinary response to such evils—avoiding them—certainly makes good 'sense' (for example, Köhler-Rollefson, Perezgrovas, Schillhorn van Veen).

Applied/development topics in ER&D

Technology development As the chapters in this volume attest, ethnoveterinary medicine includes a wide spectrum of techniques that are effective and that work well 'as is' under local management systems. Many botanicals and other traditional medicines offer valuable alternatives for the treatment of wounds, skin diseases, parasitism and poisoning. A number of traditional immunization techniques also have value. Numerous local surgical, manipulative/mechanical, husbandry and herding techniques can also be confidently and readily applied and extended. And as noted just above, even some medico-religious beliefs and procedures that may seem bizarre or irrelevant to outsiders can have practical medical value or promote rational responses to disease threats.

Furthermore, ethnoveterinary medicaments, practices and understandings are often amenable to enhancement through techno-blending, frequently in a way that adds little or nothing to their cost or complexity. Roepke's participatory experiments with Sukumu stockraisers of Tanzania are illustrative of techno-blending in its most basic and cost-effective form. He merely contributed 'outsider' insights on pharmacological activity, dosages and treatment schedules to his local co-researchers' knowledge in an effort to make some of their useful home remedies even more effective. McCorkle and Bazalar report similar ER&D experiences in the Andes, including an instance of techno-blending that entailed the rescue of an indigenous topical treatment for bovine and equine ectoparasitism and its reformulation as a reliable and cost-effective sheep dip.

But technology development based on ER&D findings is not limited solely to circumscribed rural contexts in the Third World, nor even just to livestock. Ethnoveterinary pharmacognosy and pharmacology, for example, can help discover or re-discover (Roepke) and disseminate knowledge about the medicinal value of plants and other *materia medica*. As a rule, plants employed in traditional medicine worldwide are two to five times more likely to test out as pharmacologically active than any random sample of plants (Daly 1983:226); and worldwide, nearly all the same botanicals used with livestock are also employed for humans (Anjaria, Malik *et al.*). Thus pharmacological findings from ethnoveterinary medicine can be shared between countries or regions, and often between animals and humans. (For a recent example of a rigorous trial involving the testing and transfer of an ethnoveterinary treatment to humans, see van Puyvelde 1994.)

Modern science has also drawn upon local knowledge of animal healthcare and husbandry in other realms, to the benefit of both Third and First Worlds. For example, traditional immunization methods in part gave rise to the idea of protecting livestock by exposing them to a 'cocktail' of local disease strains combined with controlled treatment.[5] And the value of cross-breeding for disease resistance with local breeds—which has long been known to many stockraising peoples—is now receiving considerable formal experimental attention (WIIAD 1992). Studies like Ibrahim and Abdu's, which detail local people's knowledge of livestock varieties and breeds, can point the way to invaluable but as-yet-untapped animal genetic resources. In the global search for more sustainable production systems, still other non-pharmacological aspects of ethnoveterinary medicine offer clues for the design of environmentally sound techniques of integrated pest and disease management (see Environmental topics, below).

Enterprise development Another topic in ER&D is the creation or reinforcement of local services, trade and industry based on ethnoveterinary knowledge and practice. In addition to the development or strengthening of privatized local healthcare delivery services (see below), particularly promising is the possibility of establishing, reinforcing or expanding local and national enterprises that produce packaged or manufactured versions of ethnoveterinary medicines. In rural market-places around the world, local residents and traders can be seen buying and selling medicinal plants and other traditional *materia medica*. Of course, livestock healers also often realize earnings in cash or kind from the preparation and administration of ethno-pharmaceuticals. In addition, in some regions (notably Asia), small firms produce trademarked veterinary drugs based on traditional botanicals. In India, for example, there are between 60 and 80 such firms (Anjaria). Besides supplying the national market, some of these products are exported internationally to satisfy the growing demand for drugs that are believed less expensive or more natural than Western commercial ones.

Large or small, all such enterprises provide employment and income-generating opportunities. With additional R&D input to validate or enhance the efficacy and uses of traditional treatments, there are tantalizing prospects for further enterprise development and expansion. Of course, as Anjaria points out, there are some potential testing, quality control, pricing and other problems in commercializing traditional drugs; but as he also notes, some creative solutions are possible.

Environmental topics Although little discussed in the present volume, some ER&D efforts have experimented with protecting biocultural diversity by actively encouraging the environmentally sensitive use and enterprise development of ethnopharmaceuticals. Maintenance of biological diversity has been promoted by assisting herders or traditional livestock healers to establish home gardens for medicinal plants that are fast disappearing in the wild, or by helping communities to organize into co-operatives for the protection, controlled harvesting and sale of sylvan botanicals. At the same time, maintenance of *cultural* diversity is encouraged, in the form of renewed status, increased earnings and new entrants for the practitioner groups who hold and apply the ethnomedical knowledge of biodiverse resources.

Indeed, much of ethnoveterinary R&D is motivated by concerns for environmental health, either alone or as it relates to human health. Like Ibrahim's chapter, the larger literature on ethnopharmacology suggests that traditional treatments based on natural materials and prepared and administered according to time-tested prescriptions and regimens tend to be environmentally more benign than their Western commercial equivalents.[6] They may be less effective but also pose less danger of seriously polluting local water supplies, lands or animal-based foodstuffs. For example, treatment based on or modelled after ethnoveterinary techniques might offer alternatives to the industrial pesticides used in dips (Heffernan *et al.*, Ibrahim, McCorkle and Bazalar, Shanklin) or some of the pharmaceuticals used in livestock production (like broad-spectrum antibiotics, hormones and steroids) that have triggered widespread fears about pollution, chemo-resistance and dangerous residues in food.

The relative benignity of traditional drugs and pesticides can make them even more attractive when stockraisers have comparatively little understanding of the use of potent Western pharamaceuticals (Grandin and Young, Heffernan *et al.*, Stem). And it bears repeating that many ethnoveterinary responses to disease involve no chemotherapy whatsoever. They instead rely on the non-pharmacological practices described earlier, many of which produce bonuses for environmental and human health. For example, as described by Perezgrovas, the Tzotzil habit of bucket-watering sheep not only wards against ovine fasciolosis; it also protects riparian habitat (and its often unique flora and fauna) from degradation or disturbance by trampling and grazing, and it keeps livestock from fouling streams or wells from which humans may also obtain their water supplies. To take another example, ethnoveterinary methods for controlling disease-bearing pests of livestock can have pay-offs for human health insofar as the same pests host etiological agents or transmit diseases of humans, too (for example, fasciolosis, malaria, schistosomosis, trypanosomosis).

Healthcare delivery ER&D has experimented with some promising alternatives or complements to Western models of top-down delivery of veterinary care and information. These consist of programmes to train local healers, producers or producer organizations and suppliers of veterinary inputs (like community storekeepers and itinerant traders) in the provision of basic healthcare information and of both modern and traditional drugs and treatments. The goal of such programmes is for trainees to become economically self-sustaining community-based healthcare workers or extensionists (Grandin and Young, Heffernan *et al.*, Schwabe, Stem). Worldwide, perhaps nearly 100 such 'paraveterinary' projects have been initiated to date (McCorkle and Mathias, in progess).

As Schwabe points out, there are also possibilities for the joint delivery of human and animal healthcare. This is because, everywhere, much the same remedies and treatment techniques are applied to both livestock and humans (for example, Anjaria, Ibrahim, Roepke); and in many Third World societies, the same healthcare practitioners often deal with both human and non-human patients.[7] One example among many such multi-species practitioners described in the larger literature are the Dinka *atet* discussed by Schwabe.

Public health Another area in which ER&D findings have been applied is public health. In particular, several authors point to some innovative possibilities for local people to support hard-pressed government agencies in the job of epidemiological surveillance and disease control. To launch effective and cost-efficient programmes of disease control, planners need timely and detailed information about a country's or region's livestock disease situation. ER&D has shown that paravets and stockraisers themselves can be instrumental in systematically recording and reporting the incidence of livestock disease, especially in remote areas that might otherwise go unmonitored (Grandin and Young, Stem). Their field-level information can provide a much-needed corrective to data that otherwise are often obtained only by research institutes on experimental farms.[8] This corrective makes for more tightly targeted public health responses, which are consequently more effective and less costly (Schwabe). Delehanty further notes that structured data on ethnoveterinary knowledge and vocabulary may save on expensive laboratory diagnostics and, via improved communication with producers, can facilitate campaigns to control any disease threats identified.

Education Several contributors to this volume explicitly highlight education as a social-sector topic that should be addressed by, and benefit from, ER&D. As Bonfiglioli *et al.* observe, primary schools and functional literacy programmes throughout the Third World suffer from a paucity of practical subject matter and reading materials that are relevant to rural students' cultural heritages and everyday life. The result is low student motivation. These authors describe several experiences in which findings from ER&D were directly useful in responding to these problems.

In like vein, Ibrahim and Abdu note that in Nigeria, as in many Third World nations, agricultural curricula have few roots in the country's own culture. Echoing similar sentiments by Roepke, they urge the insertion of ethnoveterinary information into secondary-school, university, and vocational training in veterinary medicine and animal science. In these contexts, ER&D findings can greatly improve present and future researchers' and extensionists' communication with clients, increasing their respect for useful ethnoveterinary practices and beliefs while at the same time providing a clearer understanding of what kinds of help clients most need.[9]

Socio-cultural and socio-economic topics As the prefix 'ethno' (from the Greek for 'people', 'culture') suggests, ER&D views local social mechanisms for implementing animal healthcare and husbandry practices as equal in importance to the practices themselves. These social structures vary across cultures and can be classified into many different biosocial (McCorkle 1994a) activities (herding, milking, healing, trading, storekeeping), or other kinds of groups with responsibilities in animal care, product handling or management of the natural resource base upon which stockraising depends. The social dynamics and distribution of healthcare/husbandry knowledge, roles, skills, labour availability and communication networks are topics that receive attention in almost any field-level work in ER&D. Groups may differ in these attributes according to sex, age, wealth, ethnicity, healer-specialist or other occupational status, depth of stockraising tradition and experience at rearing a particular species (Brisebarre, Delehanty, Grandin and Young, Heffernan *et al.*, Lawrence, Schwabe, Shanklin, Stern).

Still other socio-cultural considerations can influence producer decisions and actions in their animal healthcare and husbandry: sacred or secular cultural values ascribed to one or another species (Perezgrovas, Shanklin); notions of human-animal relations and moral standards pertaining to the welfare of animals as sentient social beings (for example, Ibrahim and Abdu, Lawrence); the stigma or prestige attaching to different treatment types (see Brisebarre); proprietary control over ethnomedical knowledge (ibid., Ghirotti); and of course numerous economic and production-system factors (see below). Grandin and Young's Ethnoveterinary Interview Guide provides a tool for investigating such decision-making issues; and Ghirotti's chapter on recourse to traditional versus modern medicine for people and livestock in the Sidama region of Ethiopia represents one of the few studies to make a start at quantitatively tackling some of them.

All such socio-cultural intelligence is vital for the success of both basic and applied work in ER&D. Some examples of where such information is needed include: identifying the most knowledgeable groups, from whom to collect expert ethnoveterinary information; conversely, determining which groups are most lacking in healthcare and husbandry savvy (ethno- or otherwise); determining how such knowledge is differentially acquired, refined and transmitted; selecting the best candidates for participation in field trials or for training as paraveterinarians; targeting and transferring technologies and information to the appropriate recommendation domains; and still more.

Given that one of the paramount practical goals of ER&D is the provision of cheaper (as well as more socio-culturally appropriate and accessible) veterinary options, many contributors to this volume mention economic implications of ER&D. They may do so in broad terms (Anjaria, Ibrahim and Abdu, Malik *et al.*, Roepke). Or they may discuss rough economic pros and cons of ethno- versus Western veterinary approaches in specific socio-economic and agro-ecological settings for a particular health concern (Köhler-Rollefson on camel trypanosomosis, McCorkle and Bazalar on ovine parasitoses, Stern on helminthosis and avitaminosis A) or for particular species (Shanklin on sheep versus cattle, Vondal on ducks). Another recurrent theme is the budgetary advantage of governments' drawing upon local human resources for healthcare delivery, extension and epidemiological surveillance (Delehanty, Schwabe, Stern). Schwabe describes several preliminary economic analyses of the kinds of surveillance-and-selective-action and intersectoral programmes mentioned above under Healthcare delivery. But in the present volume, only Stern reports on any rigorous research to measure relative treatment costs and benefits of local ways of handling a disease versus those advocated by Western-trained veterinarians or extensionists.

Planning, policies and institutions In ER&D as in development generally, participatory approaches have been increasingly acknowledged as critical to successful planning and implementation. A 'knowledge of local knowledge', practices, concepts and vocabulary is a necessary first step in facilitating true participation. In this respect, even simple semantic and taxonomic investigations in ER&D have multiple direct and indirect uses: gauging different producer groups' knowledge and concern about different livestock diseases (Grandin and Young, Shanklin); winning stockraisers' interest, trust and willingness to participate in field trials (Stem); and obviously, facilitating communication between producers and developers for planning, extension, training and still other purposes (Delehanty, Grandin and Young, Heffernan *et al.*). At a broader level, all such methods and tools for stimulating people's participation in livestock development constitute a topic for ethnoveterinary research in themselves (Bonfiglioli *et al.*, Delehanty, Grandin and Young, Stem). Experiences to date clearly suggest that the sustainability of development efforts can be improved by bringing local stakeholders and their knowledge, skills and social organizations into the planning cycle.

At least one author (Anderson) also sees a need for greater producer influence on livestock-related policymaking. Although not discussed in the present volume, a policy arena of growing concern is that of intellectual property rights in relation to the commercial development of technologies and enterprises based directly on local know-how (see especially Swanson 1995).

Indeed, findings from ER&D have implications for almost innumerable policy and institutional arenas. (See again the discussions of healthcare delivery, public health and education.) In general, technological, sociological, and epidemiolocial data derived from ER&D often suggest the advisability of re-examining the policies and the institutional practices and structures of livestock research or extension agencies to check that they are geared to develop and deliver truly appropriate technology and information. Such agencies can increase their effectiveness and decrease their costs by establishing policies and procedures that build upon ER&D findings, for example, by taking R&D cues from existing ethnoveterinary knowledge and practice (a majority of the chapters in this volume, but perhaps especially Ibrahim and Abdu's, McCorkle and Bazalar's, Perezgrovas', Roepke's and Vondal's), by identifying and addressing clients' expressed desires for certain types of research assistance or extension information (Anderson, Brisebarre, Stem), and by focussing on specific lacunae in local veterinary knowledge (Grandin and Young, Heffernan *et al.*).

Although not all are treated in the present volume, other pertinent policy arenas include: drug control and import/export laws; food safety regulations; agricultural or agribusiness subsidies; government incentives or disincentives for different entities (NGOs, for example) to undertake ER&D legislation concerning the organization of local self-help groups; and certification policies for paraveterinarians. Anderson, Anjaria, Grandin and Young, Heffernan *et al.* and Ibrahim touch upon some of these issues, illustrating how ER&D findings can be translated into better policymaking and more effective use of scarce institutional resources on behalf of stockraisers, consumers and national economies.

Future directions in ER&D

As the first of its kind, the present volume can only hint at the many potential benefits of studying and applying ethnoveterinary knowledge and practice. Table

2 summarizes these benefits as outlined above and as so far suggested by ER&D overall. Although attention to ethnoveterinary medicine has increased exponentially over the last decade or so, a great deal of urgent and exciting work still lies ahead for new generations of 'ethnoveterinarians'. (For a more comprehensive overview of work needed in the study and application of local knowledge generally, see Mathias 1995.)

Awareness-raising and recording

As already acknowledged in human ethnomedicine, most urgent is the recording—but always in holistic context—and preservation of the world's rich but highly endangered store of ethnoveterinary knowledge and practice (IIRR 1996). Heretofore, much valuable local savvy has been discarded or denigrated as mere oddity, superstition or nonsense. ER&D has an important role to play in changing such attitudes. Many researchers and developers face the challenge of 'un-learning' pseudo-scientific dogma that modern must always and everywhere

Table 2. Potential benefits from ethnoveterinary research and development

○ Increased animal healthcare choices for a wider range of producers as a result of identifying, validating and perhaps techno-blending cheaper or more accessible alternatives.

○ Technologies, practices, practitioners and healthcare delivery systems that are more user-friendly (more familiar, comprehensible, socio-culturally acceptable) than conventional ones.

○ Discovery of new drugs, treatments and healthcare concepts useful not only in veterinary but also human medicine.

○ Stimulation of rural and/or national economies and industries through income-earning opportunities and job creation in the areas of medicinal plant production, product development and sales, and localized practitioner services.

○ Encouragement for the maintenance of biocultural diversity.

○ Improved environmental health and reduced health risks to humans as well as animals.

○ Cost savings and improved quantity, quality, and timeliness of information in epidemiological surveillance and disease-control programmes.

○ Development spinoffs and synergisms in other sectors such as education and human healthcare.

○ Greater respect among scientists, developers and extensionists for their clients and for their clients' existing expertise.

○ Better development planning and implementation, policymaking and institution-building, resulting from improved communication with producers and their active participation and input.

○ Renewed respect among producers themselves for their own veterinary know-how; re-invigorated social structures and practitioner statuses; and through participation, transfer of R&D skills to the local level—all of which empower people to take greater control of their own animal healthcare development needs and agendas.

replace traditional (Brisebarre, Roepke). Likewise for producers who have internalized outsiders' negative assessments of their ethnoveterinary know-how. As Bonfiglioli *et al.* recount, producers' participation even in something as basic as recording this know-how can restore confidence in their ability to take a proactive role in tackling development problems themselves. At the same time, participatory recording exercises and *in situ* conservation initiatives (Agrawal 1995) help halt the erosion of local healthcare alternatives that often make very good sense.

For applied/development purposes, however, room must be also made in the recording process for systematic attention to lacunae in ethnoveterinary knowledge (Grandin and Young, McCorkle 1995). There is also need for socio-linguistically more sophisticated recording methods, like those designed by Delehanty. With rare exceptions (one is Bonfiglioli *et al.*), researchers have lacked the formal semantic training—and often, too, the cultural grounding—that would forestall simplistic judgements as to the etic equivalents of emic terminology and concepts.[10] This can engender negative assessments of valuable ethnoveterinary savvy. Conversely, as all these authors point out, the production of carefully researched vocabulary lists, texts, field manuals and computerized data bases can elucidate, enhance and extend the use and usefulness of such savvy.

Validation and methodology design

While recording and translating local knowledge and practice can be an empowering and informative experience, for ethnoscience to be broadly and ethically put to use, ultimately some means of sorting what works from what doesn't work, and under what conditions, is required (see the discussion in McCorkle and Bazalar). Although ethnoveterinary practices by and large have withstood the test of time—in effect, undergoing extensive empirical field trials by local people—such informal testing typically has been limited to specific regions, species, socio-economic conditions and production systems. In addition, traditional dosages and safety standards may be vague. Also, local knowledge is imperfect. Sometimes ethnoveterinary treatments are ineffective or even detrimental for certain of the health problems to which they are applied; and a few may be outright harmful.

Thus, researchers and developers have a clear responsibility to ascertain the general efficacy, safety and cost-effectiveness (or at a minimum, the relative health and economic risks *vis-à-vis* doing nothing at all) of local or techno-blended ethnoveterinary options before widely promoting them—just as they would do with any other medical technologies. Otherwise, ER&D risks harming the very people it seeks to serve. Furthermore, validation is necessary so as to avoid perpetuation of the 'dual knowledge' syndrome in which local know-how is automatically labelled second-rate (Lalonde and Morin-Labatut n.d.) or is seen as somehow innately primitive or non-analytical (Agrawal 1995), with the implication that its inventors and bearers are second-rate and primitive, too. Yet by comparison with human ethnomedicine, scientific validation of ethnoveterinary know-how has been limited. Much of the larger ER&D literature is only descriptive, anecdotal or exploratory.

Unfortunately, such testing as has been done has sometimes been methodologically sloppy. In screening ethnoveterinary botanicals, for example, studies have sometimes failed to take into account important variables in local drug preparation that can influence phytochemical balances and processes, and hence pharmacological effect. On occasion, these oversights have led to 'false negatives' concerning ethnoveterinary treatment efficacy and even to livestock deaths.[11] To take another example, in testing ethnoveterinary parasiticides, sometimes trials have not followed all the fundamental scientific procedures (establishing control groups, conducting necropsies as well as egg counts, making multiple measures of parasite populations across the whole of the parasitic life cycle) that would allow for accurate treatment assessment.

Beyond such basic issues of proper (but straightforward) scientific research, however, there is also the question of whether conventional scientific methods may always be suitable for assessing ethnoveterinary treatments that are somewhat unorthodox. Examples include the medicinal bouquets described by Brisebarre, or unusual preparation techniques like human mastication of the pharmaceutical materials. Furthermore, experiences in human ethnomedicine suggest that conventional methodologies may overlook some of the mechanisms by which natural medicines produce their effect, due to a blinkered view of what qualifies as therapeutic action.[12] Finally, tests of ethnoveterinary treatments under laboratory or experimental conditions using animals with fixed diets in controlled environments may not give reliable readings of treatment efficacy under real-world conditions—where animal nutrition and husbandry regimes are more varied.

The last two observations also hold for the study and validation of many non-pharmacological practices—especially some husbandry, herding, pest/parasite/predator control, and medico-religious procedures. Conventional scientific testing of such interventions as mixed grazing, habitat modification and companion species has yielded sometimes ambiguous results as to the extent and economic impact of their benefits. But rarely have such interventions been evaluated holistically as part of the totality of local healthcare techniques keyed to sensitive shifts in seasons, general livestock condition or nutrition, and parasite life cycles. When all such factors are accounted for in validation—perhaps along with considerations of human and environmental health—it may be found that non-pharmacological techniques have far more significant strategic, additive or extra-veterinary payoffs than is yet appreciated.

Finally, there is some debate in the ethnomedical literature as to when what type and rigour of biomedical validation are called for. Many authors opine that exhaustive isolation of active ingredients and definitive description of physio-chemical mechanisms should not be an automatic precondition for validation of ethnopharmaceuticals. Indeed, by these standards, aspirin (another drug of ethnomedical origin) would have to be withdrawn from the market! Not only is such research costly and time-consuming; as just discussed for non-pharmacological practices, it may also be reductionistic (Bodeker 1994). For immediate applied/development purposes, a persuasive argument can be made that if simple but scientifically correct on-farm trials support a treatment's positive benefits with no or acceptable side-effects, and if collaborating stockraisers *cum* ethno-scientists deem it satisfactory and practical, then this should be sufficient for all but 'ivory tower' purposes. In this respect, the trials described by McCorkle and Bazalar for Andean ethnoveterinary medicines are instructive.

However, to meet its overarching goal of providing cheaper yet effective veterinary alternatives that more stockraisers can readily access, ER&D must include socio-economic as well as biomedical validation. Unfortunately, the paucity of proper socio-economic assessments of ethnoveterinary alternatives in this volume appears representative of ER&D as a whole, at least to date. In fairness, though, it should be noted that the same complaint can be levelled at much of conventional veterinary medicine as well (see McCorkle 1995 and the references cited therein).

In part, this is because socio-economic assessments can be very data-intensive and methodologically complex. For example, merely comparing per-dose prices of a Western commercial drug with a nationally trademarked equivalent and with the home-made counterpart is insufficient. Transport and opportunity costs must be factored in for all three treatment types, and these costs will vary from place to place and even from household to household. If the different drugs can be demonstrated equally effective (itself not an easy task, as noted above), economic assessment might end there. But even if a local treatment proves only 70 to 80 per cent effective in comparison to potent, 90 or 100 per cent effective Western-commercial equivalents, cost/benefit analysis based on market prices and outlets may still show that it makes better economic sense.

Moreover, additional socio-economic variables need to be considered. For one thing, cash profit may not be the sole or even primary production goal of smallholder stockraisers. As noted at the outset of this chapter, typically they are managing their often multiple-species 'stock portfolios' for a complex mix of both market and non-market goods and services. For this or for other, socio-cultural reasons (discussed earlier), stockraisers may not always be willing to invest in expensive store-bought drugs or professional veterinary services. Or they may do so only belatedly, when such interventions can do little good. But with cheaper yet reliable local alternatives, people may be more likely to treat their animals promptly, thus ultimately incurring lower livestock or productivity losses. For another thing, as a number of contributors to this volume suggest, it is easy and tempting for producers to misuse certain potent but expensive Western drugs in such a way (for example, under-dosing) that animals' natural immunity is compromised and/or chemoresistance encouraged. In sum, the outcome of considerations like the foregoing can be an economic rate of return for ethnoveterinary treatments that, in practical terms, equals or even betters that for Western equivalents.

A further methodological consideration is that if any meaningful headway is to be made in getting significant numbers of validated technologies and practices into the hands of significant numbers of local practitioners and/or producers, then both biomedical and socio-economic R&D approaches must be inexpensive and readily 'do-able' (McCorkle 1994b). Otherwise, they cannot be widely implemented by national-level or NGO agencies. In addition to participatory on-farm trials with stockraisers' or traditional healers' own animals whenever possible (McCorkle and Bazalar), cost-effective methods can include: systematic prior search and comparison of the oral ethnoscientific literature with the written scientific literature (Roepke); intra- and inter-regional comparisons of ethnoveterinary prescriptions in order to identify 'best bets' for validation (Grandin and Young; see also Wanyama 1995); and Delphi-style or expert panel assessments for the same purpose or as a tentative form of validation (IIRR 1994). Elaboration of such methodological approaches has already been undertaken by several organizations, most notably the Intermediate Technology Development Group and the International Institute for Rural Reconstruction; and this task is attracting interest from still others such as Heifer Project International (Nuwanyakpa *et al.* 1990) and Oxfam (Stoufer and Ohja 1993).

Application

It is important to re-emphasize that ER&D does not mean glorifying ethnoveterinary knowledge and practice, promoting or transferring them indiscriminately or to the exclusion of Western-style medicine. Rather, the larger aim in ER&D is to identify a menu of conventional, local and techno-blended options that maximizes a given group's ability to solve animal healthcare problems whenever and wherever they arise, ideally doing so in whatever way is most accessible, cost-effective and environmentally sound. Having options is vital because all veterinary approaches are subject to limitations of one sort or another.

For example, the requisite plant materials for ethnoveterinary treatments may be locally or seasonally unavailable, or insufficient for the numbers of animals to be treated. Or the work of gathering and preparing the materials or of then administering the home remedies may be excessive relative to available household labour at the time of the health problem. (Anjaria suggests that some of these difficulties might be overcome by pre-packaged traditional medicines, however.) Relatedly, ethnoveterinary techniques that work well in one production system may not be appropriate for other systems. For example, Perezgrovas cautions that labour-intensive practices like the Tzotzil's bucket-watering and muzzling of sheep would probably be unfeasible for larger-scale producers with more diverse production or employment opportunities. In like vein, ethnoveterinary responses that have evolved under extensive, rangestock regimes are often ill-equipped to deal with the different array of diseases that arises under intensive, 'modern' husbandry. Moreover, as a number of authors point out (Anderson, Delehanty, Heffernan *et al.*), traditional systems of stockraising may be undergoing rapid technological and/or sociological change. This can make ethnoveterinary understandings and practices that were useful in the past no longer feasible or appropriate 'as is'.[13] Based on the larger ER&D literature, additional limitations that appear to characterize ethnoveterinary medicine more so than conventional medicine are: poor standardization of preparations and dosages for home remedies; a paucity of effective therapies for infectious epidemic diseases; and occasionally the existence of harmful practices.

Of course, conventional veterinary medicine has limitations, too. As Brisebarre recounts, even in the First World, it can encounter drug supply and labour constraints. And as documented throughout this volume, especially in the Third World, conventional approaches are plagued by limitations such as their prohibitive cost, difficult access, unfamiliarity or socio-cultural unacceptability, and sometimes relative environmental insensitivity. Meanwhile, the effectiveness of all medical interventions is dependent upon practitioners' or users' diagnostic skills.

All of the foregoing is by way of saying that ethno- and Western veterinary medicine have much to learn from each other when it comes to their practical application. As Last (1990:353) observes for medical systems cross-culturally, 'In theory . . . all systems may "work"; in practice, all have successes and failures, with some systems scoring much higher in particular areas of medicine' depending on the social, cultural and economic context in which they are applied. Indeed, it would be naïve to think that either ethno- or Western science alone is likely to provide a sufficient prescription for all development ills in today's rapidly changing world. The aim is not to impose one medical paradigm on another but rather to create contact points between them (Salih 1992). In contemporary problem-solving, *all* potentially helpful knowledge bases should be brought to bear in a negotiated fashion, as knowledge is always 'in the making' (Thompson and Scoones 1994).

Looking ahead
In light of Table 2 and given the exploding interest worldwide in alternative medicine for all species, work in ER&D seems certain to accelerate. This is particularly true for ethnoveterinary pharmacognoscy and pharmacology, in view of the still-dominant chemo-therapeutic paradigm plus the intensifying search for drugs to combat frightening new diseases of humans (like AIDS or the highly publicized Ebola disease) as well as increasing or mutating ones (cancer, malaria). However, ER&D should pay attention to non-pharmacological techniques, which have so far been relatively little studied. These may offer especially important, holistic approaches and insights into what seems to be, in essence, a global search for fresh paradigms of healthcare that are more responsive to today's demographic, environmental, and economic realities.

Certainly, future students of ER&D can look forward to some stimulating challenges (but also some rich rewards) in devising and implementing creative new methodologies at all levels and stages of the validation process—whether biomedically or socio-economically, at the lab bench or in the field, in research or in development. Also sorely lacking in ER&D is a critical mass of studies on the comparative advantages of ethno- and conventional veterinary responses under different constellations of exogenous factors. Moreover, ER&D findings need to be linked into the vast body of both theory and praxis in medical anthropology/sociology and healthcare extension for humans, so that findings from each can enrich the other. Particularly exciting are possibilities for the intersectoral delivery of healthcare in which formal-sector/modern and informal-sector/traditional treatment alternatives could be offered jointly to both human and animal patients, thus increasing healthcare options for all species and expanding coverage through cost-sharing across sectors (McCorkle, in press–a).

For all of the foregoing to occur and for alternative healthcare approaches to be implemented, there is also need for policy analysis and reform. For example, policies that favour funding only conventional medical R&D and delivery systems will quash research into potentially valuable ethnomedical options. Policies that make for free or subsidized provision of high-tech Western drugs, vaccines and services will inhibit uptake of valid ethnoveterinary techniques both by producers and the healthcare workers who serve them. And policies that refuse recognition to or are overly controlling of localized and privatized practitioners who can deliver validated alternative or techno-blended (as well as conventional) treatments and husbandry strategies will deprive the very public who most require such services.

As work along all the foregoing fronts progresses, kits and guidelines will be needed for assisting national-level and NGO agencies to decide what validation methods to use and how to implement them, what mix of conventional and validated ethnoveterinary techniques to extend to different client groups and how best to do so, how to handle intellectual property rights, whether to combine human and animal healthcare delivery, and more.

This volume will have served its purpose if it stimulates scientists, healthcare workers and extensionists, educators, and policymakers to take up these challenges, futher exploring and applying the demonstrated potential for wide-ranging benefits to humankind that is embodied in ethnoveterinary knowledge systems and their associated human resources.

Notes

1. Much of this introductory chapter draws upon earlier work by its co-authors (see references cited). For this volume as a whole, the editors would like to acknowledge the assistance and support across many years of the Small Ruminant Collaborative Research Support Program's (SR–CRSP) Sociology Project and of the University of Missouri–Columbia's Department of Rural Sociology, where the project was at that time housed. Additional support was provided by the SR–CRSP Veterinary Medicine Project of Colorado State University and by the Center for Indigenous Knowledge in Agricultural and Rural Development (CIKARD) of Iowa State University. The authors are grateful to Dr Paul Mundy for editorial comments and other valuable suggestions. Finally, very special thanks go to Karla Schillhorn van Veen for her unstinting assistance during the final stages of this volume's parturition. Without her help, the book could not have been successfully birthed.
2. As acupuncture is now widely accepted in conventional veterinary and human medicine, it is not treated in the present volume. Indeed, the US Office of Alternative Medicine of the National Institutes of Health has raised the question whether it should even be included under the rubric of 'alternative' (NIH 1995).
3. Producer participation may take many forms. In research design, it includes suggesting promising solutions based on local practice or on ethnoveterinary treatments. In trial implementation and monitoring it might include preparing different strengths and mixtures of local prescriptions to be tested on-farm (McCorkle and Bazalar), sampling pre- and post-test populations of the pests or parasites that an experimental treatment or practice is designed to ward against, or monitoring treatment effect in other ways, such as recording clinical observations or milk yields on written or pictographic forms. Stockraisers have also been enlisted in the job of doing faecal egg counts on-site using reflecting microscopes.
4. The jury is still out on some supernaturally related practices. While certainly such practices comfort the worried stockowner, the question is: how might extra-medical or -nutritional care and attention to (especially highly social) animals affect their physical well-being? Acts such as stroking, talking to, or even just staying by the 'sickbed' of a suffering creature may have positive somatic effects. Benign effects on animal physiology (such as slowing and regularizing of heart rate) have been scientifically demonstrated as a result of stroking and petting. Ethological studies are also suggestive in this regard. Many social animal species will lick, groom or stand watch over their sick or wounded young or herdmates. Finally, it bears repeating that supernaturally related ethnomedical acts must be thoroughly investigated. For example, might a fetish bundle hung around an animal's neck contain some pest-repelling substance?
5. For example, this method is now used to adapt cattle to trypanosomosis or East Coast Fever in East Africa, with the components of the 'cocktail' varying by region (Dolan and McKeever 1992). Editors' note: The names of parasitic diseases in this book are in general conformity with the *Standardized Nomenclature of Animal Parasite Diseases* (SNOPAD).
6. Most ethnopharmaceuticals are derived directly from crude botanicals. Among other things, this means that, in their normal use, they may tend to be less toxic, less bio-stable, and thus less bio-cumulative, both in the environment and in the body. For greater discussion of these points, see McCorkle (1995) and the references cited therein.
7. Indeed, the boundary between human and animal medicine and their practitioners is essentially an artificial one (Schwabe 1993, Ward *et al.* 1993), drawn mainly by Anglo-American cultures. A partial exception to this statement is public health epidemiologists worldwide; many are veterinarians because of their better training in population medicine and their ability to deal with complex interactions, rather than concentrating on individuals. This boundary is much less pronounced in parts of Europe, and almost non-existent in many Third World countries where the one-

medicine concept is often a quite logical and pragmatic adaptation to shortages of trained practitioners, infrastructural difficulties, and other factors (McCorkle, in press a, Schwabe, this volume; Ward *et al.* 1993).

8. Prevalent in the Third World, this bias is also not uncommon in the First World, where research tends to concentrate on a limited number of diseases even though their importance may not have been demonstrated by field data (see also Ward *et al.*, 1993).

9. In fact, suiting word to deed, Nigeria's Ahmadu Bello University now offers a course on ethnoveterinary medicine, as does the University of Chiapas, Mexico. In Eastern Europe and Germany, many schools of veterinary medicine have continued to provide training in traditional herbal and other treatments that stockraisers can readily employ on-farm. And some colleges of veterinary medicine in the United States now offer courses in acupuncture and other alternative treatments.

10. Such judgements are particularly likely in multifactorial diseases.

11. This despite the fact that research protocols for the formal pharmacological and clinical study of botanical treatments have been well codified at least since the turn of the century. Variables that must be considered include, e.g.: the precise parts or form and quantitites in which botanical materials are used, but also the local conditions (for example, soil quality, microclimate) and developmental stages at which the plants are collected; the way in which they are compounded (including additive, synergistic, antagonistic or bioavailability effects in polyprescriptions); the tools employed in drug preparation (e.g., metal versus bamboo); treatment schedules; and naturally, the species, age, weight and overall health and reproductive status of the patient(s). For some examples, see McCorkle (1995).

12. Many ethnomedical treatments are intended to have several simultaneous or synergistic actions. These may span site-specific attack on the pathology, enhanced immune response, increased cellular uptake and repression of side-effects. Bodeker (1994) gives a striking example from cancer research of how these and other therapeutic effects may be overlooked.

13. This is especially the case when nomads settle (Schillhorn van Veen and Loeffler 1990). But even then, the principles behind traditional healthcare practices remain valid, and thus can sometimes be modified to operate under the new conditions.

2. Sense or nonsense?
Traditional methods of animal disease prevention and control in the African savannah

TJAART W. SCHILLHORN VAN VEEN

FOR MILLENNIA, STOCKRAISING has formed a vital part of the livelihood and culture of many African peoples—especially those of the savannah zone of sub-Saharan Africa. Livestock are also a mainstay of the economies of today's savannah countries. Given the importance of stockraising to both household and national economies, African herders' long-standing concern with the well-being of their animals is understandable. Livestock disease, in particular, plays a perhaps more prominent role in Africa than elsewhere; the five most important diseases (ruminant trypanosomosis, contagious bovine pleuropneumonia or CBPP, rinderpest, East Coast Fever or ECF and heartwater disease) occur only rarely on other continents. Thus, Africans are confronted with more, and unique, livestock health problems. This may help explain herders' considerable attention to disease prevention and control and the lengths to which they have been known to go to protect their animals.[1]

Prevention and control of livestock disease have long been a critical concern in Africa, as testified in early Egyptian papyri (Schwabe 1978, and this volume), numerous Biblical references, and later in the works of thirteenth-century Arab scholars such as Yaqut, Ibn Sa'id, and Abu Zacaria (Cuoq 1975, see also Köhler-Rollefson, this volume). Indeed, in the early Middle Ages, Arabia was a world centre of veterinary and other medical knowledge.[2] With the spread of Islam, some of this knowledge made its way into Africa, where stockraisers adopted, adapted, refined and combined it with local (and later, European) knowledge and practice in their efforts to ward against the many diseases afflicting their herds.

For the African savannah areas, the majority of traditional practices in this regard can be classed under two broad types of adjustment to disease pressure, following the distinction drawn by Ford (1971) in his classic work on trypanosomosis: ecological and physiological. The former is commonly used when disease pressure is intermittent, localized, and to some extent avoidable. The primary objective of the ecological approach is to forestall exposure to fatal diseases, such as tsetse-transmitted trypanosomosis, CBPP, rinderpest, anthrax and blackleg. A classic example of an ecological method of disease prevention is moving herds so as to avoid contact with sources of contagion. In contrast to avoid such exogenous strategies (that is, external to the animal), the physiological approach seeks to prevent or control disease by modifying endogenous processes. A good example is vaccination. The objective of such mechanisms is to 'season', immunize, and strengthen animals so as to avert major losses if a disease strikes when herds are already subject to other stresses. Physiological responses to disease threats tend to be used when contact between host and pathogen is fairly constant and unavoidable, that is, when a disease is enzootic.

African stockraisers also employ strategies that represent something of a mix between ecological and physiological approaches, as well as still other practices—such as magical and religious procedures—that defy classification under either rubric. Nevertheless, the ecological/physiological distinction provides a useful framework for organizing an overview of traditional African methods of disease prevention and control.[3] Below, traditional responses to disease threat and the rationale behind them are presented in terms of this framework. Wherever possible, they are also assessed in light of current scientific veterinary knowledge. In describing and documenting these responses, in evidence of traditional strategies' continued use and applicability under current conditions reference is generally made not only to the early colonial literature but also to recent reappraisals and reviews and to the author's own field experience. Finally, while the focus here is on herders of the savannah zone, other groups are also mentioned where relevant.

Ecological approaches

Isolation
Perfect isolation is a common strategy of disease control in industrialized livestock production (particularly of poultry and swine). Isolation is achieved by raising animals in confinement. Although this practice has been challenged on grounds of animal welfare, it has greatly diminished the risk of most of the epizootic diseases so common only a few decades ago[4]. An essentially equivalent strategy is found in some parts of Africa, notably in remote montane or forest habitats that are not frequented by nomadic or transhumant herds. For example, systems of raising or fattening cattle in isolation are found in the Mandara mountains of Cameroon (Thys *et al.* 1986), on the island of Madagascar (Serres 1960), and in the forest zone of Central Africa. It is unlikely that disease control is the conscious reason for raising animals in these isolated areas; traditionally, a more important consideration has been protection from rustling and raiding by other tribes. Nevertheless, disease control has been the outcome. Interestingly, such areas are also home to many of Africa's more ancient breeds of cattle (see later sections).

Quarantine, defined as the separation of healthy animals from those with contagious disease, can be considered another form of isolation—albeit at the level of individual animals rather than the whole herd. Herder responses to rinderpest are illustrative. This disease was introduced into Africa only in the late 1800s, just before colonization. In view of rinderpest's recent advent and rapid progression (which leaves the stockraiser little time to study its development before the animal expires), its etiology was initially a mystery to African herders. In consequence, stockraisers often could (and sometimes still) offer only supernatural explanations for rinderpest, such as malevolent spirits, evil winds or the wrath of gods (for example, Ba 1982, Bocquen 1986, St Croix 1972). Nevertheless, pastoralists were quick to note the contagiousness of this plague. And groups such as Fulani and Twareg instituted a rule of quarantining the first cases so as to halt the spread of the disease at watering points and other places where livestock congregate (Bonfiglioli *et al.*, this volume, Dupire 1962, St Croix 1972).

Herd movements
Isolation is possible, however, only in delimited habitats or under special circumstances. In Africa, an alternative, and far more common, strategy to

achieve essentially the same goal of disease avoidance is moving animals through time and space in such a way as to preclude contagion. Where the geographical and seasonal prevalence of a disease is known, such movements are regular, leading to a broadly systematic nomadism or to a transhumant pattern in which herds spend certain seasons at one camp but move about at other times of the year.

A good example is the seasonal migration of livestock in the savannahs of West and central Africa. Herders move their animals north during the rainy season, to avoid the risk of tick- and fly-borne disease (especially trypanosomosis) in the more humid and forested south.[5] During the dry season, they take them south in search of better pasture. Detailed accounts of such migrations (for example, Dupire 1962, Ford 1971, St Croix 1972, Stenning 1959) indicate that herders are well aware that the risk of exposure to tsetse flies and other disease-bearing arthropods is much greater in the wet season and that these pests concentrate in certain, often wet and/or wooded areas. To take another example, savannah herders also employ seasonal movements to prevent liver-fluke disease (fasciolosis or hepatic distomatosis) in cattle and sheep. This disease—which is far more common among sedentary animals—is transmitted by aquatic snails. Thus, many herders correctly link it to grazing in swamps and flood plains.[6] Unless drought intervenes, they generally try to avoid such areas or at least to minimize the time spent there (see also Perezgrovas, this volume).

Whether wittingly or not, pastoralists' efforts to avoid disease-bearing insects and infested wetlands can have the added bonus of breaking the cycle of parasitic infection (Schillhorn van Veen 1978). A corollary strategy is the care that some pastoralists exercise in not allowing newly acquired stock into their herd during the wet season (for example, Knight 1974) and, more generally, in not mixing their own animals with others of unknown provenance.

A further consideration in the annual itineraries of some nomadic or transhumant groups is the need to supply their stock with an optimal diet (Breman *et al.* 1978). Herders universally appreciate the relationship between good nutrition and good health. Most also recognize specific deficiency diseases such as the night blindness that results from avitaminosis A (see also Heffernan *et al.*, this volume and Stem, this volume) or phosphorous deficiency, which manifests itself as depraved appetite (for example, eating bones). Vitamin and mineral requirements naturally vary by region, depending on the type of forage available and other factors (Schillhorn van Veen and Loeffler 1990).

Just as African wildlife migrate long distances to reach certain minerals (Weir 1972), so may pastoral herds.[7] For example, throughout much of Africa, pastoralists seasonally drive their herds to salt-licks or pans, salty wells, or halophytic pastures (for example, Ba 1982, Bernus 1979, Dupire 1962, Jousselin 1950). In addition to forming part of herders' regular regime of disease prevention and control, such migrations often form an integral part of pastoral social life, when otherwise isolated groups take the opportunity to gather for rituals and festivities. A good example is the annual *mondée*, which takes place in the late wet season among the Fulani of the Fouta Jalon of Senegal and Guinea (see Diallo 1989 or Larrat 1939 for detailed descriptions). Herders recognize the therapeutic benefits of this kind of salt supplementation—or *cure sallée*, as it is generally known in the literature.[8] But they also make these seasonal moves with an expressly prophylactic purpose, to stave off certain emically (usually, ethnically) defined disease syndromes. These syndromes go by different names among different peoples, for example: *daaso* or *wilsere* among Fulani in Francophone

West Africa, *samore* in Nigeria and Cameroon, and *ngana* in south-east Africa. All these terms largely translate as 'poor doing' and likely gloss a variety of ills (including trypanosomosis, liverfluke disease and general undernourishment) that mainly manifest themselves via a generic unthriftiness.

For decades, African stockraisers have also used tactical (as distinct from seasonal) movements to prevent serious attacks of disease. As noted above, herders recognize that flies are more active, numerous and widespread in humid places and in the rainy rather than dry season; likewise for certain times of the day during different seasons. Herders put this practical ecological knowledge to work in their herd movements. For example, if it is impossible for them to avoid moving their stock through known fly belts then, especially during the rainy season, they traverse these areas by night when the flies are inactive; watering schedules and the length of time spent at watering-places, too, are adjusted to take account of fly activity (see also Köhler-Rollefson, this volume).

A particularly dramatic example of herd movements in order to prevent or control disease is some pastoralists' response to foot-and-mouth disease (FMD). FMD can be fatal to animals that are stressed by pregnancy or work. And especially during the wet season, stock with open lesions on the mouth or feet are at greater risk of flystrike and hence myiasis and other health problems (author's field observations). To avoid FMD, herders may move their animals upwind of an infected herd. Conversely, however, they may purposely move them downwind, in the knowledge that exposing the animals to a mild case of FMD confers immunity. In essence, the latter technique constitutes a form of indirect vaccination. The practical epidemiological wisdom behind such tactics is remarkable in view of the fact that only after the 1967 outbreak of FMD in Britain did veterinary scientists give serious consideration to the transmission of FMD by wind (Smith and Hugh-Jones 1969).

Tactical herd movements may also be made in order to avoid locales in which diseases have occurred previously. Many African stockraisers skirt places where animals are known to have been exposed to, or died from, anthrax, clostridial diseases and malignant catharral fever, among other ills. Herders are not always able to enunciate a scientifically recognized rationale for their strict avoidance of such areas. Sometimes, they can explain only that 'evil spirits' haunt such places (for example, St Croix 1972:54). Nevertheless, this tactic makes sound epidemiological sense. Anthrax and clostridial diseases are caused by bacteria whose spores can survive in the soil for long periods. And African malignant catharral fever has been shown to spread by contact with the placenta of wildebeest. In the latter case, again, although herders may not recognize the specific mechanism of transmission, they have long known to avoid the calving grounds of wildebeest (Daubney and Hudson 1936).

More broadly, African herders know that the general risk of disease increases in campsites or grazing grounds under constant use. They note, for instance, that tick populations can build up under such circumstances—and with them, the risk of tick-borne diseases. To forestall such problems, pastoralists change campsites frequently; and like the Fulani of Cameroon and Central African Republic, they may also vary their migrational itineraries every few years (Boutrais 1988).

Other herding strategies
African stockraisers employ still other herding strategies that contribute to disease prevention and control. Some of the most important of these relate to

daily grazing patterns. For example, a common tactic throughout Africa is to delay turning stock out to pasture in the morning until the dew has dried (author's field observations; St Croix 1972). Ticks and nematode larvae tend to concentrate at the top of the damp blades of grass; but when the sun rises and the dew dries, they descend. Delayed turn-out thus reduces the risk of animals' picking up ticks or ingesting infective larvae. A related tactic is grazing animals at night, before the dewfall. This practice is most frequent during the hot season in West Africa, where night-time predators are few. Part of the rationale for both these tactics is nutritional: wet grass is less nourishing than dry; and most stockraisers recognize that fodder intake declines in the extreme daytime heat of the hot season. But disease prevention is likely also to figure in these grazing practices.

Another helpful herding strategy is mixed grazing of cattle with sheep and/or goats. Many of the economically significant livestock diseases in Africa are fairly species-specific. Thus a species that is resistant to or unaffected by one disease can dilute or 'graze down' a considerable part of the disease agents that would sicken another. In particular, mixed grazing reduces the build-up of intestinal parasites, which are rarely shared by ruminants. For example, cattle will ingest the infective stages of ovine, as well as bovine, parasites; but the former will not develop to maturity in cattle. Grazing cattle with sheep therefore reduces the total on-pasture population of ovine parasites and, consequently, the sheep's risk of infection. At the same time, sheep do likewise for cattle. Mixed grazing makes good sense in nutritional terms, too. Because different species have different forage preferences and feeding and flocking habits, it allows herders to extract the fullest possible benefit from the available pasture.

Given that one species may be resistant or immune to the diseases of another, keeping a mixed-species herd is itself a useful disease-control strategy. For example, rinderpest rarely affects small ruminants, and cattle do not catch sheep pox. African stockraisers purposely diversify their herds so that in case of an epidemic of one disease, they will not lose all their animals. Likewise for the common practice of splitting herds into several subherds and dispersing them among different grazing sites or villages (for example, Scott and Gormely 1980, Evans-Pritchard 1938, Dupire 1962, Pélissier 1966, Schwabe 1978).

Management strategies
Arthropod-borne diseases are numerous in Africa, and most stockraisers are well aware of the relation between certain diseases and the flies, ticks, mites and mosquitoes that transmit them—as well as of the general worry, discomfort, restlessness, and hence production losses that such pests engender. Herders' knowledge of the relationship between tsetse flies and trypanosomosis has already been discussed. An additional example from the humid savannah is stockraisers' correct association of the *Amblyomma* tick with heartwater disease and with the bacterial skin disease streptothricosis (Boutrais 1988, see also Delehanty, this volume on 'tick disease'). It is therefore no surprise that strategies to control flies and ticks constitute typically an important part of African stockraisers' response to this pervasive health risk in their ecology.

For example, recognizing that insects often concentrate in woody areas, herders may deliberately overstock pastures so as to keep vegetation down, thus destroying potential tsetse habitat (Hornby, cited in Allan 1965). However, it should be noted that in certain woodland savannah ecozones, such deliberate overgrazing could ultimately produce the opposite effect by diminishing the frequency of the bushfires that check the growth of woody vegetation (Gerrit Uilenberg, pers. comm.). On the other hand, pastoralists sometimes purposely set fire to range lands and/or chop down offending vegetation in order to control fly and tick populations (Ford 1971, 'Fulahn' 1933).

In addition, African stockraisers have long used home-made fly repellents, especially before entering a tsetse belt (Ibrahim, 1986). Repellents are prepared from a wide variety of substances in the form of ointments, oils, gums/resins/saps, lotions, washes and powders. A few examples of ingredients employed in the savannah zone of Nigeria include soap, tobacco and roots of the violet tree (see Law 1980; for additional examples, consult Mathias-Mundy and McCorkle 1989 or McCorkle and Mathias-Mundy 1992). Repellents may also take the form of protective hedges planted around compounds or animal quarters. The emic rationale for such hedges may be stated as one of warding off evil (Chavunduka 1976); but some plants used in this way may in fact have some practical repellent effect. Examples include the toxic *Boophane disticha* (English 'sore eyes') cited by Chavunduka, and certainly tobacco (Ajayi 1990). Mechanical means are also enlisted to ward against pests, such as strips of leather similar to those used in Western countries today, to screen horses' eyes from flies (Law 1980).

Other weapons in the battle against insect pests are smoke and fire. Smudge fires are a common sight in most cattle camps and corrals (for example, Bah 1983, Evans-Pritchard 1938, Ford 1971, Law 1980, St Croix 1972). During times of especially heavy fly activity, fires may be kept going day and night (Denham *et al.* 1826: Köhler-Rollefson, this volume). The smoke not only relieves fly worry but also helps prevent transmission of many serious fly-borne diseases of both cattle and horses. Sometimes, fires of insecticidal plants are lit to fumigate cattle camps and quarters (Bonfiglioli *et al.*, this volume, Ibrahim *et al.* 1983). Fires are also useful for disposing of manually removed ticks (Dupire 1962). This is a common practice throughout West Africa, where tick-borne hemo-parasitic diseases are enzootic and functional dip tanks are rare. Tick removal is performed by men, women and children at daily intervals in the wet season, and less frequently in the dry season. The ticks are generally tossed into the fire or fed to poultry. In East Africa, where tick-borne diseases (for example, ECF) are more severe, people may also have recourse to modern technologies such as insecticidal dips and sprays (Raikes 1981; see also Delehanty, this volume).

Careful attention to skin abrasions and wounds is another strategy in African stockraisers' battle against disease-bearing pests. Although wound healing is generally thought of as a therapeutic rather than a preventive act, open wounds can attract flies that feed or lay their eggs in the wounds. In the latter case, the eggs hatch into maggots and cause a condition known as wound myiasis. During the fly season, herders therefore take pains to cover any open wounds. They may dress them with cobwebs, mud, rags that have been 'sterilized' in smoke, ashes, leaves of certain plants and still other materials (author's field observations; for more examples, again consult Mathias-Mundy and McCorkle 1989 or McCorkle and Mathias-Mundy 1992).

Physiological approaches

Breeding
One physiological mechanism useful for disease prevention and control is selective breeding to improve herd resistance or tolerance to pest and disease attacks, as well as to other environmental stresses. St. Croix (1972) and others note that Fulani who migrate into a new area always purchase local bulls (even if they are of another breed) with the express purpose of enhancing their stock's adaptation to local conditions. Coupled with natural selection, such long-standing and long-recognized 'seasoning' strategies have produced some unique local breeds of disease-resistant livestock in Africa.

For cattle, examples include the Kapsigi of northern Cameroon and the dwarf breeds of the West African forests, such as the Ndama, Muturu, and Baloué. All these breeds are relatively resistant to the diseases characteristic of the forest zone, particularly trypanosomosis (ILCA 1979) but also in some cases heart-water disease (a tick-borne disease that is fatal to exotic cattle).[9] Among sheep, the Djallonké and Maasai breeds show some resistance to ovine intestinal parasites. Since the first studies in the 1970s on the genetic basis of trypano-tolerance in African cattle (Roberts and Gray 1973), further research by two major African animal research institutes (ILRAD and ILCA) has highlighted the resistance mechanism behind African stockraisers' seasoning-through-breeding strategy and led to worldwide scientific interest in the genetic bases of resistance to a variety of diseases, including foot-rot, mastitis and intestinal parasitism as well as trypanosomosis (Albers and Gray 1987, Dineen and Outteridge 1984).

Provision of colostrum
Feeding of colostrum—a lactating animal's first milk—constitutes a form of natural immunization. It contains antibodies that protect a new-born against many of the diseases survived by its dam. The antibodies are transferred to the offspring if it suckles during the first day after birth. Although herders may or may not be aware of the one-to-one link between colostrum and neonate health, they recognize that young animals are usually unaffected by certain diseases (more than 30 for cattle alone). In any case, most African stockraisers endeavour to ensure that neonates do in fact suckle within this time period.

Vaccination
Historical records suggest that the Chinese developed the first crude vaccine. They used a technique known as variolation—inoculation with a small piece of infected material from a mild case—to vaccinate for human smallpox. Knowledge of variolation spread westward from China and was known in Europe by the early 1700s (Hopkins 1983). Towards the end of the century, based on contemporary 'folk' knowledge, an English (Benjamin Jesty) and a Dutch (Geert Reinders) farmer demonstrated the feasibility of vaccination against, respectively, smallpox in humans and rinderpest in cattle (Bruins 1951). The European smallpox vaccine was based on cowpox materials, and derived from the long-standing recognition of the benefits of contact between humans and cattle, as evidenced by various references to 'pretty milkmaids'. It was not until 1796 that Edward Jenner scientifically tested this cowpox-based vaccine.

African herders have experimented with and used vaccination techniques for at least as long as their European counterparts. When two new diseases struck the

African continent (CBPP in the mid-1700s and rinderpest just before coloniza-tion), stockraisers there developed useful home-made vaccines in the relatively short space of only 30 to 50 years. An understanding of the value of vaccination requires several very astute, empirical observations. The first is noting that, once exposed to a given disease, a surviving individual is thereafter immune. This principle is not easy to derive in that it does not apply to all diseases and may hold only for a limited time. Second is the observation that the virulence of etiological agents can be attenuated via various procedures such as heating, drying, diluting or fermenting. This fact, too, is not immediately obvious, especially for diseases that are often fatal. Third, noting that certain diseases do not strike nursing or young animals also requires some thought. It is clear, however, that African pastoralists learned and applied all these lessons in what is one of their principal traditional physiological strategies of disease prevention and control: vaccination.

For diseases with high mortality rates, the goal of vaccination is obviously to *prevent* the disease. For ills that are rarely fatal, however, the goal is to *control* the problem by inducing a mild case of the disease at will. That way, herders ensure that it is contracted at an opportune time when animals are in good condition, thereby forestalling more serious outbreaks later on, when herds are migrating or are otherwise stressed.

An example of the control function of vaccination is African herders' vacci-nation for FMD, employing a well-known method termed 'aphtisation'. With a thorn or other sharp item, they inoculate their stock with unchanged infective material (secretions or tissue) from the udder, feet or tongue of animals with a mild case of FMD. This procedure confers immunity for about a year (author's field observations). Similarly, to ward against brucellosis, some West African herders insert unchanged material from an aborted foetus into a shallow incision in the tail of the animal to be immunized (ibid.). The success of this brucellosis vaccination is variable (see below) and it is used rather infrequently, perhaps because the prevalence of brucellosis varies by region. Nevertheless, some African stockraisers have long recognized the link between brucellosis and abortion in cattle, even though outbreaks of the disease generally seem to be fairly localized.

To control camelpox, some African camel raisers have been known to use a method similar to that found in Asia and Arabia (Bernus 1969, Curasson 1947, Monteil 1952, Köhler-Rollefson, this volume). Doutressoulle (1947) describes a technique in which crusts from infected animals are pulverized in milk and the resulting vaccine is given in the lips with a needle or a thorn. Generally only a few animals need be inoculated because the infection easily spreads by itself. The crusts are stored from one year to the next, given that this disease is especially prevalent during the rainy season, when increased fly activity pro-motes its spread. Employing a very similar method and one that is still in use among shepherds in many parts of the Western world today, Africans sometimes also vaccinate their small ruminants against contagious ecthyma (Larrat 1940).[10] Both these vaccines are effective and pose little risk to the animals.

As noted above, African herders also devised their own vaccines for CBPP. When CBPP was introduced to the continent by cattle imported into Southern Africa, colonial governments initially made no efforts to develop a vaccine. Not surprisingly, therefore, by the late 1800s various native methods of CBPP immunization were in wide use in both West and East Africa. (No data are available for southern Africa.) Briefly, these consisted of variations on the following procedures: lung lymph or tissue from an animal dead of CBPP is inserted into an incision on the muzzle, forehead, nostrils or ear of the animal to be inoculated; the wound may then be dressed with mud or other materials; after it reacts, the infective tissue is excised and the wound is debrided and cauterized. (For greater detail, consult Bernus 1981, Government of Nigeria 1929:24–5, Larrat 1940, Maliki 1981, Schinkel 1970:255–6, Schwabe 1978, Bizimana 1994.) These crude CBPP vaccines reportedly are effective if properly prepared and administered (see below). However, there is considerable risk of mortality from complications attendant upon the surgery and/or from the induced case of CBPP itself (Bonfiglioli *et al.*, this volume, Mares 1951, St Croix 1972). Because of this risk, not all herders were/are eager to use such vaccines. Where a specialist skilled in vaccine preparation and administration was available, their use may have been more common. For example, most such vaccinations in southern Senegal were performed by a single healer (Larrat 1940), not unlike the work of the Dutch healer/farmer Reinders a century earlier in the northern Netherlands (Bruins 1951).

In contrast to CBPP, when rinderpest struck Africa just before colonization, the new colonial governments were quick to initiate work on a vaccine. Nevertheless, African pastoralists devised inoculations of their own, as well. One method consisted of drenching with an aqueous suspension of dried faecal material from a mildly affected calf. Another involved the oral or intra-nasal administration of an infusion made with a piece of dried intestine from an animal dead of rinderpest; this material was first macerated in milk for two to three days. Still other methods are described in the literature (Larrat 1940, Mares 1951, Schinkel 1970:255–6). The last author reports that, in northern Somalia, indigenous vaccination sometimes led to outbreaks of rinderpest, but that overall it considerably reduced losses to the disease. In West Africa, only calves were inoculated, based on stockraisers' empirical observation that nursing calves were less susceptible to rinderpest—a correct assessment for the young of dams with protective antibodies. On balance, in light of the continuing epidemics of rinderpest in Africa, however, these native vaccines seem unlikely to have been very effective.

Some pastoralists also use controlled exposure as an indirect method of immunizing calves against rinderpest; they deliberately mix their calves in with diseased cattle (St Croix 1972). This technique makes sense only where the disease is enzootic, however. It is risky, in that there is no way to mitigate the virulence of the infection. As many as 50 per cent of the calves could well die. Still, where no other alternatives are known or available, presumably saving half one's calves is better than losing them all when an epidemic strikes. In an innovative 'combination' strategy, Baggara pastoralists of the 1950s quickly worked out that they could permanently protect an animal against rinderpest by having it immunized once with a commercial vaccine and then, within two years, intentionally exposing it to the disease (Gillespie 1966).

Finally, Kavirondo herders have been reported to 'vaccinate' against blackleg by sprinkling the blood of an animal that has succumbed to the disease over susceptible cattle (Wagner 1970). The efficacy of this procedure seems very uncertain, however. The blackleg bacteria—which are indeed found in the blood of affected cattle—could conceivably enter the bloodstream through skin abrasions. Assuming this were the case, depending on a number of factors, this procedure could have highly variable effects ranging from none, to a mild infection and subsequent immunity, to a severe case of blackleg, and death.

In summary, some of Africans' home-made vaccines were and are generally effective—notably those for FMD, poxes and ecthyma. The efficacy of others is dubious (blackleg, rinderpest) or most likely variable (CBPP, brucellosis) depending on a number of factors in vaccine preparation and administration. Such factors include: the virulence of the vaccine, the proper dosage for animals of differing ages, the general condition of the animal, and the mode of administration with respect to risks such as secondary infections or other complications. However, it is noteworthy that African stockraisers appreciate and use four recognized methods for attenuating a vaccine's virulence: desiccation, petrification, dilution and fermentation. In addition, they often by preference vaccinate less susceptible animals, such as calves that may still may carry maternal antibodies or that are for other reasons less severely affected.

Today, traditional vaccination techniques are less widely used—or in the case of rinderpest, no longer used at all—because modern vaccines are less risky, more reliable, and in the case of rinderpest, now more generally available thanks to immunization campaigns. However, for prevention and/or control of certain livestock diseases, traditional vaccinations were—and in some places, still are—the best available option for many African stockraisers under prevailing social, economic and political conditions.

Sense or nonsense?

Whether or not for explicitly verbalized, 'sensible' reasons—that is, reasons recognized and accepted by conventional medical science—many African stockraising societies have traditionally employed an array of strategies to avoid or mitigate the threat of disease in their herds. As this chapter has endeavoured to show, many of their ecological and physiological approaches to disease prevention and control make good epidemiological sense.

Africans' ecological approach is especially noteworthy. Indeed, the art of herding is one of the most important tools in managing livestock disease. In addition to good judgement, it requires considerable practical understanding of ethology, entomology, botany, geology, soil science and other disciplines. African stockraisers put this ethno-ecological savvy to work in preventing livestock disease by strategically moving, dividing, maintaining and acquiring multiple-species herds across both time and space. They also apply this knowledge to improve the immediate habitat of their stock, using a variety of tools—physical-chemical (in the form of fire), ethno-pharmacological, mechanical, and more (Curasson 1947). Herders' physiological methods of disease control—like selective breeding and traditional vaccination techniques—also attest to the acuity of stockraisers' empirical observation and reasoning (Schwabe 1978, Schwabe and Kuojok 1981).

At the same time, however, an overview of the literature shows that African herders perform and/or conceptualize many disease-control and other veterinary procedures in non-scientific, social and religious contexts or idioms.[11] Examples given earlier include, respectively, salt supplementation and ascribing diseases to the action of evil spirits or winds. In the latter regard, however, for all practical purposes stockraisers may often be correct. Certain locales may well be infested with 'evil spirits' in the form of persistent pathogens such as bacterial spores. And like FMD, a number of diseases can indeed be spread by 'bad air', 'evil' winds, or other pseudo- or semi-aerial modes of transmission (for example, on dust particles or the bodies of insects). In any case, an overview of the literature likewise suggests that magic or ritual alone—unaccompanied by naturalistic methods of healthcare—is usually employed only for poorly understood, little-known or newly introduced diseases, plus other kinds of calamities over which people have no control.[12] Even so, as the history of rinderpest in Africa attests, this does not prevent herders from trying to find naturalistic causes or solutions too.

The fact that much practical veterinary (as well as human medical) acumen may be couched in supernatural, social or other non-conventional terms or contexts has sometimes blinded researchers and developers to the effectiveness and the sound scientific bases of African herders' approaches to the prevention and control of livestock disease. Indeed, outsiders' lack of appreciation of African veterinary knowledge in the twentieth century is remarkably reminiscent of the misunderstandings between farmers and veterinary academicians in late eighteenth-century Europe (Bruins 1951). It is time to discard the notion that stockraisers' own practices and perceptions are mostly nonsense. Quite the contrary, they often make good veterinary sense.

Notes

1. For example, a Nigerian Fulani once travelled nearly a day to ask the author and his colleagues to come treat his herd, some 70km distant, for trypanosomosis (which we did).

2. As early as 1800 BC King Hammurabi of Babylon laid out laws concerning the fees veterinarians could charge for treatment of cattle and donkeys. In contrast, veterinary science was not well established in Europe until the seventeenth century. Even then, it was initially concerned only with equine medicine, mainly because of military interests. Bovine and small ruminant medicine was not even taught in the early European veterinary schools.

3. This overview is based on an extensive review of the literature and the author's experience as a veterinarian in Cameroon, Ethiopia, Nigeria and Senegal for more than a decade.

4. Under such intensive production systems, however, an array of so-called 'emerging' diseases (such as coccidiosis, tuberculosis, mastitis) have arisen to take the place of the 'old' ones.

5. Interestingly, West African cavalry units of the eighteenth and nineteenth centuries often operated only during the dry season because of the risk of fly-related mortality during the rains (Law 1980).

6. Some Fulani groups erroneously link liverfluke disease to leeches in animals' drinking-water. People base this association on the considerable similarity in shape, size, colour, and body tissue of flukes to leeches. In fact, given that both these pests require moist habitats, in a sense leeches may serve as a proximate indicator for the presence of the disease.

7. This nutritional strategy of disease prevention could also be classed under physiological approaches. But given its association with seasonal movements and features of the natural environment, for purposes of this discussion it is classed as ecological. In areas without natural mineral sources, stockraisers perforce obtain salt or natron through purchase or exchange, or they feed their animals ashes.

8. Some pastoral groups value the salt cure more as a purge than as a part of good nutrition and disease prevention (Benoit 1982). Reports of sand colics in horses and camels suggest that it may be necessary to purge the sand that accumulates in the intestinal tract throughout the long dry season. The high sulphate content of some salts could in fact effect such a purge (author's field observations).

9. These breeds, however, have rarely been exposed to the newer epizootic diseases of the savannah, to which they are therefore highly susceptible.

10. It is not known whether ecthyma existed in Africa prior to colonization. There are no descriptions of the use of this vaccine in pre-colonial times, so it is unclear whether it was introduced by colonial veterinary services or whether it was derived locally by analogy with the camel-pox procedure.
11. This is even more true among traditional healers. For instance, accounts of the skills of the renowned Cameroonian/CAR animal healer Alhaji Ori stress his 'power over the Spirits' and his devoutness as a Moslem in addition to his knowledge of medical botany and livestock diseases (Bocquen 1986:350). Many traditional healers' factual knowledge and techniques are masked by the use of ritual and witchcraft, which enhance their reputation. The combination of magical and religious acts with naturalistic aspects of animal healthcare is hardly unique to Africa—as many of the chapters in this volume attest.
12. For a discussion of this principle in human ethnomedicine in Africa, see Miller (1980).

3. Ancient and modern veterinary beliefs, practices and practitioners among Nile Valley peoples

CALVIN W. SCHWABE

THE NILOTIC PEOPLES comprise several million cattle-culture pastoralists of north-eastern Africa who speak languages of the Eastern Sudanic branch of the Nilo-Saharan phylum (Ehret 1982, Greenberg 1963). They are divided into three main linguistic groups: the eastern or plains Nilotes, exemplified by the Bari, Turkana and Maasai; the southern or highland Nilotes such as the Nandi; and the western or river/lakes Nilotes represented by such peoples as the Shilluk, Nuer, Luo and the group highlighted here, the Dinka. Dinka pastoralists number an estimated two to three million. They represent the largest ethnic group in the southern region of Sudan, Africa's largest country. Their territory extends from east of the Nile River westwards along the southern edge of the Sudd, an immense swampy excrescence of the Nile. As with the neighbouring Nuer, among Dinka:

> . . . the only labour in which they delight is the care of cattle (Evans-Pritchard 1937: 209) . . ., cattle and their kin-owners are symbiotic (ibid.:211) . . ., [these pastoralists] tend to define all social processes and relationships in terms of cattle. Their social idiom is a bovine idiom (ibid.:214) . . ., *cherchez la vache* is the best advice that can be given to those whose duty is to understand [their] behaviour (ibid.:209).

This chapter describes Dinka veterinary healers, beliefs and techniques for cattle, along with some of their parallels in ancient Egypt.[1] The value of such comparative ethnoveterinary research is two-pronged. Information from and about modern-day peoples can help interpret the ethno-archeological record (Kramer 1979); at the same time, it can suggest practical alternatives for Third World livestock development.

Drawing upon the study of ethnoveterinary knowledge and practice among Dinka pastoralists of today, the chapter seeks to understand and interpret the 'mindset' of pre-dynastic cattle-culture Egyptians with respect to the emergence of the rudiments of biomedical science from healing magic in the ancient Nile valley (Schwabe 1990a). In this regard, two major hypotheses are explored. First, that some of the more rational roots of Egyptian medicine lay in a comparative biomedical process that drew analogies to humans from observation, inference and experimental demonstration in bull sacrifices; and that Egyptian priest-healers had opportunities to apply these findings in practice, both to bulls destined for sacrifice and to gods incarnated as living bulls (Schwabe 1978). Second, analysis of the findings from this synchronic/diachronic comparison suggests that some types of ethnoveterinary practitioners, beliefs and methods in the Nile valley may be of great antiquity. This fact may help explain their enduring credibility and acceptance. Finally, the chapter discusses ways to take advantage of such long-standing skills and human resources in extending both animal and human health services to pastoral peoples in Africa and other parts of the Third World.

Types of healers and concepts of comparative medicine

In many indigenous medical systems, human and animal healing are not differentiated. Both are done by the same persons. Examples of such healers among the Dinka include certain individuals, generically called *tiet*, who are able to communicate with the divine. Some *tiet* have more specific titles and/or exalted standing, like the *bany bith* 'priest of the fishing spear' (Ater 1976, Lienhardt 1961) or the *ran de Ring* 'man of flesh' (Schwabe 1987). Some of these individuals plus other *tiet* known as *ran cau* are believed to possess the power to heal by exorcism. Still others known as *ran wal* control secret herbal remedies. According to Western-educated Dinka veterinarians, some *ran wal* remedies are quite effective, particularly those for snake bite and scorpion sting. Dinka have yet another class of practical manual healers called *atet*, a generic term that translates as 'specialist'. *Atet* perform wound and abscess surgery, bone-setting, horn surgery, castration and obstetrics—all but the last three on both people and cattle (Schwabe 1991, 1984a, 1984b:171–4, Schwabe and Kuojok 1981).

In ancient Egypt, healers had similarly varied designations and tasks (Ghalioungui 1983, Jonckheere 1958, Leca 1983, Lefebvre 1956). A group of healers called $wr-ḥ^c.w$ (literally 'great of the flesh') were especially associated with the priesthood of Sais (Ghalioungui 1983: 5–6), whose *Per Ankh* 'House of Life'[2] enjoyed considerable medical repute. Priests called *ḥm-k3* 'servant of the *ka*' were responsible for feeding the soul or the animating double (*ka*) of a deceased pharaoh; they also performed circumcisions (Ghalioungui 1983: 11). In certain respects, these two classes of healers resemble Dinka *ran de Ring*, who are endowed with the magic of 'living flesh' (see below). Healing magicians similar to *ran cau*, called *s3w*, possessed special amulets. Egyptian *ḥrp.w srq.*, associated with the scorpion goddess Serqet, are reminiscent of the Dinka *ran wal*.

Certainly, the priests of the lion goddess Sekhmet—who could cause and prevent plagues—practised both veterinary and human medicine.[3] While many Egyptian priests probably administered some forms of therapeutic magic, priests of Sekhmet—mentioned in both the Ebers and Smith medical papyri—enjoyed a special reputation as healers over a very long period. Some priests of Sekhmet had an additional and more frequent Egyptian medical title, *swnw*.[4] However, not all *swnw* healers were identified as priests. It is not known whether *swnw* also treated sick animals, but it is clear that some of the priests overseeing and certifying the act of bovine vivisection/dissection (that is, sacrifice) were *swnw*.

Both Sekhmet's and other Egyptian priests probably devoted considerable attention to keeping bulls destined for sacrificial dissection 'free from blemish', that is in good health (Herodotus, translated by Rawlinson 1952). In fact, the Kahun veterinary papyrus—the only Egyptian medical papyrus written in the first person by a healer—is unequivocally a religious document. This fragmentary veterinary text is one of the two oldest surviving medical papyri. It offers prescriptions for treating cattle, dogs, birds and fish—in other words, comparative medicine. A number of human ailments are mentioned in other Egyptian medical papyri (Schwabe 1984b:256, Walker 1964). By Ptolemaic times, most healers of humans bore Greek names; but animal healers (*hippiatros*) still had Egyptian names (Nanetti 1942). This fact further indicates that the even earlier Egyptian healers did not neglect the health of their vitally important animals (Schwabe 1994). Thus, in the ancient Nile Valley, human and animal medicine were not separated conceptually. And as with Dinka healers today, early Egyptian healers probably practised comparative medicine.

Lessons learned from bull vivisection and dissection

This finding of a comparative medical approach is of historical importance in that it helps explain how Egyptian healers obtained the rudimentary knowledge of mammalian anatomy, physiology and pathology that they used in practice. Many historians of ancient medicine have side-stepped this issue or have adduced inadequate arguments that Egyptians' experience with mummification formed the basis of their medical acumen (Gordon 1990).

Certainly, among Dinka medical-veterinary *atet*, bull sacrifice has been indispensable to the accumulation of a corpus of rudimentary biomedical knowledge that is also applied to people (Schwabe and Kuojok 1981). The central religious, social and cultural act in Dinka society is bull sacrifice (Lienhardt 1961, Schwabe 1987). Dinka never kill and eat cattle except as a symbolic act of communion during sacrifice.[5] An elder carefully dissects the animal. Designated anatomical portions are then distributed to specific individuals or social groups. Each bone or type of bone has its own name; and different musculo-skeletal assemblages are assigned to certain classes of persons. In illustration of the extent of anatomical classification involved, the spine is considered to consist of the atlas, called *yiith thaar*, the axis *ngok*, the cervical vertebrae *yeth yuom*, the thoracic vertebrae *duolnhom*, the lumbar vertebrae *reel*, the sacrum *piec* and the coccygeal vertebrae *anguek nguek ke yol*; the entire musculo-skeletal assemblage of the tail is *yol* or *anyieng*.

In their vivisection/dissection rites, Dinka *atet* and other elders also make observations of physiology. From such observations, they have drawn certain correct or incorrect inferences. For example, blood is regarded as originating in the liver; and urine is believed to arise from 'dirty' blood in the kidneys. Similarly, they observe pathology; combined with clinical signs, observations of pathology are used to classify a number of disease entities (Schwabe and Kuojok 1981 and below).

In Egypt, bull sacrifice was common from pre-dynastic times onwards. It was central to important religious rituals—especially those having to do with the preservation of life, resurrection or other funerary practices (Eggebrecht 1973). As already noted, the officiating priest was sometimes also a *swnw* or, healer. One text accompanying a depiction of the religio-veterinary act of bull sacrifice indicates that such priests were responsible for certifying the purity of the sacrificial animal's 'blood', i.e. its health (Sauneron 1960b:78).

Not surprisingly, therefore, most Egyptian hieroglyphs for the internal organs of both humans and animals are based on models of bovine (or possibly other ungulate) organs (Erman and Grapow 1957, Gardiner 1957). The only surviving detailed anatomical list is a bovine one (Gardiner 1947). Moreover, the second Egyptian pharaoh was said to have been a healer and to have written an anatomy book (Waddell 1971). At that early date, such a book would necessarily have been on bovine anatomy. In sum, as Ghalioungui (1973:47) notes, '. . . knowledge of animal anatomy must have long preceded that of human anatomy. Every [Egyptian] physician was more or less a veterinary surgeon, and the *wabw*, the "pure priests" . . . entrusted under the Ancient Empire with ritual inspection of the sacrificial beasts, must have possessed a fair knowledge of that art.'

Physiological theory

The body's animating force According to Dinka beliefs, two vital elements depart the bodies of cattle and people upon death: *atiep* 'shadow' and *weei* 'breath'. Along with *Ring* 'flesh' and *riem* 'blood', these are considered essential to life (*wei*). At death, the *wei* goes to the sky. The *wei* of a sacrificial bull may serve as a messenger from the sacrificers to the 'spiritual force in the sky' or to the spirits of their ancestors.

Ring, which is a manifestation of spiritual force or divine power (*jɔk*), is the animating force in muscular tissue; it may persist for some period after death. When Dinka *ran de Ring* priests are possessed by *jɔk*, *Ring* is evidenced by an uncontrollable muscular trembling. This trembling is usually exhibited when they perform a sacrifice. *Ring* is likewise manifested in the sacrificial animal by post-mortem fasciolations (tremors) in cut or uncut muscle fibres (Schwabe 1987). Such fasciolations may be spontaneous, or they may be induced by the priest or healer striking the muscles and limbs of the sacrificed bull. In modern terms, *Ring* is ATP (adenosine triphosphate), the biochemical that is in large part responsible for muscular contraction in all mammals (Schwabe 1986a). Dinka *ran de Ring* priests believe they can replenish their own supply of *Ring* by consuming the raw, twitching, 'living flesh' of a sacrificial bull. This act of communion nourishes the priest's *Ring* via chyme, which also possesses sacred properties.

In ancient Egypt, shadow likewise departed the body at death, as did another element called *ba*. Interestingly, *ba* also meant 'ram', though it was often portrayed as a bird. *Ba* is sometimes likened by Egyptologists to the Christian notion of soul and thus somewhat resembles Dinka *wei*. A possibly ancient parallel to Dinka *Ring* was the property the Egyptians called *ka* 'bull'. Its hieroglyph consists of arms raised above the head in probable imitation of the horns of a bull. *Ka* has been likened to the double or the animating principle of a deceased person or bull. *Ka* could be nourished in the afterlife by feeding the deceased's 'body': its mummy or statue. For the pharaohs, this task was performed by the servants of *ka*, the paramedical *ḥm-k3* priest–healers.

One of the first and most important Egyptian rituals of resurrection was 'opening of the mouth'. This rite was performed both for human beings and for the living incarnation of the Apis bull god upon the creature's death. The rite involved touching the mouth of the deceased with the sacrificial animal's severed forelimb (always the first part removed) and/or with the adze used in the dissection (Schwabe *et al.* 1989). Numerous historical depictions of this ritual plus laboratory reenactments of its surgical procedures (ibid., Schwabe 1986a) clearly indicate that—just like their Dinka counterparts—the Egyptian priests who oversaw bovine sacrifice not only observed the resulting postmortem muscular tremors and the contractions of whole muscles in the severed forelimb; they also induced such phenomena by percussive stimulation with the sacred adze. They thereby demonstrated the irritability or contraction of excised muscles ('flesh'). They then tried to transfer the responsible animating principle (*ka* ?) to the deceased human (or bull god). Their goal was to revivify the deceased. Conceptually, revivification would constitute the ultimate form of medical intervention.

From prescriptions in three early Egyptian medical papyri calling for 'living flesh' or 'flesh from a live bovine animal' (Buchheim 1960), it is clear that this knowledge of muscular function was later used in other, more conventional therapeutic situations. Thus, as with Dinka priests, it is probable that Egyptian priest–healers (especially practitioners such as the *wr-ḥᶜ.w* 'great of the flesh') first applied to human therapy such rudiments of biomedical science that they derived by analogy from bull sacrifice. In the case of both Dinka and ancient Egyptians, this process and the lessons extracted from it can be regarded as primitive examples of comparative medical research.

The source of semen and life Observing that bulls with spinal injuries cannot breed, Dinka assert that semen arises in the brain and spinal cord (Schwabe and Kuojok 1981:235). Thus the spinal cord of a sacrificial bull may be given to an uncle of the sacrificer to ensure that the uncle's daughters will be fertile. To prevent backaches—which Dinka attribute to insufficient or excessive sexual activity—the sacrificer may wear the bull's dried penis as a belt or he may roast the organ and drink its melted 'fat'.

Ancient Egyptians believed that semen originated as bone marrow, especially in the thoracic spine. The spinal cord was considered to be the vertebral skeleton's marrow (Sauneron 1960a, Yoyotte 1962). They believed, too, that the penis was attached to the spine and that together these organs comprised the male reproduction system. Textual and orthographic evidence for these beliefs goes back to the earliest dynastic literature; and they are stated explicitly in later texts (Gordon and Schwabe 1989, Schwabe 1986b, Schwabe *et al.* 1982, Schwabe and Gordon 1988, 1989). To acquire this magic of the gods, the pharoah consumed the vertebrae and decoctions of bones from sacrificial bulls (Schwabe *et al.* 1982). This pharaonic communion rite is seemingly akin to the Dinka *ran de Ring's* consumption of the twitching flesh of sacrificial victims.

This early physiological theory was apparently based on priest–healers' empirical observation that the bull's penis attaches to the first coccygeal vertebrae of the spine by the white, non-striated retractor muscles of the penis (Schwabe *et al.* 1982:446). Coupled with the fact that semen and bone marrow resemble one another, such observations led priests to a series of inferences that together provided an explanation for the reproductive role of males, whether bovine or human. Thus this was another early application of the analogical principles of comparative medical research—that is, the use of animal models to answer human biomedical questions.

Knowledge of cattle diseases

Centuries of such empirical observation and experience have resulted in a rich storehouse of ethnoveterinary knowledge and technique among Nilotic cattle-culture peoples. Elsewhere, the depth, detail, and accuracy of such practical veterinary acumen have been analysed for Dinka healers' and herders' diagnostic criteria for anthrax, contagious bovine pleuropneumonia (CBPP), rinderpest, foot-and-mouth disease, tuberculosis and fasciolosis (Schwabe and Kuojok 1981). Additional, heretofore unreported information about Dinka knowledge of disease includes the following.

Dinka diagnose trypanosomosis (*liei* or *luac*) by a rough coat, hair loss beneath the tail, dry nose and clear eyes, followed by death. At necropsy the flesh and fat are watery and no blood flows from cut vessels. Blackleg—called *abanyjier* 'disease of the shoulder' or *macou*—is diagnosed by swollen and fevered forelegs and thorax, lameness, seepage of fluids from muscles containing patches of clotted blood, and death.

Ticks are removed to prevent a disease called simply *jong acak* 'tick disease' that is characterized by fever and anaemia. Dinka say this condition results from the heads of ticks being left in the skin. While Dinka appreciate the value of tick birds, they know that the birds often leave the tick's head behind. Whether for human infants or for calves, diarrhoea is known as *alaakic* (or in Bor Dinka, *yac*), meaning 'stomach'. Dysentery is distinguished by the term *yac riem* 'stomach of blood'. People or animals with dysentery are often quarantined.

Ethnoveterinary applications

Problems of delivering veterinary, public health, and other basic services to pastoralists are far more complex than for settled peoples (see also Stem, this volume). From colonial times, numerous attempts have been made to attach government veterinary assistants to transhumant and nomadic groups in Africa. But such efforts have generally met with little success, for a variety of reasons (Baumann 1990).

For one thing, even where veterinary assistants are from the same ethnic group as their clients, young people with little community standing are usually selected. Moreover, the assistants are typically relatively 'modernized' in that they have received elementary and technical education, often in a foreign language. Many are thus reluctant to return to traditional ways of life. In any case, because of their youth and lack of status, such health assistants do not command the authority that recognized indigenous healers do. The latter are often men of prestige with considerable power. Relationships between such healers and youthful medical assistants have typically been confrontational rather than cooperative.

To offset such tensions and to improve the delivery of government veterinary services to pastoral peoples, appropriate indigenous healers could be incorporated into official veterinary and/or human health organizations (Schwabe 1980, Schwabe 1984b:171–4, Schwabe and Kuojok 1981). Of course, these healers must be selected on the basis of their skills and their traditional areas of experience. Most cultures have several types of indigenous healers, not all of whom would be appropriate. Illustrating from the Dinka case, *atet* would be a logical choice because they already possess many skills that modern veterinary medicine recognizes as useful. Using the native language, basic training could be given to the selected group of healers so as to: confirm their abilities to recognize important diseases; improve what they already do and teach them a few other valuable techniques, for example, of wound care; correct any dangerous errors in belief or practice; and instruct the healers *cum* veterinary assistant and their communities in their proper role *vis-à-vis* government health services.

This proposal derives from the author's decades of experience with indigenous health beliefs and practices among Dinka, Turkana and Maasi (Schwabe 1990b, 1991). Certain types of indigenous healers within such communities could play a useful part in meeting a number of critical primary healthcare needs. This approach capitalizes upon community respect for traditional healers while eliminating potential frictions over role responsibilities with Western-trained practitioners. Also, by using existing human resources for service delivery wherever practical, the approach minimizes the risks of the uninformed introduction of alien, culturally disruptive medical beliefs and practices.

Equally important, trained healers could serve as a grassroots organization for the disease surveillance systems that are essential to implementing and evaluating well-informed and efficient programmes of disease intervention (Schwabe 1984b:171–4, 304–5). Numerous mass vaccination campaigns mounted throughout Africa have proved prohibitively expensive and ineffective in the face of meagre human and financial resources and recurrent political-economic instability. One example of past failures and future prospects comes from southern Sudan. Because of civil war, this region belatedly joined in pan-African efforts to eradicate rinderpest (JP-15) and CBPP (JP-28). But given Sudan's limited veterinary resources, only a small percentage of the region's cattle were ever actually vaccinated under these programmes (World Bank 1978). As a result of these initial failures, a bilateral Sudanese-German (GTZ) effort undertook the first systematic survey of cattle diseases in southern Sudan (Zessin and Baumann 1982).[6] Epidemiological analyses of the survey data on rinderpest and CBPP have been completed (Majok *et al.* 1991, Zessin *et al.* 1985) and those on trypanosomosis, various tick-borne infections, brucellosis, fasciolosis and several other helminthosis are in progress (Carlton 1991, 1992, Majok 1991). Overall, these studies suggest quite different distributions of some diseases than had been previously assumed on the basis of very little factual field evidence. They also suggest improvements that should be adopted in field procedures for similar surveys elsewhere and be incorporated into all aspects of on-going epidemiological surveillance as the core of veterinary service (Schwabe 1980, 1984b:393–492).

In delivering healthcare services, most poor countries confront a basic quandary. Money for costly conventional interventions such as mass vaccination is scarce, but so is money for the disease intelligence that would allow interventions to be more effectively targeted. In the absence of adequate disease intelligence, mass vaccination is so expensive because it must reach and inoculate animals that may not be at risk. To address this quandary, Zessin and Carpenter (1985) conducted a preliminary comparison of the benefit/cost feasibility of a conventional mass vaccination scheme as versus a surveillance-and-selective-action system of disease control in southern Sudan. The latter also incorporated traditional healers as important collectors of primary data (Schwabe 1980, 1984b:295–308, 393–429). Analysing the CBPP figures from the aforementioned survey in combination with economic data, Zessin and Carpenter concluded that an on-going surveillance-based programme that included local healers would be more cost-effective than conventional schemes.

Although renewed civil war has stalled implementation of such a programme in Sudan, a more comprehensive pilot project of surveillance using improved survey design elements gleaned from the Sudan work has since been implemented by the same GTZ team in central Somalia (Zessin *et al.* 1988). This project (later also interrupted by civil war, however) enlisted and trained nomadic animal health auxiliaries (NAHAs) to assist the government veterinary service. While traditional *atet*-like healers are lacking in this region of Somalia, the NAHAs selected were all nomadic herders who enjoyed local reputations for their knowledge of animal disease and husbandry. These individuals were nominated by committees of their pastoralist peers. Analyses have been initiated to ascertain whether the NAHAs' diagnoses are close enough to those of regular veterinary teams' as to make them valuable disease surveillance adjuncts. These studies will provide recommendations for continuing, discontinuing or modifying the NAHA training programme as part of a surveillance-based disease control strategy for pastoral Somalia, once peace is restored (Baumann 1990).[7]

Still further practical and economic advantage could be taken in pastoralist Africa of the fact that human and animal ethnomedicine often overlap. These overlaps could be used to facilitate co-operation between veterinary and public health branches of government, for example, in zoonoses control or in joint vaccination campaigns for both people and their animals (see also Ghirotti, this volume). Defence of professional turf and other barriers to co-operation among different government agencies account in part for the relative inefficacy and high cost of present programmes (Schwabe 1981, Schwabe and Schwabe 1990, WHO 1982).

It is important to note that if any government service *does* reach pastoral peoples, it is almost invariably animal, rather than human, healthcare. Among contemporary Nilotic Mundari, for example, animals have typically benefited more than their masters from Western medicine. Herders who have themselves never visited any type of government clinic, much less a hospital, nevertheless bring their cattle for inoculation (Buxton 1973). In many developing countries today, the veterinarian is still the service agent most likely to cross the threshold of rural homes. Hence, developers concerned with human health and other highly desired social services could profitably link into an innovative expansion of existing systems of rural veterinary extension (Schwabe 1981, 1984b).

Southern Sudan offers one example of such intersectoral co-operation. There, the UNICEF- and WHO-assisted Expanded Programme of Immunization (EPI) for vaccinating children against readily preventable diseases was grafted on to pre-existing cattle vaccination programmes in Bahr el Ghazal and Eastern Equatoria provinces among, respectively, Dinka and Mundari pastoralists. The goal of this joint effort was—even under disruptive wartime conditions—to achieve higher rates of vaccination coverage for both children and cattle than human and veterinary health programmes had previously been able to reach independently (Schwabe 1989). A preliminary assessment of this joint initiative (Schwabe and Schwabe 1990)[8] found that, despite current inadequacies, veterinary services have an exceptional capacity to act as a focus for cost-effective intersectoral efforts over broader development arenas within poor pastoral areas.[9] Indeed, as the 1989 study revealed, the price that Mundari cattle raisers were willing to pay for cattle vaccination alone was sufficient to finance the total effort. Significantly, too, the Mundari scheme has used paravet personnel (albeit not traditional healers).

Such intersectoral opportunities are especially germane for the least-developed countries, that is, the 'Third World's Third World'. With few exceptions, these nations are largely or entirely pastoral. Many have no alternative land-use possibilities (Pratt and Gwynne 1977, Schwabe 1984b:55–122). Especially at the local level in very resource-poor pastoral nations, delivery of health and other services could be greatly increased by basing modern outreach programmes on indigenous and other pre-existing institutions. In particular, human health initiatives that are linked to and promoted by veterinary services could be especially effective among African pastoralists, where traditional beliefs and practices about healing may be inextricably enmeshed in a totally fused (Riggs 1973, Schwabe 1994:Table 1) system of religion, health and animal husbandry that is central to human–animal symbiosis and survival.

Notes

1. It is not known whether the pre-dynastic and dynastic Egyptians (who spoke a language of the Afro-Asiatic phylum) were in contact with the ancestors of the Dinka. But the Egyptians did interact with some ancient black cattle-keeping peoples—identified by them as Wawat, Irtet and people of Yam—who inhabited the Nile Valley south of the first cataract, that is present-day Aswan (Adams 1977). We know,

too, that the A-Group and C-Group inhabitants of ancient Nubia, at least some of whom were no doubt these same peoples named by the Egyptians, were also cattle keepers (Adams 1977:152–3, 159, 197, 203, 330). Apparently so were the inhabitants of Egypt's pre-dynastic, pre-literate Badarian, Amration and Gerzean periods, as well as the early dynastic Egyptians. All these groups' archaeological remains suggest they lived lives not unlike those of today's Dinka (Adams 1971:111, 126, 139, Aldred 1965, Childe 1957, Frankfort 1948, Schwabe 1984a, Schwabe and Gordon 1988, Seligman 1932).

2. *Per Ankh* were sites in Egypt established, initially, for bull sacrifices and accompanying communion(?) rituals for the pharoah. Later, these sites became associated with healing, the keeping of papyri, and learning generally.

3. One priest of Sekhmet, Aha-Nakht is shown with the following text: 'I was a priest of Sekhmet, powerful and gifted in his craft, who lays his hands on patients, and thereby knows their condition, gifted in examining with his hand, who knows oxen' (Ghalioungui 1983:10). A later tomb text states 'Your herds are numerous in the stable thanks to the science of the priest of Sekhmet' (Ghalioungui 1983:12). Sauneron's (1960b:161) interpretation of the priests of Sekhmet is ' . . . [he] is renowned for his medical knowledge, specializing however in animal illnesses; one would consider him rather a veterinary'.

4. The Egyptian medical papyri mention *swnw* more often than they do priests of Sekhmet. Of the 50 Old Kingdom *swnw* known by name (Ghalioungui 1983:16–23), one is shown performing an act possibly related to human healing. This is Ghalioungui's No. 52, who is depicted squatting by the bed of the tomb's occupant. Three others—Irenakhty (No. 6), Wenen Nefer (No. 16) and Iry [?] (No. 51)—are also identified as priests and are shown presiding over the sacrifice and dissection of a bull, that is, a veterinary act. Wenen Nefer is further identified as a priest of Sekhmet.

5. Because for many pastoralists cattle *are* wealth (not simply a source of wealth) and because meat-eating among some of them is a religious act, this poses a problem in planning for capital formation through export of meat from parts of pastoralist Africa (Zessin 1991). To help overcome strong community reluctance to slaughter cattle expressly to eat, a palsied *ran de Ring* was employed several years ago in the municipal abattoir of Rumbek in Dinkaland to assure that every steer going to slaughter was blessed for some particular religious purpose, for example, for the marriage of so-and-so, for the recovery of so-and-so's child and for settling a dispute between two families.

6. The survey described here was done in the Bahr el Ghazal province. Further surveys were planned for other provinces in southern Sudan, but with the renewed civil war they were suspended.

7. Combined epidemiological and economic analyses are also in progress of the total disease, reproduction and husbandry data obtained from this project, as well as the outcomes of some simple but novel veterinary interventions tested by the project (Zessin 1991).

8. A fuller account entitled 'Vaccination of Children and Cattle in Pastoralist Africa: Practical Intersectoral Cooperation' is in preparation by C.L. Schwabe, C.W. Schwabe and S.S. Basta.

9. This subject is being examined in considerably greater detail in on-going work by Majok and Schwabe (1992). Significantly, similarly pioneering veterinary initiatives resulted in the first governmental outreach to rural peoples in Europe some 200 years ago (Schwabe 1984b:165–6; see also Schillhorn van Veen, this volume).

4. Recourse to traditional versus modern medicine for cattle and people in Sidama, Ethiopia[1]

MAURO GHIROTTI

Traditional veterinary practices have for long been treated like trees on savannah farms—not formally cultivated, yet valued and used.
(Paraphrased from Chavunduka and Last 1986)

IN MOST TRADITIONAL societies, there is no clear division between veterinary and human medicine (Schwabe 1978). Both contribute continuously to the development of local theories of and therapies for health and illness, just as they do in Western medicine. For example, in Africa and elsewhere, many of the same plants are used to treat both livestock and people (for example, Ibrahim, this volume, Ibrahim *et al.* 1984, Sofowora 1982). This symbiosis is even more evident in pastoral societies. Because of the vital economic and cultural functions of livestock in such societies, animals provide the model for medical knowledge (Evans-Pritchard 1940, Lewis 1961, Schwabe, this volume).

With the incursions of Western peoples and cultures, however, traditional Third World communities have encountered new pathologies; most have also changed their perceptions of illness and reduced their reliance on traditional medicine (Foster 1976, Wirsing 1985). Part of the acculturation process, these phenomena vary from society to society according to the cultural profundity of certain customs and the degree of Western-world pressure. Comparative studies aimed at analysing the post-contact use of traditional versus modern medicine in livestock and human healthcare are rare. This chapter offers one such analysis.

The research setting and methods

The Awraja
Located in the northern part of Sidama Province, the Sidama Awraja occupies some $5\,900\text{km}^2$, with a human population of 1.5 million (Figure 1). The Awraja is one of the most densely inhabited areas of Ethiopia, with 254 people/km^2, in contrast to the national average of only 32 people/km^2. As part of government policy, the territory's scattered population is being organized into nucleated settlements. This 'villagization' process is designed to facilitate the provision of basic social services and the organization of political activities.

The region is divided into three main ecozones, each with different agricultural systems and development potential (Figure 1). The lowlands are situated in the Rift Valley and range between 1100m and 1600m in altitude. Because of poor soil and an average annual rainfall of only 400mm in the lowlands, the main human activity in this zone is pastoralism. The next belt, the midlands, ranges from 1600m to 2000m and averages more than 1500mm of precipitation annually. Most of the Awraja's human population is concentrated in this very fertile zone. It has sustained rapid population growth because it furnishes a favourable environment for agriculture and development. The farming system, a combination of horticulture and animal husbandry, is characterized by the cultivation of false banana (*Ensete ventricosum*), which is the principal staple

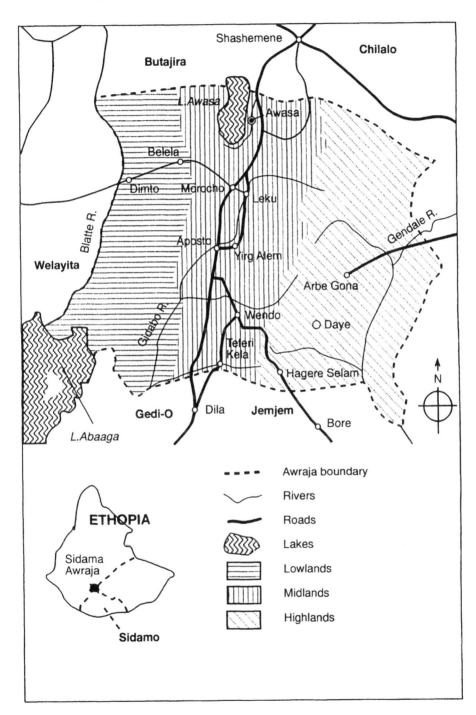

Figure 1. *The study region of the Sidama Awraja*

food, and by cash crops. Major cash crops include coffee (*Coffea arabica*, a wild shrub indigenous to southern Ethiopia) and *qat* (*Catha edulis*, whose leaves are chewed as a stimulant). Various fruit trees also contribute significantly to household income. Incomes in the midlands are higher than in the other two zones (Anonymous 1984). A tarmac road and the majority of the Awraja's dirt roads are found in the midlands, as are the main health services and the regional and district capitals. The territory above 2 000m constitutes the highlands, whose potential for cereal production has not yet been fully exploited. At present, abundant pasturage allows highland farmers to raise large numbers of live-stock, including the horses that provide most of the transport in this zone.

The comparative study reported here was conducted in the coffee-growing midlands. The principal ethnic group in this zone is the Sidama, a Cushitic-speaking people. The Sidama are divided into clans (*gherey*) that were governed in early times by a monarchy (Ayele 1975). Nowadays, however, they live together with the Oromo pastoralists (the Guji) who used to be their traditional enemies. 'Sidama', which means 'foreigner', was the name used by the Oromo during their expansion from the eastern Ethiopian highlands into the Awraja (Biasiutti 1959). The label has come to be applied to the Awraja as a whole, as well as to the province.

The Sidama are traditionally cattle raisers. But especially in the midlands, their way of life has changed as cultivation has invaded grazing areas. With a burgeoning population, people now prefer cropping to stockraising (Ayele 1975). Today, an average family of six to seven members must survive on a plot of approximately 0.4ha; 94 per cent of midland farmers own less than 1ha. Such small plots do not justify keeping draught oxen; instead, land is tilled by hand. Herd size is limited mainly by the scarcity and low carrying capacity of the range land, and some 48 per cent of local herds are made up of breeding cows (Ghirotti 1988). For both cultural and economic reasons, cattle are the principal domestic species. They provide prestige, extra income from sales of butter and sometimes bullocks, and manure for horticultural production. Milk and milk products are important components of the family diet. Whenever farmers are able to do so, they invest part of their coffee earnings in cattle.

Very little is known about Sidama medicine. But Sidama have a good know-ledge of medicinal plant properties[2] and special terms for various illnesses and symptoms in both humans and livestock (Ayele 1975, Central Statistical Office 1971, Ghirotti 1988).

Methods

The data presented below were collected as part of a household-level study of farming systems and child malnutrition. A questionnaire was administered to 102 heads of household from four Peasant Associations (that is, rural communities or villages) in the area. Two of the four associations were 'villagized' and two were not. The total population of each community ranged from 2 400 to 5 600, with a mean of 4 400. The questionnaire collected information on livestock ownership, veterinary problems encountered, and recourse to both traditional and modern veterinary or human medicine throughout the past year. Interviews took place in August 1988, during the rainy season. This period corresponds to the beginning of the traditional Sidama year and the end of the Ethiopian calendar. Thus, it was easier for farmers to recall events of the past year.

Household income was estimated by inventorying the previous year's agroforestry and livestock ownership and production, plus other sources of family income such as seasonal and casual labour, public work, handicrafting and trade. This inventory was then converted into monetary figures, in terms of Ethiopian Birr (Ghirotti 1988).[3] At the end of each interview, selected data (such as the number and species of animals owned) were verified using house condition as an indicator of wealth. All interviews were conducted in the local language (Sidamigna) through a trained interpreter during house-to-house visits.

Healthcare choices for cattle and people compared

The questionnaire results indicated that 96 per cent of the interviewees owned livestock, and approximately 89 per cent had cattle. About 10 per cent of households owned equids; 29 per cent kept small ruminants, mostly goats; and 61 per cent raised chickens. Goats and chickens are kept as a source of cash in case of emergency, but poultry are raised for home consumption as well.

During the year surveyed, 44 per cent of the farmers owning livestock needed veterinary assistance, mostly for cattle. The main problems they encountered in their cattle husbandry were, in order of priority: *haricho* 'diarrhoea'; *woramtu* 'cough, diarrhoea and emaciation', probably due to internal parasites; *butanu* 'cough'; and mastitis. There is no veterinary assistant in the four communities sampled, however. The few veterinary field staff are mostly engaged inadministrative work and the vaccination of cattle against major diseases. In the study sites, traditional livestock remedies are available. Also, modern drugs can be obtained from pharmacies, drug vendors, health centres, or more rarely, community agricultural agents. The proportion of farmers using indigenous, modern, or both types of medicine is shown in Figure 2.

Farmers' choice of veterinary treatment was not influenced by the type of disease. Neither was there any significant difference between the estimated income of farmers using traditional veterinary treatments and those choosing modern medicine. For the former, their average income was E. Birr 1 246.3 with a standard deviation of 439.7; for the latter, these figures were 1 120.1 and 487.9 (P > 0.1). Recourse to Western medicine, however, was higher in the villagized Peasant Associations (P < 0.005). Treatment success was independent of treat­ment choice (P > 0.1). In fact, eight of the farmers using traditional medicine and six of those using Western drugs reported that the animals they treated died.

For family health problems, farmers go to the nearest health station, buy drugs directly from a pharmacy or dispensary, or both (see Figure 3). Alternatively, they may use traditional treatments. No one in the sample reported using *both* traditional and modern health services for family members. Poor farmers—those with an estimated income of E. Birr 975 (SD = 542.2) for the year studied—more often chose traditional medicine (P = < 0.01). This figure contrasts with an average income of E. Birr 1 258 (SD 555.1) among the farmers who used modern medical systems and drugs.

Table 1 shows the numbers of interviewees who used traditional and/or modern veterinary medicine and compares them according to the type of healthcare they chose for family members. All but one interviewee reported seeking some type of assistance with human medical problems during the study period; but more than half (59) did not use veterinary treatments of either sort during this time. Although none of the interviewees reported using *both* traditional and modern medicine for family members, six did so for their livestock.

We might expect that families who use traditional medicine for themselves

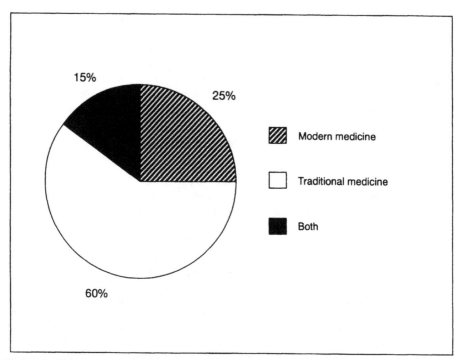

Figure 2. *Recourse to traditional versus modern medicine by Sidama farmers seeking veterinary assistance during the year studied (N = 42)*

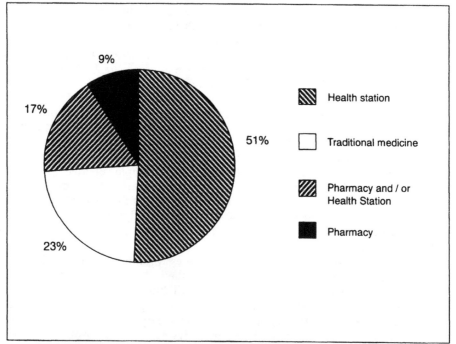

Figure 3. *Sidama farmers' recourse to traditional versus modern medicine for people during the year studied (N = 101)*

Table 1. Interviewees' recourse to traditional versus modern medicine for live-stock and people

Human treatments used	Veterinary treatments used					
	Traditional	Modern	(Subtotal)	Both	Neither	Total
Traditional	6	2	(8)	1	15	24
Modern	19	9	(28)	5	44	77
Total	25	11	36	6	59	101[a]

[a] A total of 102 farmers were interviewed. One farmer used traditional veterinary medicine but did not have recourse to any form of human medical care during the study period.

will also choose traditional treatments for their livestock. But Table 1 indicates that this is not the case, at least during the period studied. Thirty-six households exclusively used one or the other type of veterinary medicine (the third column in Table 1). Six of the eight households (75 per cent) who resorted to traditional medicine for family members and who also treated livestock chose only traditional veterinary treatments. But 19 of the 28 households (68 per cent) who employed modern medical treatments for humans also used only traditional veterinary medicine. A chi-square test reveals that the choice of types of veterinary and human healthcare is unrelated (chi-square not significant at P < 0.1 level).

Discussion

The Ethiopian government has made tremendous efforts to provide rural areas with basic community infrastructure and social services, particularly in health and education. In 1975 and 1978, the government mounted educational campaigns that included basic human healthcare delivery. After the WHO/UNICEF Alma Ata Declaration of 1978, it instituted a national primary healthcare programme. This programme sought to strengthen community involvement in healthcare and to promote co-operation among the different sectors working in human health and development, including indigenous healers. Adopting China's 'barefoot doctor' model, the Ethiopian government has trained selected farmers in basic health concepts and then returned these individuals to their rural communities.

Yet only a limited proportion of the population uses the national medical service. Instead, traditional medical systems meet most community needs for healthcare via a network of local herbalists (the *kabira* or the *debtara*), mystic healers (the *zar* doctors of the Amhara culture, the Islamic *sheikh*, or the *qala*) and birth attendants (Young 1979). In the highlands of eastern Ethiopia, for example, traditional practitioners handle almost 53 per cent of all human healthcare. Modern medicine is used in only 26 per cent of cases, and the remaining 21 per cent of patients take a pluralistic approach. As might be expected, coverage by government services is higher in urban than in rural areas (Slikkerveer 1982). But where roads are poor and household incomes low, as in the neighboring Arsi region, recourse to modern health services is still under 30 per cent, even near provincial centres (ISS/ICU 1986).

In the coffee-growing midlands of Sidama, traditional medicine is more widely used for livestock than for people. A number of factors may explain this. For one thing, all Sidama elders and experienced farmers are knowledgeable about indigenous veterinary remedies, and this knowledge is widely shared. Local veterinary practices are not kept secret. Thus, people probably have much more confidence in ethnomedicine for animals, since its efficacy has been proven for so long by so many.

In contrast, traditional healers of humans form an organized class that jealously guards its professional knowledge, handing it on from father to son or to a chosen apprentice. Their ethnomedical practice is still an important source of income and prestige. Traditional healers see the modern health system as a competitor. In spite of all the government's efforts, cooperation between traditional doctors and civil servants is very limited,[4] with the exception of the traditional birth attendants.

Another factor is that, in the study area, modern veterinary assistance is less readily available than are human healthcare services.[5] As in most of Africa, veterinary services are constrained by national budget problems. The limited availability of modern veterinary care also reflects the fact that stockraising is no longer the principal economic activity in Sidama households. In any case, when cattle fall sick the Sidama farmers have few alternatives. They must make their own diagnosis, possibly with help from an elder, and then either use folk remedies or buy modern drugs. But commercial drugs are quite expensive. They are much easier to justify in cases of family illness. This is borne out by the fact that households with higher incomes more commonly use modern medicine for family members.

Conclusion

The situation in the Sidama midlands may be somewhat special. The region enjoys favourable conditions for high-yielding agricultural production and cash cropping, and it has good roads, communication systems, schools, hospitals and health centres. The average income in Awraja coffee-growing zones is one of the highest in Ethiopia; and it is two to three times greater than incomes in the highland or lowland zones (Anonymous 1984). One of the most frequent complaints of highland farmers is the great distance they must travel to reach markets or public services (Ghirotti 1988). It is likely that in the highlands and lowlands, as in other rural regions of Ethiopia where communications are poor and incomes low, modern healthcare for both animals and people is much less accessible than in the coffee-growing midlands.

Especially in regions where formal veterinary assistance cannot be readily provided, a better understanding of ethnoveterinary medicine might allow government authorities and developers to strengthen traditional systems of animal healthcare. More research needs to be devoted to traditional systems because they embody an inestimable cultural and technical heritage elaborated across centuries of experience. Many Sidama elders are quite willing to share their local veterinary knowledge. As Ibrahim (1986) has observed in Nigeria, collecting reliable information on veterinary, as versus human, ethnomedicine is much easier because it is freely exchanged. Moreover, such information can lead to a better understanding of human ethnomedical concepts and techniques, too (Ibrahim, this volume). With a more profound appreciation not only of herbalism but also of the whole emic perception of illness, it should be possible to design better forms of collaboration between veterinary and human, and traditional and modern, systems of healthcare.

Notes

1. This study was conducted during fieldwork for the International Course for Primary Health Care Managers at District Level in Developing Countries, organized by the Istituto Superiore di Sanitá, Rome, and supported by the Italian Ministry of Foreign Affairs. The author is very grateful for the assistance of: Drs R. Guerra and P. Warren, course supervisor and anthropologist, respectively; Mr T. Estefanos of the Ethiopian Nutritional Institute; the staff of the UNICEF/WHO Joint Nutritional Support Programme, Sidama; Dr S. Sanford of ILCA; Ms S. Z. Babsa, typist; Ms A. Sophie, ILCA librarian; Mr G. Beccaloni, Agricultural documentation, FAO; Ms Zebenay I., interpreter; and Dr R. B. Griffiths, who provided valuable commentary on the manuscript. In addition, the co-operation, patience, dedication and knowledge of Sidama farmers and of local medical and agricultural field staff provided the author a great lesson in humanity and civility.
2. On the other hand, traditional healers are not always able to control the side-effects of some of their botanical remedies. Examples are the local drugs *kosso* (*Hagenia abyssinica*) and *enkoko* (*Embelia schimperi*). These are used to treat *Taenia saginata* in humans (which is quite frequent in Ethiopia because of the custom of eating raw meat) and other gastrointestinal infections. These indigenous taenicides are responsible for severe diarrhoea that, particularly for children or the old, can be fatal.
3. At the time of research, one Ethiopian Birr equalled US$2.05; or, US$1.00 equalled E. Birr 0.49.
4. The many difficulties of achieving such co-operation so as to establish a syncretic health system have been detailed for Cushitic and Bantu Africa by Last and Chavunduka (1986), Oyebola (1981) and Slikkerveer (1982, 1990).
5. However, only two of the 43 interviewees who sought some form of veterinary help viewed this as a problem. Nearly all of them instead considered the lack of pastureland and cash as major constraints to livestock production (see also Stem, this volume).

5. Ethno-toxicology among Nigerian agropastoralists

MAMMAN A. IBRAHIM

IN ORDER TO survive, human beings throughout history have had to discriminate between poisonous and non-poisonous materials (Trease and Evans 1978). Poisonous materials are especially abundant in rural areas, where the natural environment has been left more nearly intact than in urban environs. Moreover, in most of the developing world, many plants regarded as poisonous are also used as food and healing drugs, in addition to their more dramatic uses in homicide or trial by ordeal (Dalziel 1937, Fraser and Mackenzie 1910). Thus it is hardly surprising that rural peoples have acquired a knowledge of natural toxins and other drugs. Their practical understanding of toxicology extends not only to themselves but also to their domestic animals.

Curiously, though, ethno-toxicology has received little systematic scientific attention, despite its far-reaching implications for R&D from a variety of disciplinary perspectives, including (among others) veterinary and human medicine, pharmacology, the environmental and agricultural sciences, and anthropology. Unfortunately, ethno-toxicological and ethno-pharmacological knowledge is dwindling among the younger generation in many countries. Also, knowledge is lost and the risks of poisoning further increased by the resettlement of people and their herds in new places where both the natural and human-made environment is unfamiliar to them. (See Keeler 1975 for a telling example from the western US.)

This chapter records some of the ethno-toxicological knowledge still held by Hausa and settled Fulani agropastoralists of Nigeria. Although the focus is on ethnoveterinary toxicology, concepts and examples are also drawn from human ethnomedicine in rural Nigeria, since many apply equally to people and animals.[1] First, Hausa terms for and types of vegetable, animal and other poisons are described, along with their uses, treatment and control. Special attention is given to neglected poisons of animal origin. Then, agropastoralists' ethno-toxicological concepts (and development workers' inattention to them) are analysed for their implications vis-à-vis the introduction of potent Western drugs as part of veterinary or human healthcare development in nations like Nigeria.

Terminology, types, uses and control of toxic substances

In rural Nigeria, there are many opportunities for livestock poisoning. This threat is exacerbated by factors such as an extended dry season, frequent droughts, overgrazing, nomadic and other movements of animals, and certain husbandry practices. However, most agropastoralists are well versed in the dangers, as well as the benefits, of toxic vegetation found in their environment. A herd's well-being depends in large part upon its owner's astute use of forage resources. During the dry season, for example, stockowners often provide their animals with extra feed in the form of crop residues and/or cuttings and loppings from wild plants. And during the cropping season, in areas where the law requires most animals to be confined, stockowners must carefully select and supply *all* their herds' feed.

In addition to plants, Hausa and Fulani recognize various animals and other organic or inorganic materials as toxic. Nigerian agropastoralists' ethno-toxicology also includes non-physical or supernatural agents such as spirits, curses, hexes and the evil eye. These 'poisons' are believed to act at a distance, sometimes with tangible materials such as charms serving as their vehicle.

The generic Hausa word for poison is *guba*; the word for 'antidote' is *makari* 'the breaker'.[2] Poisons of vegetable or animal origin are called *dafi*, and any deadly poison administered by mouth is called *ma'dashi* or *ma'das*. Emically, *guba* also includes the curses, hexes, evil eye (*baki, 'kofi, sammu*), and so forth noted above. Often the term *magani* 'medicine' is used to denote the non-physical components of such intangible poisons (Abraham 1958). Beyond this generic vocabulary, specific toxic substances often have distinct names. The names of especially toxic items often reflect their effect. An example is the *kashe kaji* 'kill fowls' plant (*Psorospermum guineense*; Dalziel 1937). There are also special terms for other sources of poisoning such as snake bites (*cizo*), snake strikes (*sari*) and insect stings (*harbi* 'to shoot').

In Hausa communities, the traditional authorities on poisons and their antidotes include circus performers (*gardawa*) and the indigenous guilds of hunters (*mafaruta* or *'yan baka*) and blacksmiths (*ma'kera*). However, difficult cases of poisoning—particularly those involving substances of animal origin—are by preference referred to the blacksmith. This is because of his unique expertise in preparing *gunguma*, the potent poisons for arrows and spearheads (Fraser and Mackenzie 1910). These include *tururubi* and *tunya*, respectively prepared from *Gnidia kraussiana* and *Euphorbia posonii*, plus other ingredients. These poisons are also used in fishing (Dalziel 1937).

Types of toxins
Toxins of vegetable origin For historical reasons, the study of indigenous poisons, drugs, and foods in Nigeria has centred on botanicals. British colonial forces naturally paid particular attention to the poisons tipping the arrows and spears launched at them (Baker 1970), but they were also interested in other native drugs and foodstuffs that were toxicologically active (Rosevear 1976). In addition to the colonial literature, there is a sizeable contemporary literature on poisonous plants of Nigeria (Nwude 1981, 1982a, 1982b; Nwude and Parsons 1977; Singha 1965). This literature almost invariably consists, however, of studies of toxic plants as defined by scientists, rather than by local people. Yet local understandings of toxic plants differ from scientists' in several important ways.

For example, Nigerian agropastoralists view only a few plants as so toxic that they are employed solely as poisons—notably those used in warfare, hunting and fishing. With these limited exceptions, most toxic plants are employed for beneficial medicinal or nutritional, as well as poisoning, purposes. Even some of agropastoralists' food staples (such as sorghum and bitter cassava) are toxic. In general, plants that have only insidious or cumulative toxic effects are not generally recognized by rural Nigerians as poisonous (Ibrahim *et al.* 1983, Nwude 1982a).

Like traditional stockraisers everywhere, however, Hausa and Fulani agropastoralists are quite knowledgeable about the toxic forages in their environment.

They know that the leaves of *baska* (*Erythrophleum guineense*) are highly toxic
to sheep (Nwude and Chineme 1980).[3] Herders also know that different varieties
of the same plant species can differ in toxicity; that the active agent often
concentrates in a particular part such as the roots or seeds; and that certain
factors such as moisture may increase the risk of poisoning. For these reasons
Fulani do not graze their stock on the dew-soaked forage of the early morning.
The stated rationale behind this practice is to prevent diarrhoea in their herds.
However, herders may also recognize that moisture encourages less-discriminate
grazing or that it makes some poisonous plants more palatable, as has been
shown for certain species elsewhere (for example, *Halogeton* spp., Brunner and
Robertson 1963, cited in Nwude 1976). As a general precaution, in the vicinity
of human habitations or corrals and cattle camps, Hausa and Fulani eradicate all
plants known to be poisonous. Herders also take pains to see that their animals
do not graze in any other places infested with such plants.

Whether for livestock or people, poisonous plants used as foods and medicines
are subjected to various extraction and detoxification procedures beforehand.
Such procedures sometimes include pH adjustments using ash and potash
(*kanwa*) or botanical acids. Ash from the burnt bark of *jiri* (*Stereospermum
kunthianum*) and *gogai* (*Striga senegalensis*) is also included in oral antidotes
for plant poisoning in livestock. Striga is used specifically for sheep and goats
poisoned by excess consumption of freshly harvested sorghum (Nwude and
Ibrahim 1980). Hausa and Fulani also appreciate the role of catalysts, activators
and other drugs. For example, *chitta aho* (*Zingiber officinale*) is used to delay the
action of internal poisons. Milk, eggs, and sugar are given as demulcents to
retard the absorption of poisons. '*Gya' da* oil (from *Arachis hypogaea*) serves as
a cathartic to enhance elimination of toxins (Nwude 1982b, Nwude and Ibrahim
1980). Prescriptions involving drugs such as purgatives and emetics, which are
known to produce undesirable side effects, are usually accompanied by their
antidote or deactivator.

Toxins of animal origin Among the approximately 100 species of snakes
found in Nigeria, 40 are venomous and 10 are deadly (Nwude 1982b). But
Hausa and Fulani regard *all* snakes as poisonous, along with some species of
gecko and skink lizards.[4] Unaware of the significance of fangs in distinguishing
poisonous from non-poisonous snakes, rural people generally believe that venom
is produced and stored in the tail and then transported to the mouth during
envenomation. Neither do most rural Hausa and Fulani realize that a snake
that has lost its fangs cannot deliver its venom.

Some snakes are considered to possess, or even to be, spiritual powers.
Malevolent spirits in particular are said to manifest themselves as snakes. Folk
belief holds that such snakes may transform themselves back into spirits and
exact vengeance upon anyone who molests or kills them. Thus people are careful
not to offend these snakes *cum* spirits by avoiding annoying behaviours such as
whistling, hissing, or destroying the reptile's abode. Similarly, it is not wise to
mention a snake by name, for it may respond with an unwelcome night-time visit
to the speaker or his herd. To be on the safe side, most people speak of *abin
'kasa* 'the thing on the ground' rather than *maciji* 'snake'.

To remove powerful spirit-snakes without incurring their wrath, people sometimes call in a snake-charmer. A charmer may also be called upon to keep snakes
away from poultry—as the Poultry Department of a Nigerian University recently
did. Alternatively, Hausa and Fulani may surround their poultry coops with
slices of garlic (Ibrahim and Abdu, this volume) or plant certain species of

Euphorbia and lemon grass around them to repel snakes. People also take care to keep such areas clear of twining vines like *ciwo* (*Landolphis florida*), which they believe attract snakes. Snake bite in livestock is treated by feeding the soaked bark of *jan yaro* (*Hymenocardia acida*) or by drenching with an infusion of *Annona senegalensis* leaves.

Sometimes correctly and sometimes not, Hausa and Fulani agropastoralists also regard a vast number of arthropods as poisonous. These include wasps, bees, spiders, caterpillars, millipedes, earwigs, biting ants, scorpions and ticks. To take one example, a malodourous green locust is believed to be poisonous when eaten by livestock—possibly because it is usually found in association with *tumfafiya* (*Calotropis procera*), a poisonous weed. When an animal is stung by a scorpion, fresh leaves of *kalkashin 'korama* (*Heliotropium indicum*) are squeezed and rubbed on the hide at the site of the sting. Hausa and Fulani believe that ticks (*kaska*) produce venom, but agropastoralists are generally unaware of ticks' precise role in disease transmission. Nevertheless, Fulani are always careful to remove the large *Amblyomma variegatum* (Fulful'de *kooti*) from their animals because this species is believed to be more dangerous than the smaller *miri* (Bayer and Maina 1984).

Manufactured toxins Rural Hausa and Fulani encounter few manufactured or inorganic poisons in their environment. However, they are familiar with the toxic properties of paraffin, which they use as a cheap and effective insecticide against termites, mosquitoes and other household pests, and as an acaricide for livestock. Paraffin is used both as a foot-bath for sheep and as a wash for ectoparasites of cattle, although the latter practice sometimes causes chemical dermatitis.

Non-physical toxins Nigerian Hausa and some settled Fulani practise a form of voodoo known as *bori*, which calls upon evil spirits (see also Ibrahim and Abdu, this volume). Perhaps the most feared of such spirits is the malevolent *Gajimari*, who is said to cause many mysterious deaths among both domestic animals and people every year.[5] It turns out that this 'spirit' is in fact a mixture of toxic biogases produced in unexpected places (Ibrahim 1990). People use the leaves and roots of *tazargade* (*Artemisia maciverae*) to ward against voodoo attacks. Whether burnt as incense or worn as an amulet, the smell of the leaves is believed to drive off evil spirits. In addition to the supernatural (and in the case of humans, psychosomatic) action of spirits, curses and hexes, there is some evidence that slow poisoning may play a role in the so-called voodoo deaths of livestock and people in Africa (Jensen 1970).

Implications for development

As many researchers and developers have observed, a frequent problem in introducing Western-style veterinary medicine in rural areas is stockowners' injudicious use of commercial drugs (see Grandin and Young, this volume, Mathias-Mundy and McCorkle 1989). Stockraisers are prone to misdosing with such drugs or to administering them indiscriminately, sometimes thereby aggravating the health problems of their animals. Development workers and other outsiders tend to lay all the blame for such behaviour on the ignorance of the local population. Seldom do they stop to consider that their *own* ignorance of local toxicological, pharmacological and related ethnomedical knowledge, practice and terminology may be part of the problem. In fact, while a review of the literature for Nigeria suggests that indigenous posological concepts and regimens are perhaps the least-developed aspect of the ethnomedical system

(Ibrahim *et al.* 1983), it also suggests that such concepts and regimens are the least understood by Western-style researchers. Several factors are involved in this mutual ignorance, each with different implications for the extension of Western pharmaco-therapies and agro-chemicals.

First, the therapeutic objective of local practitioners is clinical improvement rather than complete elimination of the causative agent. Consequently drugs are given 'to effect'. Of course, for certain ailments, incomplete treatment of intoxicating or infectious agents can be beneficial insofar as it encourages development of tolerance or premunity. But Hausa and Fulani apply their therapeutic objective of clinical improvement to *all* health problems, including those treated with Western drugs. Thus, people often discontinue prescribed treatments or medications just as soon as they or their animals show signs of recovery.

Second, Nigerian agropastoralists' ethnomedical system includes only limited concepts of carrier status; the idea of culling apparently healthy animals based on invisible evidence such as serology is totally alien. This is perhaps understandable in light of the fact that rural Nigerians have little access to the technology necessary to detect micro-organisms, complex parasitic life cycles, or other invisible or subtle agents of disease.

A third factor is rural people's multidimensional use of poisons and other drugs. To take just one example, a study of 107 plants employed in Hausa therapies for gastro-enteric disorders in humans found that about half these plants also served as food for people (Etkin and Ross 1982) and animals (author's field experience). Even indigenous materials employed as insecticides are also sometimes eaten by humans and livestock. In short, for rural people, the line between poison and food or feed is thin.

A fourth factor in Nigerians' apparent disregard for posology is that their own, local drugs are mainly crude botanicals. Thus their pharmacological action varies greatly according to such factors as place and time of plant collection, storage methods and season of the year. Crude botanicals are also easily degraded in the Nigerian environment, and they are typically more readily biotransformed *in vivo* than are commercial drugs. Under such variable conditions and in the absence of analytical techniques other than bio-assay, perhaps people's failure to fix dosages makes sense.

Rural people have applied the toxicological and pharmacological concepts and practices they have derived through experience with their crude botanicals of low potency, toxicity and persistence to the vastly more purified, potent, toxic or persistent commercial pharmaceuticals and agro-toxins. Yet development professionals have made little effort to understand this quite logical analogy. They have been even slower to grasp the implications of this process for human and animal health.

To illustrate the results of this analogy, Nigerian merchants, for example, see nothing wrong with keeping flies away from meat and fish offered for sale in the market-place by spraying their wares with potent commercial insecticides. As noted above, some of the plants that provide indigenous insecticides also serve as foodstuffs. Likewise for Nigerian fishermen who, on analogy with their traditional fish poisons, have been known to dump DDT and other chemicals into the dams that supply cities, villages and livestock with drinking-water. To take another example, Nigerians pay little heed to the Western-style slaughter clearance periods instituted for livestock treated with commercial drugs. Since their traditional pharmaco-therapy mostly involves drugs they believe to be safe enough to eat as food, people have little notion of harmful residues in meat or other animal products. Moreover, traditional culling practices dictate slaughter and consumption of sick animals that fail to respond to treatment. In any case, given Nigeria's current economic crisis, the health risks from protein deficiency are doubtless greater than those from drug residues. Consequently, even trained veterinarians and physicians ignore the slaughter clearance rules.

Development workers' ignorance of even basic ethnomedical vocabulary, too, can contribute to the misuse of introduced drugs. For example, Hausa and Fulani are somewhat stoic in their attitude towards pain, and really have no precise word for 'analgesic' or 'pain-killer'. While some traditional remedies in fact consist of local analgesics applied primarily to reduce the pain, they are named according to the problem they are used to treat. An example is *maganin kunama* 'scorpion medicine'. Unfortunately, the Hausa word chosen by pharmacological advertisers as the translation for 'analgesic' also means 'tonic' or 'stimulant'. Traditional tonics are culturally highly valued and approved, and people take them frequently. This mistranslation has led to the widespread misuse of Western analgesic drugs, not only among rural Nigerians but also among the educated élites. People now take such drugs as paracetamol and acetylsalicylic acid (aspirin) before going to work each day or whenever they feel tired, which can be several times daily. Government edicts to prohibit the generalized sale and use of these drugs have had no effect. But the entire problem could almost certainly have been avoided if the trouble had been taken to first learn some simple facts about the vocabulary of traditional pharmacology.

In sum, whether for purposes of livestock development or improved human health, study of a people's ethno-medical system can help predict how they will respond to the introduction of new medical options. If governments or change agents choose to blunder ahead with development 'plans' in ignorance of the corresponding ethnoscience, then they really have no one but themselves to blame for the outcome.

Notes

1. A fuller and more integrated discussion can be found in Ibrahim's study of the rainbow spirit (1990).
2. All non-English terms are from the Hausa unless otherwise noted.
3. This is also the toxic plant of choice for unhappily married Hausa wives who want to do away with their husbands. Chemical analysis reveals that *Erythrophleum guineense* contains a variety of alkaloids, of which norcassaidine is the most toxic (Watt and Breyer-Brandwijk 1962).
4. Ibrahim's study on human and animal toxicology (in progress) offers greater detail on Hausa and scientific names of snakes and other species deemed to be poisonous, their distribution in rural Nigeria and local beliefs and proverbs pertaining to them.
5. Other names for this evil spirit are *masha ruwa* 'the water drainer', *maje sama* 'the one who goes up', *bakan gizo* 'rainbow', or simply *babba* 'the great one' (Ibrahim n.d.).

6. I stand for my horse:
Equine husbandry and healthcare among some North American Indians[1]

ELIZABETH ATWOOD LAWRENCE

To be alone with our war-horses . . . teaches them to understand us, and us to understand them. My horse fights with me and fasts with me, because if he is to carry me in battle he must know my heart and I must know his or we shall never become brothers. I have been told that the white man, who is almost a god, and yet a great fool, does not believe that the horse has a spirit [soul]. This cannot be true. I have many times seen my horse's soul in his eyes.
(Chief Plenty-coups, cited in Linderman 1930:100)

THUS DID THE most respected chief of the Crow Indians describe a vital aspect of his people's relationship with their horses. In North America the advent of the horse resulted in the flowering of a distinctive horse culture during the eighteenth and nineteenth centuries among tribes such as the Apache, Arapaho, Arikara, Assiniboin, Blackfoot, Cheyenne, Comanche, Cree, Crow, Hidatsa, Kiowa, Navaho, Nez Perce, Omaha, Pawnee, Ponca, Sarsi, Sioux and Ute. Besides providing formerly pedestrian peoples with such practical benefits as transport and traction, horses became the most prized of all possessions among equestrian Indians. Horses were the measure of wealth, the standard for trade and payment, and a symbol of prestige and power. Additionally, as Plenty-coups' words suggest, the horse dramatically expanded mounted Indians' mental as well as physical horizons. Indeed, these swift, powerful and responsive creatures became an intimate part of every aspect of equestrian Indians' psychological, spiritual and aesthetic lives. The result was one of the closest human–horse relationships known in history.

This relationship extended across the whole of an Indian's life and continued even after death. Among Apache or Navajo, for example, the central importance of horses to a new-born child was established shortly after birth. An infant's umbilical cord was tied to a horse's mane or tail or buried in a horse track to assure future fortuitous interactions with horses; and infants were fed mare's milk to make them grow strong. Puberty rites involved horse songs, horse symbolism and invocations to equine beings. In numerous tribes, a gift of horses to the bride's family was vital at the time of marriage. As adults, hunters and warriors felt a deep sense of unity and identification with their mounts. When a Navajo took his horse into war, for example, he would 'whisper the message he really intended for himself: "Be lively; you and I are going into a dangerous business, my horse. Be brave when you go to war and nothing will happen; we will come back safely"' (Clark 1966:160). Finally, a favourite mount often accompanied its master into death, by means of a widespread funeral custom in which the animal was ceremonially sacrificed so that horse and rider would be eternally linked in the spirit world, just as they had been on earth.

Such was the intimacy between Indians and their mounts that, among Apache or Navajo, if a horse injured its rider, when pacified the animal could heal the very injuries it had caused in anger. It was assumed that the injured person must have offended the animal. So a shaman would be hired to perform a curing rite begging the horse's forgiveness and invoking its help in healing. In one such Navajo rite, a song to the Horse Spirit correlates the health and well-being of horse and human: 'Let the means that keep your body in health also keep my body in health!' (Clark 1966:176). In the Navajo Beauty Way and Water Way ceremonies, the help of White Water Horse is invoked for curing people. Similarly, in the Blessingway ritual Turquoise Horse is believed to restore peace and order to the mind and body of a Navajo who feels out of harmony with his surroundings. A song of invocation indicates that the spirit of this equine entity 'belongs to the patient, the turquoise horse with lightning feet, with a mane like distant rain, a black star for an eye and white shells for teeth, the horse spirit who feeds on the pollen of flowers' (Clark 1966:171). The words of the song indicate the importance of aesthetics, as well as power, in healing—here expressed through the beauty of the horse, who partakes of the universal splendours of nature.

Most equestrian tribes believed that horses possessed supernatural abilities and that certain animals held a secret power evidenced by their great feats of endurance, miraculous escapes or recovery from mortal wounds; dead horses could even return in spirit form. Lakota Sioux refer to horses as *wakan*, 'holy' or 'sacred', 'Because what is *wakan* constitutes the very ground of being, it is the basis for important interrelationships among life forms' (DeMallie and Jahner 1980:147, 168). *Wakan* is also associated with healing. Many tribes believed that horses could bestow some of their special powers upon favoured men and women, making them expert in curing and other rites and skills. For example, a Crow story relates how, in exchange for a young woman's solicitous care of an old pregnant mare, the mare endowed her with exceptional expertise as a midwife.

Such notions of inter-species reciprocity generally permeated traditional Indian–horse relationships. According to the treatment it received, a horse could intervene in a corresponding way to bring benefit or misfortune to its owner or others. For example, an old-time Crow warrior who treated his mount well was rewarded with supernatural knowledge for obtaining many more horses. As he recounts:

I was a poor boy. I had one mare and I cared for her like a babe. I took her to water and to places where the grass was fresh. I had a vision in which she transformed herself into a spirit-man and made known to me the secrets of multiplying the herd. You see the great drove I now have. If you are patient and care for the horses as you would a child, the spirit-horse will pity you and you will become prosperous. (cited in Curtis 1970:60)

Or as a Hidatsa father instructed his son:

These horses are gods, or mystery beings. They have supernatural power. If one cares for them properly and seeks good grazing and water for them, they will increase rapidly . . . if you will remember my words and observe them when you are older, your horses will increase . . . These horses . . . have minds and understand. I once had a stallion and did not guard him as I should, so he wandered away to another herd of horses. Even then, I did not go to get him, but let him go as if I did not care. One night I dreamed that the stallion stood before me. 'You did not care for me as you should have done,' he said. 'You would not give me good water and grass, so I went to another country . . .' Not long after that, some enemies came and stole that stallion from me.

So the dream came true. He went to another country and I lost him. Ever since that time I have taken good care of my horses. (cited in Wilson 1924:142, 145)

Apache likewise believed that a horse poorly cared for or mistreated would take revenge by causing the perpetrator to fall sick. Only a shaman specializing in the ceremony of the horse could cure such ills. Lakota Sioux expressed a similar sense of reciprocal interaction (see DeMallie and Jahner 1980:147, 167–8). Similarly, Cheyenne horse doctors and their families were constrained by strict rules of behaviour and taboos that, if broken, would bring harm to themselves or their herds. Horse doctors who struck a horse on the head, for example, would never again receive horses in payment for their services. It is especially noteworthy that 'no horse doctor would eat horseflesh, and no horse doctor would shoot a horse, wild or tame' (Grinnell 1923–2:143).

Modern-day Crow likewise believe that abusing, harming, or killing a horse will bring illness, injury or misfortune to humans. Many Crow still honour this tradition by refusing to injure or kill any horse. Reportedly, two Crow Indians who participated in a government slaughter of reservation horses in the 1920s soon afterwards 'drank, beat people, had no luck with their families, and went to early deaths. Both men died from horse accidents.' Crow children are still admonished that 'Cruelty to horses backlashes in your face. If you run your horses all the time, something bad will happen to you sooner or later.' Out of gratitude for the many benefits that horses conferred upon their people, Crow also continue to observe their tribal taboo against eating horsemeat.

Healthcare practitioners[2]

Because of equestrian Indians' high regard for horses, special knowledge and procedures developed to help increase herds, cure their diseases, heal their injuries, restore their vitality, protect them from harm, and control their actions during racing, hunting and warfare. Various tribes held that such knowledge and skill were acquired, used, and rewarded in different ways. Traditions also varied within tribes as to whether healthcare was the job of specialists (either as members of a cult/guild or as individual shamans or horse doctors) or whether ordinary horse owners could treat their own animals.

Certain tribes had a horse medicine cult comprised of an exclusive group of practitioners who possessed powerful horse medicine. Because of the secrecy associated with these organizations, relatively little is known about them. They have been documented most fully for Crow (Lowie 1924) and for Blackfoot and certain related groups such as Piegan (Ewers 1969). But horse cults also appear to have existed among other tribes, such as the Arikara, Arapaho, Assiniboin, Cree, Kiowa, Oglala Sioux and Sarsi.

A central feature of both the Crow and Blackfoot cults was the Horse Dance, a ceremony in which new members were initiated and secret knowledge about equine medicine was exchanged. Drumming, singing, and dancing with sacred paraphernalia, at times imitating equine gaits and motions, were part of the ritual, which featured an altar decorated with horse motifs cut from rawhide. Among Piegan, such a cult originated from a dream of its founder, in which horses he had treated well imparted to him special curative powers, along with details of the Horse Dance. Only individuals who owned horse medicine could dance. Such medicine was sometimes originally obtained through communication with other animals. For example, one Crow medicine man (presumably a cult member) stated that a blackbird taught him how to capture horses from the enemy. The grandfather of one of the author's Crow informants also 'received his horse medicine from this bird, which gave him special ability to control horses'. Cult membership and knowledge were generally transferred along familial lines to a brother or son; but a non-kinsman who aspired to the power could exchange gifts and/or money for a member's esoteric information and instruction.

Although Apache and Navajo lacked such cults, certain shamans possessed special powers over, and from, horses. They knew medicines, rituals, songs, prayers and other procedures to increase herds, geld stallions, break mustangs, win races, teach horsemanship to young boys, and endow their protégés with the ability to perform dangerous equestrian feats without mishap, as well as to prevent and cure disease and injury. Along with the precious gift of horses and the art of raiding, rules for equine husbandry and healthcare were originally taught to Apache and Navajo by culture heroes who instructed people to keep their horses holy as well as healthy. Specific medicines and rituals were directly imparted to horse shamans by a Holy Being, a horse, or an agent of a horse.

Among Apache, for example, a 'horse could take a fancy to an individual and bestow its magic potencies upon him' (Clark 1966:100). One Apache thus favoured acquired his power through horses who addressed him as follows: 'Grandchild, you know our ways. We belong to you now' (Clark 1966:101). The kinship term signified that man and horse would henceforth share an intimate relationship. Another Apache received his power from an old sorrel who gave him the capacity to cure a seriously injured companion, plus songs that led the man to become a prominent horse shaman. Yet another shaman obtained his extraordinary abilities to track and heal horses from a cowbird, who had in turn received this power from a horse. The powers of some Apache horse shamans also extended to their own herds, such that they possessed 'fit horses all the time'. For example, one shaman was known for having horses that 'were nice and fat because she knew songs for them', and 'the ceremony of the horse' enabled her to 'take wild horses and saddle them up. They were always gentle to her' (Opler 1965:296–7).

Other tribes, such as the Cheyenne, had neither guilds nor shamans that devoted themselves exclusively to equine husbandry and healthcare. Instead, 'the doctor [either male or female] who possessed the power to heal men exercised this power as well on horses', and instruction in human medicine included 'the secrets of doctoring horses' (Grinnell 1923–2:139–40).

Specialists in equine healthcare typically were paid for their services. For multiple castrations, for example, a Blackfoot medicine man might earn a horse; for only one or two operations, less valuable objects such as blankets, shirts and arrows were paid. For exercising their racing medicine, Apache and Navajo shamans were recompensed with items like saddles, blankets and bridles. Among Blackfoot, Crow and other groups, membership in the Horse Dance Society was much sought after because members were reputed to become wealthy not only from the fees they earned but also by means of supernatural assistance. As one Crow medicine woman recounted:

. . . considerable property was acquired by me and my family since we got the medicine bundle—plenty of horses and other valuables. Sometimes there was a rumor that all medicines were to be taken away by the Government; then I could never sleep for fear of losing this horse medicine. I do not consider myself holy, but attribute my success to this medicine.   (Lowie 1924:333).

Another adoptee into the Crow Horse Dance society described how he became wealthy. He related that one night he and his wife sang horse society songs and '. . . the next morning . . . as soon as I got to my herd I saw two new [Sioux] race horses among mine with brand-new saddles and blankets'. Another time, singing brought him three more horses. On yet another occasion, after singing with his wife, 'The following day there was a big fight and I captured the prettiest horse ever owned by a Sioux, a red-eared pinto, and in addition a perfectly white horse . . . I also got the root for restoring horses [see next section] . . . When people were about to race, they paid me . . . to . . . make him [the racehorse] win. Sometimes a horse was given in payment for this' (Lowie 1924:333–4). In contrast to Crow medicine men and women, Cheyenne horse doctors took whatever they were offered (horses, blankets, saddles, arrows, robes, sometimes a 'good fat buffalo') rather than a fixed fee. (Grinnell 1923–2:139).

As noted earlier, equine healthcare specialists dealt with more than just disease and injury. Oglala Sioux medicine-men, for instance, were hired to lure away enemy horses during a raid, to make horses swift, to revive exhausted mounts, to calm balky animals, to handicap rivals' racehorses, and to ensure that brood mares produced fine offspring. Some specialists possessed still other powers. Among Blackfoot, for example, horse medicine men had the ability to capture wild horses by rubbing secret substances on their hands, feet and ropes, and then circling the wild horses upwind so that they would be attracted by the odour, subdued and lassoed. One celebrated 'old-time' Cheyenne horse doctor would 'spit horse-dung from his mouth' and sometimes a colt's hoof would come part way out of his mouth and then retract again. To call his favourite horse in from the prairie, he held his medicine bag in his hand and sang. He declared that his horse 'helped him in his doctoring' (Grinnell 1923–2:143).

Specialists were not required for all procedures relating to equine health and behaviour, however. Horse owners of some equestrian tribes carried out many healthcare regimens, preventive and therapeutic interventions, and rituals and other procedures to influence the reproduction, well-being and performance of their horses (next section). Apache and Navajo families, for example, had their own ceremonies to protect and multiply their herds. Someone in every Navajo family usually possessed good-luck songs for these purposes, passed down through the generations. According to Navajo myth, the gods gave each animal a secret, sacred name when they created it. A fortunate few among horse owners knew these words and by uttering them could protect their horses from danger or help them recover from illness or injury. These names were kept a carefully guarded secret; only when close to death would an individual finally will this special knowledge to a relative or worthy successor.

Husbandry and healthcare practices[3]

Husbandry
Supervision and quartering Hunters and warriors seldom let their swiftest or favourite mounts out of their sight. Like other equestrian tribes, Cree 'tenderly cared for and jealously guarded' their horses, who grazed under surveillance during the day. 'At night, valuable horses were picketed to the tipi door. When there was danger of an enemy raid, the owner of a good horse would tie its halter to his foot or wrist as he slept in his tipi. Other horses would be hobbled by

binding their forelegs with rawhide thongs' (Mandelbaum 1979:63). Blackfoot and other Plains tribes also observed these precautionary measures, especially for their finest war and buffalo mounts.

Navajo traditionally surrounded their hogans with four tie-posts—one for each cardinal direction—and buried ritual items in the post holes. Saddle horses were tied to the post facing the direction from whence they had been ridden. The posts magically improved equine behaviour, reproduction and health. Among traditional Navajo, to ensure good luck and health, buildings for horses must face east because the sun rises there and because wind and storms seldom come from that direction. Corrals and fences should never be built of lumber from a building where a death has occurred, lest misfortune befall the animals quartered there.

Nutrition Both Apache and Navajo appreciated the relationship between good equine health and rich forage—especially with regard to the nutritious grama grasses found throughout their territorial range. Whites who travelled through Apache country during the nineteenth century attributed the extraordinary endurance of Apache ponies to this forage's 'singularly strength-giving properties', noting that it was 'this plentiful distribution of the most strengthening grass in the world' that allowed the Apache to 'maintain his herds, make his extraordinary marches, and inflict widespread depredations' (Clark 1966:142). On the other hand, toxic plants such as burrowweed, Jimson weed (*Datura stramonium*) and locoweed (possibly *Oxytropis* spp.) were also common. Locoweed represented such a serious threat that Navajo tradition explained its existence as a deity's way of regaining animals: 'When there are too many horses coming upon the earth, I will send locoweeds and the horses will die from this. That is how I will get my horses back' (Clark 1966:144).

Gelding Equestrian tribes commonly gelded stallions to keep them from breeding with mares and to make them swifter and more tractable. Many horse-owning native groups were convinced that geldings tired less easily than stallions, although the Indians of Saskatchewan felt that castration diminished a horse's 'strength and vigor' (Dobie 1950:271). Usually a specialist was preferred for this operation, and the surgery was often accompanied by ritual acts (see also Ghirotti and Woudyalew, this volume).

A Hidatsa specialist gelded a colt in the following manner. Three objects symbolizing the castrator's art were included among the 10 items comprising his fee, and were used during the operation. The surgical site was anointed with medicine made from a turnip-like root while the specialist prayed, 'Let this make your body good and strong'. The area was then rubbed with sage (*Artemisia* spp.); the testicles were severed; and the wounds were sutured. Since the gelding would have the same qualities of speed as the species whose sinews were used for sutures, the colt's owner was given a choice: the jack-rabbit runs swiftly, but stops unexpectedly; the antelope is an excellent sprinter but cannot maintain its rapid pace; the elk runs more slowly but has greater strength and stamina. (In this case, the owner chose elk, and noted that the horse in fact became a very fast racer.) Following surgery, sage was again applied to make the horse's body 'good', to heal the wounds quickly, and to make the animal 'grow and spring up like these plants' (Wilson 1924:146–9). Then the colt was faced westwards and led in a circle around its severed testicles, which had been thrown in the same direction. Finally, the owner was instructed to cast the testicles into a river from which the horse would drink, and then four days later, to let the animal enter the river to wash the wounds.

To make geldings fleet, Blackfoot specialists used deer or antelope sinew for sutures. After surgery, someone rolled one of the testicles along the horse's back, saying 'This will surely be a fast buffalo horse' (Ewers 1969:57). Next, the horse was made to run. For several days after the operation, the animal was watched closely. One expert gelder was believed to possess secret power because no post-surgical swelling ever occurred and his patients never died from the operation. He always used antelope sinew and every horse he gelded turned out to be fast. When many horses were castrated within a short interval, the tribe remained in one place until all were completely healed.

Among Apache, horses were thrown and tied for the operation, which was accompanied by essential ceremonies. One Apache castration specialist required that he be given gifts of four articles used by the horse (such as a saddle blanket, bridle or rope) in order to allow his power to work. A certain Navajo surgeon always ended the operation by drawing a pattern with the horse's own blood from the animal's forehead down its legs, concluding with a slap on the thigh. Without this ritual, he explained, the 'horse won't run fast' (Allen 1963:165).

Reproduction Medicines of both plant and animal origin were used to influence fertility and reproduction. For example, Blackfoot made pregnant mares chew cicely roots so they would drink more water, which reportedly put them in good condition for foaling. To obtain a pinto foal—the most admired colour for a mount—Blackfoot would tie the black-and-white-plumed body of a magpie around the pregnant mare's neck. Arapaho also had medicines to create foals of certain colours. Piegan used a necklace of 'big turnip' to keep a pregnant mare in fine condition and cause her to give birth to a big foal; a necklace of turnip plus a jack-rabbit's front feet would produce a fast colt.

Coupled with good-luck songs, prayers, and sometimes gifts to the gods, Apache and Navajo used several methods to obtain or avoid certain kinds and colours of foals. To insure strong, healthy foals, Navajo horse owners followed procedures prescribed by the Holy Beings: at birth, a foal's umbilical cord was tied off with string and a coloured bead (white for females, turquoise for males); later, a string with the appropriate coloured bead was tied in the foal's mouth and the animal was then left to nurse for four days with the bead in place. Navajo destroyed deformed or twin foals, as well as the dam of twins. Twins indicated that witches had ridden the mare at night while perpetrating their evil deeds; therefore it was unlucky to keep such foals or their dam.

Navajo held Blessingway ceremonies to assure the fertility and increase of their herds, as well as their horses' general health and protection from illness or witchcraft. A versatile rite that is still fundamental to the Navajo ceremonial system, the Blessingway is performed 'for good hope' and 'places the Navajos in tune with the Holy People' (Kluckhohn and Leighton 1962:212–13), ensuring health, prosperity and well-being for both humans and animals. The Navajo ceremony that is held for horses involves a medicine pouch and various horse chants. The pouch contains, among other things, tiny stone fetish-figures of horses that the Holy Beings once taught the Navajo to revere and that 'brought them [the Navajo] many fine real ones [horses] and always protected their herds' (Clark 1966:131–132). An example of the chants used in such ceremonies is the Song of the Horse. It invokes the powerful guardianship of th 'Sun's mighty turquoise horse' so that earthly horses can share his power and be safe from evil forces. The refrain 'How joyous his neigh!' illustrates the beauty of such songs (Curtis 1968:362).

Conditioning and behavioural control Virtually all Plains peoples used botanical stimulants and other substances to impart speed, endurance, protection and good luck in racing, hunting, raiding and fighting. Members of the Crow Horse Dance Society possessed a 'powerful elixir' of a certain root plus other secret ingredients that they administered intranasally, orally or topically to the hooves so as promptly to restore an exhausted animal to normal condition, 'as though he had not run at all' (Lowie 1924:329). One member of the society who had this elixir in her medicine bundle explained that, 'On the warpath when a horse was worn out the riders would point the root toward the four quarters, then place it in the horse's mouth, and this would make the horse as fresh as ever' (Lowie 1924:333). Another member of the Crow Horse Dance Society described how he put a secret restorative root that he got from his father into racehorses' mouths to make them win.

On buffalo hunts, when snow and ice made footing precarious, a Blackfoot medicine man would sing, pray and chew a black root that he then applied to the mounts' hooves to prevent mishap. This root was imported from Indians in whose southernmost range it grew, and it was still being used in the early 1900s by those who understood how to administer it. Apache mixed this root—which they called 'black medicine'—into the feed of sluggish horses. Lazy horses were also bled and turquoise was applied to the cut. Apache, Comanche, Sioux and possibly also Navajo slit the nostrils of their horses to make them long-winded.

Prior to a race, Apache horsemen rubbed their mounts' feet with certain herbs to make the animals run faster. A Navajo shaman could be employed to administer sacred datura for the same purposes—either by having the horse chew the root, by administering an infusion of the root, or by throwing it in the animal's face. Probably Apache and Navajo, as well as Comanche, made racehorses long-winded by having horse shamans blow the pulverized root or leaves of certain plants into a mount's nostrils. Medicine could also enable a horse to accomplish extraordinary feats such as leaping over a wide coulée to escape enemy pursuit.

Cheyenne horse doctors used 'two different plants' to revive and strengthen a mount when it tired. One, *Thalictrum* spp. was dried, pulverized and administered orally to make Cheyenne horses 'spirited, long winded, and enduring'. Another 'strong medicine' made from the dried and powdered flowers of a certain plant was applied to the sole of each hoof of a horse ridden into battle to make it 'enduring and untiring'. The powder was also blown between the animal's ears to make it long-winded (Grinnell 1923–2:141–2, 187–8). Grinnell describes one such treatment as follows. The horse doctor held the medicine in his left hand while placing a pinch of the substance in the right side of the horse's mouth with his right hand. With the same hand he then took a pinch of medicine in his own mouth, blew it against the horse's body behind the right shoulder, and rubbed his hand over it; then he blew another pinch on the horse's right flank and rubbed it. Passing behind the rump, he repeated these same procedures on the animal's left side, reversing the use of his hands. He then returned to the right side of the horse, blew a pinch of medicine out of his right hand four times, and rubbed his hand up the horse's head from the nostrils over the ears. Finally, the horse was turned loose; if it rolled, the medicine was 'good'. This procedure could vary in details, sometimes involving more extensive areas of the horse's body and ending with pulling the horse's tail four times.

Teton Sioux gave dried, powdered *Clematis* root intranasally to tired horses when pressed by enemy pursuit. Nez Perce scraped the end of *Clematis* root and held it in the nostrils of a fallen horse for an 'immediate stimulating effect' (Ewers 1969:277). They also revived an exhausted mount by chewing wild peony root, placing it in the horse's mouth, and making the animal swallow it. Peony seeds administered in the same fashion just before a race increased a horse's speed. Arapaho rubbed peony root on the nose of a tired mount to refresh it. Omaha, Pawnee, Sarsi and Ute also knew various botanical remedies such as sorrel and *Clematis* to stimulate mounts and give them speed and endurance.[4]

Botanical ingredients and other substances were used together with magic and witchcraft. To revive an exhausted Blackfoot war mount, medicine was applied to its nose or mouth and then its tail bone was tapped three times with medicine rubbed on the hand. Sioux and some other tribes painted their war horses with designs that conferred the qualities necessary for battle. For example, 'symbols of the lightning' drawn down the shoulder and hind leg imparted 'speed and strength', and a 'circle around the eye [was] intended to aid the horse's eyesight' (Fronval and Dubois 1985:78). Blackfoot specialists rubbed medicine on a warrior's rope to cause enemy horses to come close enough to be lassoed during a raid. Powerful Blackfoot medicine applied to a whip that was pointed towards enemies and then dropped in their tracks could make their horses falter or fall.

To stop enemy pursuit as a raiding party escaped with a stolen herd, one Apache shaman employed a species of cactus that was thrown on the trail to make the pursuers fall from their horses. Navajo believed that chewing datura root before purchasing horses helped 'get them [the horses] cheaper'. Applying pollen to the rope of a prospective purchase could make its owner almost 'give the animal away'. Four other botanically-derived medicines were used to acquire a rich person's horses and other possessions (Clark 1966:151–2).

To cause a rival racehorse to falter and drop behind, a Blackfoot jockey might touch a stick smeared with potent medicine to his rival's mount during the race. On the pretext of examining the legs of a 'sure winner', Apache and Navajo specialists rubbed a medicine made of poisonous plants such as Jimson weed or poison ivy (*Rhus radicans*) on the animal's legs (or administered it orally) to hex the favourite into losing. Conversely, to protect a racehorse against a witch's harm, coyote pollen (or dust from where a coyote had stood) could be applied at the base of a mount's tail just before the race. The pollen was considered efficacious 'because in a long time nobody has hurt Coyote' (Clark 1966:140).

Since Navajo horse raids were considered sacred missions, associated ceremonies made use of the Blessingway, which was held in order to bring raiders and their mounts good fortune and to protect the horses they would capture. Apache horse shamans sang to the corralled herd about to embark on a raid so the animals would give their riders good luck. To increase a racehorse's speed, an Apache shaman would perform a ceremony and attach an eagle feather to the animal's tail, bridle or rope, or instruct the jockey to use the feather as a whip. Apache horses that were 'scary' and 'jumped sidewise' were calmed by tying eagle feathers to their manes or bridles (Opler 1965:299). To promote fleetness, Apache or Navajo shamans might hang amulets around the racehorse's neck— hawk feathers, antelope horns or the claws of bears, mountain lions or owls. And 'anything fast like the coyote, the fox, the wind, or clouds', was 'used in songs to make a horse run fast' (ibid.). Racing rituals included singing for the horse at home on the day before the contest. This could be done by the owner; if he did not know the proper songs, another person with the necessary knowledge might be hired.

Since much was at stake in Apache and Navajo racing—money, possessions and prestige—owners engaged specialists to take elaborate precautions against witchcraft and/or to hex rivals' mounts, by means of a variety of acts of singing, rites and sympathetic magic. For Navajo, one way to make a horse lose was to 'steal his shadow' by having 'a witch perform a bad sing' over something that had touched the animal (for example, dirt from its track, hair, sweat or dust from its body, foam or saliva from its mouth, its manure or urine or something the horse had worn). The item was buried in some lonely or 'bad' spot where something evil had occurred, and a song invoking malevolence was sung to rob the real horse of the 'living part' that gave it strength (Clark 1966:140–41).

Blackfoot and related tribes used magical procedures to cause a rival mount to fly the track, buck or kick up. Among the Cheyenne, horse doctors were often engaged to make a rival racehorse step in a hole and fall. To do this, the horse doctor would surreptitiously take a handful of dirt from the track left by the animal as it was led up and down prior to the race, and place the dirt in a gopher hole. Apache, Comanche and Kiowa all later adopted this custom. Similarly, on Cheyenne buffalo hunts or large war parties, in order magically to protect the horses from falls and injuries, 'The doctor walked up and down over the horses' tracks and sang his mysterious songs' (Grinnell 1923–2:141).

Healthcare

According to reports in the literature and informant testimony during the author's field research, both healthcare specialists and horse owners enjoyed considerable success at treating a number of equine problems, including blind staggers, gunshot and other wounds, distemper, coughs, sores and lesions of various kinds, and broken bones.[5] The literature provides some dramatic examples of Indians' expertise in equine healthcare. For instance, a Blackfoot medicine man was able to save a horse shot in the chest during battle by the following procedure. First, he burned some sage nearby; then he applied medicine to the horse's mouth and to the bullet's entry and exit points, rubbed medicine on his hands, and finally tapped the horse on the kidneys several times. His patient 'began eating grass' and 'recovered completely' (Ewers 1969:271). Another medicine man treated a war mount that had been severely wounded 'above the kidneys'. The man first told the animal, 'You are a fine horse, but I am more powerful than you . . . You will not die. I shall doctor you.' He then painted the horse's breast with red earth paint; tied a plume to the patient's forehead and a rabbit's tail to its tail; rubbed his horse medicine on the horse's nose; smeared the medicine on his hands and tapped the horse four (three?) times on the back. 'The horse was cured and lived many years longer' (ibid.).

As the foregoing examples illustrate, therapeutic treatments were frequently combined with ritual acts or magic. Among Cheyenne horse doctors, even treatments 'for ordinary disease' entailed ritual acts. For example, an aqueous drench made from two unidentified plants always included five pinches of medicine—one for each of the four cardinal directions and the middle (Grinnell 1923–2:141–2). Similarly, a Blackfoot medicine man who was often called upon to treat horses that were staggering and near death would rub medicine on the patient's nose, back and kidneys, and then shake its tail four times; if the animal flinched or moved during the procedure, its recovery was assured. As with husbandry, natural and supernatural procedures were often intimately inter-linked in equestrian Indians' equine healthcare.

Pharmaco-therapy Certain practitioners of equine healthcare possessed a sacred medicine bundle containing objects such as plant materials, mane hair or the horny growths on horses' legs known as chestnuts.[6] Among Navajo, even ordinary horse owners kept a buckskin pouch of herbs, pollen, tiny stone horse fetishes and sacred shells and pebbles; these items were designed to help safe-guard the owner's herd from witchcraft and other dangers. Botanical substances and other ingredients used by specialists were generally kept secret, and thus were seldom recorded by anthropologists or other observers. However, the literature does name a number of the specific plants and other ingredients that were employed in Indians' equine medicines.

For example, Blackfoot and related tribes were known to use ground fir needles, baneberry root (*Actea rubra*) and sagebrush flowers. And they adminis-tered decoctions of snakeweed (a species of yucca), big turnip, smellfoot and bitter-root orally or intranasally to horses with colic or distemper. Reservation Piegan found coal oil to be very effective against colic. Another Blackfoot treatment for distemper consisted of throwing the sick animal, touching a red-hot wire to its nose, and then administering a mixture of sage and other ingredients intranasally. When freed, the horse sneezed; pus was discharged; and the animal recovered. Dakota, Sioux, Omaha, Pawnee and Ponca treated distemper with smoke from burning comb plant. Nevada tribes burned chips of Indian balsam on slow coals on a shovel and then covered the shovel and the ailing horse's head with a sack, thus causing the animal to cough and release the discharge. Apache and Navajo burned *camote-de-monte* to cure equine coughs.

One of the most important medicines of these last two tribes derived from antelope-sage root, a member of the buckwheat family. Besides administering it to sick mounts as an infusion or as a poultice for injuries, people chewed the root themselves in order to obtain good luck with horses. Another plant, probably white prairie-clover (possibly *Dalea* spp.), was used as an emetic to cure 'light-ning infection', an affliction believed to result from lightning striking the animal. Navajo treated equine diarrhoea and bladder disorders with night-blooming *Cereus* and they made a laxative from creosote and leaves. Another item in the Navajo equine pharmacopoeia was 'solidified sea-foam', undoubtedly coral from the Gulf of California (Clark 1966:136).

Apache and Navajo sprinkled powdered medicinal herbs on saddle sores. Navajo also used an ointment of sheep grease and red ochre for sores, and sagebrush for wounds and burns. Creosote bush furnished an antiseptic that was applied as a powder to sore eyes and open wounds, or was combined with animal fat as a salve for painful areas. The leaves, fruit or root of the sacred datura were efficacious for healing sores; but because of this plant's potential toxicity, only a shaman should employ it. Blackfoot horse owners' medicines for saddle sores included: a decoction of boiled snakeweed; dry root (alumroot, *Heuchera* spp.) mixed with buffalo fat and boiled in water; and a compound of boiled tobacco, animal fat, a bitter grass and salt, which was said to heal a sore in one month. Pawnee made a decoction of the tops and leaves of the sticky head plant for saddle galls. Shoshone used the juice of milkweed (possibly *Asclepias* spp.) for sore backs and a decoction of yarrow leaves (*Achillea millefolium*) for collar boils on draft horses. Blood Indians applied herbal medicines after pricking a swelling with a new arrowhead until the blood ran.

Apache and Navajo also employed a number of botanical and other medicines to cure or protect their mounts against illness they believed to have been induced by witchcraft. A bewitched horse might suddenly begin to sweat, lie down and roll and appear moribund. A Navajo who 'knew the plants for the horse' (Clark 1966:142) could sometimes cure the animal, however. A number of witchcraft remedies were made from plants with such names (in Navajo) as gila monster, mountain lion, and bear plant—terms that imply these species' great power. Other treatments involved Blessingway smoke rites in which the shaman burned a special preparation in the corral where the affected animal was penned so that it would inhale the fumes. This preparation included pine needles, pinyon pitch, 10 other plants and shavings from the horns of deer, elk, mountain sheep and antelope. To combat the effects of witchcraft, Apache and Navajo drenched with infusions of spruce, ponderosa pine and juniper or a solution of *camote-de-monte*, which was said to prevent most known evils. However, some Navajo felt that no treatment could cure a bewitched horse.

To treat tender-footedness, Apache applied grease and gunpowder to the hooves and then blew fire from a live coal on them; healing was rapid. Buffalo or other fats served as a general hoof medication. Comanche hardened their horses' hooves by leading the animals back and forth through a slow fire of wild rosemary–artemisia. After long journeys to salt deposits or on hunts, Navajo applied salt water to the mouths, joints and hooves of the pack horses while chanting prayers to Grandmother Salt, such as 'May my horse be strong and stand the load' (Clark 1966:148).

For snake bite, Blackfoot and Shoshone applied mashed roots of false hellebore and alum. Comb plant was also a popular snake bite remedy among many tribes. Crow repeatedly applied poultices of fresh mud to snake-bite wounds until the swelling was reduced. To protect against snake bite as well as lightning strikes and other serious injuries, Apache and Navajo drenched their horses with infusions of spruce, ponderosa pine and juniper.

Surgery and bone-setting To cure blindness, Apache cut the vein leading down from the affected eye. Navajo removed saddle galls with a knife and cleansed the wound. For lampers, they excised the sores on the horse's swollen palate with a knife. A remarkable feat of abdominal surgery was witnessed by a mid-nineteenth-century fur trader. He observed Mandan-Hidatsa treat a horse whose belly had been ripped open by a buffalo horn. The animal was thrown, 'the entrails replaced, and the rent sewed up with a sinew'. Not only did the horse recover, but it 'ran as well and seemed to be in every respect as valuable as before' (Boller 1972:239).

Some Blackfoot medicine men could heal fractured bones by rubbing them with mud. An alternative treatment consisted of singing and rubbing dirt on the shank-bone of a buffalo or a horse and then tying the bone to the affected limb. After four days' rest, the limb was washed, the bone untied and dirt rubbed on the leg; reportedly, the fracture healed and the horse walked away 'without even a limp' (Ewers 1969:271). Blackfoot horse owners treated broken legs by lancing the affected area to make the blood flow and then splinting the leg with rawhide-wrapped sticks; however, a lump remained where the break had occurred, and the horse always limped.

Other techniques For urinary blockage, Apache horse owners prayed while lightly striking the afflicted animal's back four times with a knotted rope; the horse was trotted for a few hundred yards and then returned to its original position. To keep magpies from pecking at open sores, Hidatsa tied a special headless arrow to the mane if the sore was on the back, or to the tail if the area beneath it had been abraded by a saddle thong. A stick or branch would not do for this purpose. Large wing-feathers from the spotted owl might be attached to the arrow where the magpies would easily see them and be frightened away. Cree warded off magpies by covering sores with a piece of leather or buffalo paunch sprinkled with ashes. Crow and other tribes conscientiously treated saddle sores by resting their mounts whenever possible, ideally until the sores healed. (Tribes with few horses were reportedly much less humane in this regard, however.)

To prevent or treat lameness resulting from worn hooves, Apache, Blackfoot, Cree, Crow and Navajo all shod their horses with 'moccasins' of buffalo, cow, deer or horse hide in the form of a pouch secured with a rawhide drawstring. Horse manure was packed inside the pouch and replenished from time to time. Comanche soaked the moccasins in water beforehand. Apache treated mounts with swollen feet by standing them in streams for prolonged periods.

The cultural context of equine husbandry and healthcare

To understand and interpret equine husbandry and healthcare among North American Indians, their practices must be placed within the context of tribal culture. Generally, Indians inhabited a universe that they perceived as essentially spiritual. Religion was not separate from other spheres of daily activity, but was at the core of all existence. Supernatural power flowed through every form of life, and all beings were animated by the same pervasive force. Hence, boundaries between living things were permeable, and exchanges of energy and power between species were common. This interconnection made it possible for a turnip or a magpie to impart its size or colour to an unborn foal, or for feathers, claws and sinew to endow horses with the qualities of the animals from whom they had come. Moreover, knowledge about one animal species was applicable to others, including humans. Obstetrical skills, for example, were transferred from horses to people, and sometimes fertility beliefs concerning animals were ceremonially extrapolated to humans.

In contrast to Western society's view of nature, the Native Americans' ethos included no imperative for domination of the nonhuman realm. They saw the natural world as a circle of interrelated beings, with humankind as an equal but not a superior species. The Western notion of a hierarchy of animal forms with humans at the top was utterly alien to American Indians. Hence they did not unilaterally impose veterinary and other interventions upon horses. Rather, Indians worked with both the natural and the supernatural forces present in the universe to influence behaviour and bring about healing. For example, by relating a medicine not only to the patient but also outwards to the four cardinal directions, healthcare practitioners infinitely extended the range of powers at their disposal. Of course, the beneficent forces that could bring about health and well-being had to be carefully cultivated and cajoled into cooperation. Therefore, interventions often took the form of ritual acts, songs and prayers, and involved magical objects that, as concomitants of pragmatic actions, were vital to invoking these spiritual forces. An ordinary stick, for example, could not fend off magpies from sores; the power of a special arrow was needed. And using an eagle's feather to distract a shying horse augmented the practical effect of the object by imparting the special strength of the animal from which it originated.

Reciprocal interactions between natural and supernatural realms also characterized the relationship between people and the animal kingdom. The human–horse relationship was such that not only did people take care of horses; horses also took care of people. In the words of Turquoise Boy (a Navajo culture hero instrumental in obtaining the first horses from the Sun's corral for people on earth), horses were 'that by means of which people live' (Clark 1966:123). Besides the many practical benefits they conferred on humans, horses guided and safeguarded people throughout every important stage of life. They also punished or rewarded people according to the treatment they received—just as other animals had done before the advent of the horse. Horses revealed to Plains peoples rites and medical secrets such as the Horse Dance, and horses could lend their powers to assist in human healing.

Reciprocity between humans and animals was matched by reciprocity between humans and gods. Native Americans who benefited so greatly from the acquisition of horses were mindful that such extraordinary gifts ultimately emanated from the gods. Deities were thus intimately involved in equine husbandry and healthcare; and balances were maintained, as when the gods reclaimed surplus horses through locoweed poisoning. Since horses were sacred, medical treatment involved consideration of that status, and equine specialists required supernatural power. In many tribes, whether for specialists or ordinary horse owners, to guard and protect the health and well-being of these miraculous creatures was a holy obligation as well as a personal duty.

Some observers of native life during the horse era commented on the excellent care that Indians gave their horses. Others, however, reported that Indians treated their horses inhumanely. Even today, white neighbours of Crow horse owners criticize certain Indian husbandry practices—such as not fencing horses in, or leaving them outdoors in the winter. But these traditional practices reflect an intrinsic respect for animals as independent beings and a deeply ingrained admiration for animals' extraordinary powers of survival. Equally important, 'The essential thing about the Indian's relationship with his horse' was that he thought of the animal 'as he thought of himself' (Clark 1966:160; also see Lawrence 1985:36–7). Indians' harsh and difficult existence meant that survival depended upon strength and endurance, and people demanded as much of their horses as of themselves. Thus, techniques that Westerners perceive as cruel may be in fact pragmatic procedures that toughened the animals for the difficulties and dangers they once had to endure. Still today, Crow identify with their horses' hardiness, asserting that—like other animals—horses' special power results from their ability to survive unaided by humankind and without clothing, shelter or fire.

For Crow and other tribes, this remarkable endurance is part of what distinguishes animals from human beings. It also enhances animals' roles as intermediaries between people and the Great One. Moreover, for Crow the ruggedness of their horses symbolizes their tribe's own historic ability to survive. Surrounded by powerful enemy tribes and later conquered by the white man, they have nevertheless managed to keep much of their culture intact (Lawrence 1985:49–51). The horse has played a critical role in this regard, as evidenced by the following events. In the early 1900s, a government programme was carried out to reduce drastically the number of horses on the Crow reservation by rounding up and slaughtering a great many of the animals. Such a campaign directly violated the native ethos that included a strong taboo against killing horses. As Navajo subjected to a similar programme expressed it, the Holy Beings—not 'Washington'—should decide how many horses people may possess (Clark 1966:165). Modern Crow still voice their sorrow and horror at the government's disregard for the sacredness and significance of horses; they express their hatred for the perpetrators of such brutal and sacrilegious acts; and they point out the devastating, disintegrative consequences of the loss of horses for both individuals and Crow culture. When large herds of horses were later restored to the reservation thanks to the efforts of a native superintendent who understood his people's needs, Crow spirit and tribal culture were revitalized. Today, Crow cherish the continued interaction with their mounts, whom they view as their 'long-lost brothers'. As one informant expressed it, 'The Crows came back to their original selves when they got their horses again'.

Such experiences stand as a sharp warning about the dangers of livestock reduction schemes and intrusive veterinary or other development programmes that fail to respect the beliefs, values and traditions of animal-centered cultures (see also McCorkle 1994). Indeed, for the most part, North American Indians' equine husbandry and healthcare techniques must now be described in the past tense. Gradually, acculturation and modernization are eliminating the old ways. The spread of Western science and the accompanying desacralization of life are eroding the spiritual and aesthetic dimensions of equine ownership and healthcare among North American Indians—and with them, the sense of identity, security and well-being so beautifully expressed in one Navajo horse chant (cited in Clark 1966:210).

> *Before me peaceful,*
> *Behind me peaceful,*
> *Under me peaceful,*
> *Over me peaceful,*
> *All around me peaceful.*
> *Peaceful voice when he neighs.*
> *I am Everlasting and Peaceful.*
> *I stand for my horse.*

Notes

1. This chapter represents a greatly revised and condensed version of an earlier article (Lawrence, 1988). In addition to an extensive review of the extremely limited and fragmented literature on North American Indians' equine healthcare, the chapter draws upon the author's field research among contemporary Crow of Montana between 1975 and 1980. Throughout the text, informant quotations are from the author's field notes, unless otherwise indicated. The author is grateful to the Crow people for their hospitality and willingness to share their love of horses. Special thanks also go to Mark, Priscilla and Bob for their participation in fieldwork in Crow country.

2. Due to the secrecy and sacredness that surrounded American Indian healthcare specialists and the fact that most early observers and chroniclers of Indian life paid little attention to equine medical practices, information about both is exceedingly sparse. Fortunately, a handful of frontier explorers, traders, travellers and missionaries documented their observations and a few anthropologists recorded what the last traditional tribal elders and informants still practised or remembered about the care and treatment of horses according to the old ways. The historical information

presented throughout this chapter was largely gathered from the following sources (for further detail, consult Lawrence, 1988): for Apache, Clark (1966) and Opler (1965); for Blackfoot, Piegan and related tribes, Ewers (1969); for Cheyenne, Grinnell (1923); for Comanche, Wallace and Hoebel (1972); for Cree, Mandelbaum (1979); for Crow, Curtis (1970) and Lowie (1924); for Hidatsa, Wilson (1924); for Lakota Sioux, Powers (1986) and DeMallie and Jahner (1980); for Navajo, Clark (1966) and Kluckhohn and Leighton (1962); and for certain plant remedies, Gilmore (1977) and Murphey (1987).

3. Throughout this section, Latin names of plants are not always given because rarely was it possible to determine with certainty the species or sometimes even the genus of the plants referred to in much of the literature solely by popular or native-language names. However, interested readers can consult Kindscher (1992) for possible identifications [editors' note].

4. Although plants with depressant effects such as larkspur, lupines, locoweed and death camass grew on Montana ranges, information about the medicinal use of these species among Plains and Plateau tribes is lacking (see Ewers 1969:277).

5. Reportedly, they were less successful at combating epidemic disease, however. See Ewers 1969 on the great mange epidemic of 1881–2.

6. Cheyenne horse doctors tied their medicine bundles to the handle of their whips, so that the materials would always be handy in case a horse required treatment. Another type of medicine was kept in a bag on the Cheyenne specialist's left hip or, in the case of one woman, on a belt around her waist.

7. Tradition and modernity:
French shepherds' use of medicinal bouquets[1]

ANNE-MARIE BRISEBARRE

UPON ENTERING A sheepfold in southern France's Cévennes region, one's attention is immediately drawn to a number of large, dark objects dangling from the rafters like enormous bats. In the dimness of the fold, it is often difficult to discern that these items are in fact huge bouquets of plants covered with dust and spider webs (Plate 1). These bouquets form an integral part of the traditional veterinary system in Cévennes. Along with simple surgical operations and sometimes magico-religious acts, Cévenol shepherds have long relied upon local, plant-based treatments for animal health problems (Brisebarre 1978:167–80). In fact, the practice of hanging up bouquets of plants to cure and/or forestall livestock disease is found in virtually every part of France, where it is also widely applied in human ethnomedicine. The practice enjoys a very long history dating back at least to the twelfth century. For example, the first professional manual on sheep raising in France, written in 1379, suggests hanging up henbane (*Hyoscyamus niger* L.) to combat sheep pox (Brie 1979).

Despite the widespread and long-standing use of medicinal bouquets, the classical literature on phyto-pharmacology barely mentions them, presumably because they are considered unorthodox and irrational. To correct this oversight, the present chapter overviews and illustrates the use of therapeutic and prophy-

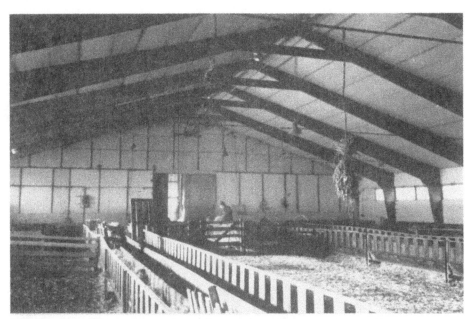

Plate 1. *Even in the most modern Cévenol sheepfolds, one finds medicinal bouquets hanging from the rafters. The large bouquet to the right of the photo is marciouré; the small round one seen hanging up and to the left is san cap.*

lactic bouquets in present-day France. First, general aspects of medicinal bouquets and related practices are discussed, including: the types of plants and other materials used; their collection, preparation, and administration; the diseases treated; and underlying ethnomedical beliefs. Second, contrastive case studies are presented of how bouquets are currently employed among traditional French shepherds versus their more modern counterparts who, dissatisfied with Western veterinary alternatives, have adopted and re-interpreted this centuries-old measure.

The information presented below derives from more than a decade of research based on: a wide-ranging bibliographic review of numerous sources such as anthologies of folkloric traditions, specialized monographs and breeders' manuals; systematic field collection and botanical identification of plants used in medicinal bouquets; and participant observation and interviews during fieldwork with stockowners, local healers, zootechnicians and veterinarians in two major sheep-raising regions of France. In Cévennes, 30 shepherds participating in two important transhumant networks were systematically surveyed about their knowledge and use of medicinal bouquets. Most of these were older men, including a number of key informants selected because of their extensive ethnoveterinary knowledge and the professional esteem and status they held among their peers. In Sologne, interviews were conducted with a small group of younger, 'modern' shepherds and the local zoo technicians who advised them. (For bibliographic and methodological detail, consult Brisebarre 1984, 1985, 1987, 1989 and 1990.)

Hanging bouquets to heal and prevent disease

Whether applied internally or externally, botanicals used in classic phyto-pharmacology usually act through direct contact. But plants suspended as bouquets can act only from a distance, as per Lieutaghi's (1983) 'open' formula. French ethnomedicine has long held that air can carry agents and vectors of disease; in emic logic, it can therefore also transmit treatments for disease (Brisebarre 1985: 21–5). French stock raisers explain that medicinal bouquets operate primarily via the aerial diffusion of substances associated with the plants' 'smell', which may or may not be detectable by humans. More rarely, there is a preliminary contact-transfer phase between the bouquet and the diseased part of the anatomy or between the bouquet's administrator and the patient. Where contact is involved, it is designed to draw the sickness out of the patient's body and into the therapeutic item.

A comparison with fumigation, another common way to administer botanicals, is helpful here. With fumigation, there is no direct contact between the plant and the patient's body, but the plant's active substances are extracted, transported and administered via smoke or water vapour. In like vein, the active ingredients of medicinal bouquets are assumed to diffuse spontaneously into the air of the fold or barn. Unlike fumigation, however, a bouquet's action is continuous—for example, throughout the entire lambing season. Informants stress this advantage.

Bouquets are sometimes also made of non-plant materials. These include animals such as vipers, toads and salamanders; and religious objects such as medals, consecrated ribbons and prayers that have been blessed by a priest and/or obtained on a pilgrimage. Vegetal bouquets must always be hung up fresh, preferably when they are in flower and hence at their peak of biological activity. Similarly, only live or freshly killed animals can be hung as medicinal bouquets

(Bouteiller 1966: 295, Collectif 1973: 149, Van Gennep 1937–58:1852–53). Religious objects should be suspended as soon as possible after they have been brought home. 'Freshness' is deemed critical to the effectiveness of all such treatments.

Variations in the use of medicinal bouquets involve the location and manner in which they are suspended, the disease or species being treated, any associated rituals and the season of the year. For example, bouquets may be placed in highly visible locations; or they may be hung secretly in a dark corner, hidden from the sight of the uninitiated. In the latter case, they can be left open to the air or, especially for animal-based bouquets, they may be suspended in a pot or sachet.[2] The branches of trees or shrubs are sometimes simply wedged under a beam of the fold or barn. Other plants are arranged into bouquets, wreaths, crosses or mixed-species faggots. The type of arrangement is a key part of the prescription.

These arrangements can be administered either individually or collectively. To treat a large animal like a horse or cow, the medicinal item is positioned directly above the ailing creature in its stall.[3] But for sheep, which are always left free in their folds, several bouquets may be suspended at various locations so that their combined odour will reach and 'cover' the whole flock. A bouquet's medicinal action can also be generalized or localized via, respectively, inhalation of the active substances in the odour versus some form of external contact with the diseased parts of the animal's body.

The stockowner or a member of his family may determine the choice and placement of the bouquet. However, magico-religious reinforcements are often involved. For example, the plants or other materials may have been collected by a healer or a shepherd–specialist; incantations or prayers may be recited over the treatment items and/or the patient; the items may have been blessed or rubbed on the statue of a saint during a pilgrimage.

Finally, the use of bouquets is often linked to the seasons. Sharp seasonal shifts in temperature or, during some seasons, the need to house animals for long periods in crowded quarters can increase the danger of disease. When such events coincide with seasonal husbandry operations like lambing, health measures are considered even more critical.

Diseases for which bouquets are prescribed
Table 1 details specific livestock ailments for which hanging plants are prescribed. (For comparable data for humans, see Brisebarre 1990.) The table excludes very general or imprecise terms (e.g., 'disease', 'epidemic', 'evil spell', 'bewitchment') that arose in the course of research. It also excludes the use of plant arrangements to ward off pests and predators (for example, serpents, weasels, wild cats) of livestock or to promote general good health and fortune (for example, the common Christian practices of hanging up box and bay laurel or nailing crosses of vegetable matter to the walls or doors of dwellings, folds and stables). Significantly, all the ills listed have dermatological signs. Most of these conditions display cutaneous lesions such as rashes, ulcerations and raw or reddened areas. Many involve the formation of scabs, crusts or squamae that later dry up and fall off. Some also have a distinctive and unpleasant odour.

Most of the conditions listed in Table 1 are well defined and differentiated in the veterinary literature. However, folk nosology often groups a broad range of animal (and human) diseases under the same all-encompassing vernacular term. (see also by Delehanty, this volume). For standard French *dartre* (*enderbis* in

Table 1. Sheep diseases[a] for which bouquets are prescribed

Disease terms[b]	Disease description[c]
bouchise (lamb thrush)	A yeast (*Candida albicans*) infection of the oral mucosa in young lambs that causes redness, spots, sores and scabs on the lips and mouth, along with a distinctive, unpleasant odour. The technical term is buccal candidosis.
ecthyma (soremouth, Doby mouth, pot)	A scabby viral infection that manifests itself mainly on the muzzle of lambs, the clinical signs are very similar to those of *bouchise*. In fact, without laboratory analysis, these two conditions are difficult to distinguish. The technical term is contagious ecthyma.
muguet (—)	A popular French term that, because of clinical ambiguity, apparently may be glossed for lambs as either *bouchise* or *ecthyma*, much as English-speaking stockowners use 'soremouth' to gloss many kinds of buccal symptoms.
dartre (ringworm, barn itch)	A mildly contagious skin disease caused by a fungus of the genus *Trichophyton*. *Dartre* is the vernacular term for the scaly, round depilations that result. In Aveyron, the name is *enderbis*. The technical term is tinea.
Piétin (footrot, foul foot)	A highly contagious disease of the feet of sheep, caused by the interplay of the bacteria *Fusarium necrophorum* and *Bacteroides nodosus*. Clinical signs include swelling, reddening, lameness and moist, necrotic inflammation of the skin in the cleft of the toes. This word
Fic (—)	designates a wide variety of dermal conditions in both animals and humans (see text).
clavelée (sheep pox)	A contagious skin disease caused by capripox virus. The principal clinical sign in sheep is the formation of skin nodules.
gale (mange, scabies)	Caused by parasitic mites that attack the skin, this condition is characterized by severe itching, scabs and depilation. For sheep, the technical name is psoroptic mange.
poux (lice)	A skin condition caused by the proliferation of lice. The major sign is itching, manifested by the animals' constantly rubbing themselves against posts and other such objects. The technical name is louse infestation.
verrue (wart)	Papillomata that form in the cutaneous epithelium. Warts vary in appearance, but their surface is usually keratinized, villous or cauliflower-like.

[a] Some of these diseases are thought to be zoonotic, or more specifically, transmissible from animals to children.
[b] French shepherds' local terms are listed first, followed by common English glosses in parenthesis. In some cases, however, no gloss is possible.
[c] Disease descriptions draw primarily upon Garnier and Delamare (1974) and Villemin (1984), with additional information from Blood et al. (1983) and, especially for English glosses, Ensminger (1970) and Tjaart Schillhorn van Veen (pers. com.).

northern Langue d'Oc) encompasses a great variety of scientifically distinct cutaneous diseases of both animals and humans. To give another, more dramatic example of how broad the semantic field of a single term can be, throughout Aveyron and Lozere, *fic* is applied to 'skin' diseases in animals, humans and even plants! One translation is 'tree canker'; for sheep, cattle and horses, *fic* can be glossed respectively as 'footrot', 'foul foot', and 'canker' or 'pox'; for both livestock and people, it is sometimes used to mean 'wart' and, in humans only, 'hemorrhoids' (Collectif 1973, Vayssier 1879, author's field research).

In any case, it is clear that French folk nosology clearly recognizes a general category of diseases that roughly translates as ailments with patent cutaneous lesions for which bouquets constitute the preferred treatment. The existence of this disease category in turn raises the question: Is there a corresponding folk category of items designated as appropriate for use in such bouquets?

Plants and animals used

Based on both bibliographic and field research, Table 2 summarizes data on 26 plant species currently or traditionally employed in bouquets to combat dermatological problems in livestock and people. The table also lists available information on the diseases each plant is used to combat and the regions or *départements* of France where its use has been observed, along with the sources of this information.

Most of the species listed in Table 2 are common throughout France and are found in areas that farmers pass daily. Only three are somewhat rare or limited in their distribution. *Caoumegno* and *san cap* (Nos. 15 and 26) grow only in mountainous areas; and *lathrée clandestine* (No. 23), a parasitic plant that grows on the roots of trees, is found only in western and central France. Several plants listed are anthropophilic; that is, they grow on old walls, among debris, in hedges, or along embankments and the edges of forests. Although all 26 are wild species, some have been transplanted around houses and gardens (for example, Nos. 16–18, 24, and in Aveyron, even No. 12, *marcиouré* 'stinking hellebore').

Where data are available, Table 2 also lists salient features that emically define a plant as appropriate for use in medicinal bouquets. These features can be glossed as odour, toxicity, aggressiveness and similarity. Odour is important because, as noted earlier, it is assumed to be the mechanism by which bouquets achieve their pharmacological effect. With regard to toxicity, informants believe that, as with odours, plant 'poisons' or 'venom' can also diffuse into the atmosphere. Aggressiveness refers to prickly or thorny plants. In numerous popular beliefs, such species can 'ward off evils' like general misfortune or the evil eye, which are believed to be associated with or causative of disease. Finally, similarity relates to any perceived resemblance (biological, physical or symbolic) between the medicinal materials and the symptoms of the diseases they are employed to treat (next section).

If plants used to combat sorcery and unspecified diseases (Nos. 1–10) are omitted, 16 remain for which bibliographic and/or fieldwork information is sufficient for category analysis. Significantly, all but one of these 16 are or were used externally in veterinary or human dermatology (Fournier 1947).[4] One-fourth of the 16 give off a strong or unpleasant odour (Nos. 11–14). Nearly half have a certain toxicity. Nos. 12 (*marciouré*), 14, and 15 are indisputably poisonous, while 11, 16, 17 and the berries of 18 are toxic in high doses. Three (Nos. 18–20) are aggressive, that is, thorny or spiney. Finally, four are used in signature medicine (see Underlying folk beliefs, below). The brown-speckled twigs of No. 21 are associated with pustules; similarly, only spotted varieties of 22 are chosen for hanging. The white scales on the trunk of 23 are suggestive of

Table 2. Plants commonly used in therapeutic bouquets[a]

Nomenclature	Uses	Distinctive features	Sources
1. Lady's mantle; *alchémille alpine*; *Alchemilla alpina* L.			Laplantine 1981, Nardonne 1981.
2. Common alder; *aulne glutineux*; *Alnus glutinosa* (L.) Gaernt.			Research by Groupement 'Santé en Aquitaine'. Lacrocq 1921.
3. Goosefoot; *chénopode Bon-Henri*; *Chenopodium Bonus-Henricus* L.			Brisebarre field research.
4. Bay laurel; *laurier*; *Laurus nobilis* L.			Van Gennep 1937–1958.
5. Ivy; *lierre*; *Hedera helix* L.			Van Gennep 1937–1958.
6. Walnut tree; *noyer*; *Juglans regia* L.			Van Gennep 1937–1958.
7. Onion; *oignon*; *Allium cepa* L.			Seignolle 1969.
8. Hornbeam; *charme*; *Carpinus betulus* L.			
9. Ash; *frêne*; *Fraxinus excelsior* L.			Seignolle 1969.
10. Hazel tree; *noisetier*; *Corylus avellana* L.			Seignolle 1969.
11. Greater celandine; *chélidoine*, *herbe de fic*, or *herbe aux verrues*; *Chelidonium majus* L.	Entire plant used for *dartre* or *fic* in both animals and humans in Aubrac.	Toxicity, odour	Collectif 1973.
12. Stinking hellebore; *ellébore fétide* or *marciouré*, *pisso-co*; *Helleborus foetidus* L.	Entire plant in flower used for *bouchue*, *muguet* and *ecthyma* in sheep in Cévennes, and in Rouergue for *enderbis/tinea* in calves and *dartre* in both animals and humans.	Toxicity, odour	Brisebarre field research.
13. Herb Robert; *geranium herbe-à-Robert* or *chancrée*; *Geranium robertianum* L.	Entire plant (in flower or not) used for *ecthyma* in Perche and southern Sologne.	Odour	Brisebarre field research.

Table 2. (Continued)

Nomenclature	Uses	Distinctive features	Sources
14. Henbane; jusquiame, tume, juscarime or henvebonne; Hyoscyamus sp.	Entire plant used for clavelée in Brie.	Toxicity, odour	Brie 1979.
15. White bachelor's buttons; renoncule à feuilles d'aconit or caoumegno; Ranunculus aconitifolius L.	Entire plant in flower used for fic in Cévennes.		Durand-Tullou 1981, Brisebarre field research.
16. Box; buis; Buxus sempervirens L.	Twigs used for eczema and psoriasis (humans) in Brittany.	Toxicity	Bouteiller 1966, Brisebarre field research.
17. Elder tree; sureau; Sambucus nigra L.	Twigs used for ecthyma in Perche.	Toxicity	Bouteiller 1966, Rolland 1896–1914.
18. Holly; houx; Ilex aquifolium L.	Twigs with fruit used for ecthyma and both animal and human dartre in Côtes-du-Nord and Mayenne, and for enderbis/dartre/tinea in both animals and humans in Cantal, Rouergue, Lozère and Béarn.	Toxicity, similarity	Delpastre 1982, Descoeur 1959, Maupas 1961, Brisebarre field research, research by Groupement 'Santé en Aquitaine'.
19. Common blackberry; ronce; Rubus fruticosus L.	Twigs used for dartre in humans in Manche.	Similarity	Seguin 1941.
20. Butcher's broom; fragon petit houx; Ruscus aculeatus L.	Entire plant used for ecthyma in Lot.	Aggressiveness	Brisebarre field research.

21. Buckthorn; *bourdaine*; *Rhamnus frangula* L.	Twigs used for *dartre* in Mayenne.	Similarity	Bouteiller 1966.
22. Elm tree; *orme*; *Ulmus campestris* L.	Twigs used for *dartre* in animals in Maine and Loire.	Similarity	Bouteiller 1966.
23. English equivalent unknown; *lathrée clandestine* or *herbe de fic*; *Lathraea clandestina* L.	Entire plant used for *fic* in animals in Aubrac.	Similarity	Collectif 1973, Vayssier 1879.
24. Privet; *troène*; *Ligustrum vulgare* L.	Twigs in flower used for infant *muguet* in Poitou and for human *chancre* in Vienne.	Possible toxicity, similarity	Bouteiller 1966, Rolland 1896–1914.
25. Wild service tree or mountain ash; *alisier*; *Sorbus torminalis* (L.) Crantz.	Twigs used for sheep *ecthyma* in Perche, leaves for *dartre* in Mayenne.		Bouteiller 1966, Brisebarre field research.
26. Plantain or waybread; *plantain holosté* or *san cap*; *Plantago carinata* Schrad.	Entire plant used for *bouchise*, *muguet*, and *ecthyma* in Cévennes.		Brisebarre field research.

---

a Plant names are given first in English, followed by formal French and, where known, vernacular French. Following Coste 1901–1906, the scientific Latin name is listed last. L. indicates that the Latin is from the Linnean system. In some cases, no English-language equivalent for the plant in question was identified.

certain dermatological pathologies. Informants say the flowers of No. 14 remind them of *muguet* in infants. Only two of the 16 plants (Nos. 25 and 26) had no discernible relationship to any of the four features.

Underlying folk beliefs

The diverse plant species listed in Table 2 do not share any one overt feature that clearly sets them apart as a group. However, they must be further analysed in terms of the medicine of signatures. Dating from the sixteenth century, this medical tradition relies heavily upon the fundamental principle of sympathetic magic that 'like implies like'. This assumption still underpins much of French ethnomedicine. The logic behind the choice of items to suspend can thus be further elucidated by analysing the characteristics and processes that shepherds ascribe to these items and comparing the findings with the folk nosology of the ailments they are supposed to cure or prevent.

Like cures like As Crollius writes in *La Royale Chimie*, 'Herbs speak to the inquisitive doctor by their signature, revealing through a few resemblances their internal virtue' (1624, cited in Lieutaghi 1983:47). This corollary of the like-implies-like principle is at work in all four of the features discussed above. Research reveals the following correspondences between the objects used in bouquets and the dermatological conditions they fight. Ailments that give off a bad odour are combated with unpleasant- or strong-smelling plants. For ills diagnosed as the result of venom or poison, toxic plants are employed as antidotes. Skin problems believed to arise from spells or miasmas are counter-acted with aggressive plants and animals, to ward off the evil. Diseases that display rashes, pustules, squamae or growths are treated with plants that have speckled twigs, spotted leaves, small flowers or scales and with animals that have spots or a pimply or blistered appearance.

The fact that most of the species listed in Table 2 possess only one of these four features does not impair their effectiveness in people's minds. In sympathetic magic, even a single similarity between the active agent and the object or condition acted upon is sufficient (Mauss and Hubert 1950). However, additional supernatural elements may be incorporated so as to reinforce the efficacy of medicinal bouquets (Brisebarre 1984). These may involve: the magic numbers three, seven, and nine; collection of the medicinal items at an auspicious moment, for example, at sunrise or during certain phases of the moon; and the involvement of a priest, healer or other specialist.

Like follows like Signature medicine also posits a causal correlation between the changing state of the remedy and the progression of the disease being treated. The fresh, flowering bouquets of medicinal plants gradually dry out, or the dangling carcasses of recently killed or expired animals mummify slowly or rot and disintegrate. Accordingly, the patient's scabs or squamae dry up and/or fall off. In folk beliefs, the coincidence between the drying or rotting time of the remedy and the disappearance of the lesions explains the phenomenon of healing at a distance.

Contact between the diseased part of the body and the remedy reinforces this relation. One example is a common cure for footrot that uses a tuft of grass on which the ailing animal has trod. While procedures vary from region to region, in Sologne the tuft is hung on the first hawthorn bush encountered. The grass dries, the hawthorn dies, and the animal is healed (Edeine 1974:566). In other cases, such transfer items are burnt after they have dried out, thus breaking the chain of transfer.[5]

Like repels like This corollary of the like-implies-like principle is most apparent in the choice of animal species employed as bouquets. Vipers, toads and salamanders all share an aggressive and venomous image in French folklore; and in fact, all three secrete venom, the latter two through their skin. People believe these creatures can project the venom into the eyes of their victims. Informants describe these species as strange, 'creeping', damp and slimy; in brief, as unsettling and repulsive.

As noted earlier, in the logic of French ethnomedicine, if air can transmit diseases then it can transport their corresponding treatments, too. Hence people may hang up repulsive animals in order to repel unpleasant or frightening organisms and elements such as flies, mites, lice, fleas, germs, poisons, impurities, miasmas and spells. In popular French belief, all such phenomena—some visible, some not—inhabit the air around us and can provoke disease. Thus people seek 'to repel malignant air' (Corbin 1982: 16) with bouquets of repugnant animals as well as with poisonous, strong-smelling or thorny plants.

Opposites mediate One further principle is embodied in the choice of plant and animal species used in medicinal bouquets. It is no accident that all such species are wild, because sometimes the wild can mediate the tame (Lévi-Strauss 1962). In combatting diseases that manifest themselves on the skin—the boundary between the individual and the external world—the logic is that wild is to tame as external is to internal.

To take one example, if prolonged and/or crowded stabling has contaminated the air of a fold, stockowners have two options. They can turn the herds out to pasture, that is, transfer them from a domestic to a wild environment, from inside to outside. Conversely, they can bring the outside to the inside by hanging restorative wild plants or animals in the fold or barn. Wild species that are symbolically dangerous or ambivalent (for example, toxic or aggressive) can be 'tamed' and made beneficial through various actions: by a priest's blessing or a healer's incantation; by carefully following the instructions for properly picking and positioning the plants; and by transplanting the wild plants to one's garden, thus semi-domesticating them (as well as ensuring they will be on hand when needed).

Case studies of bouquet usage

Traditional usages
Shepherds' use of marciouré *bouquets* A frequent skin disease of sheep is what Cévenol sherpherds term *muguet* (Table 1). Both to cure and prevent this ill, they employ bouquets of the strong-smelling *marciouré*. Informants say the flowers of this plant are 'green and pungent, they might even be poisonous'. They add that *marciouré* blossoms in early March, when no other plants do so. (This may explain its common French name.) March is also one of the two traditional lambing seasons in Cévennes and the one in which *muguet* is most prevalent; the disease is reportedly rare in the October–November lambing season.

To prevent *muguet*, *marciouré* bouquets may be hung in the fold as early as the first lambing in spring. Less foresighted shepherds may delay until they detect the tell-tale reddening of the lambs' lips. They say that, within a few days of putting up the bouquets, scabs will form on the lips and thereafter the pustules of *muguet* begin to dry up, along with the *marciouré* flowers. The bouquets are not removed from the fold until they fall of their own accord. Whether for prophylaxis or thearpy, the plant is never brought into contact with the animals.

The shepherd himself generally collects this common plant from his own pastures. The value and uses of *marcioré* are familiar to all Cévenol shepherds, and this knowledge is handed down from father to son. But sometimes another shepherd 'who knows about it' actually installs the bouquets. Such men are acknowledged by their peers to have the power to validate and empower the procedure.

A healer's use of san cap *bouquets* Much rarer than *marcioré, san cap* (*Plantago carinata* Schrad) occurs only in very specific, siliceous and/or dry-grass biotopes. In Cévennes, *san cap* means 'healthy head', in reference to the plant's role in treating *muguet*, which affects the 'head' (or more precisely the mouth) of lambs. In the lower Cévennes, *san cap* is known as 'the healing plant of St M', the home of a shepherd–healer who is able to endow *san cap* with its medicinal powers.

The healer defines his practice as 'healing with a secret' or 'conjuration'. His services are gratis. He recounts how 'If a shepherd wants to use my plant, he must bring me a lamb, generally the one most affected . . . If he has several folds, he must bring one lamb from each. I have a secret formula that must be respected and I say it over the lamb.' The healer recites his formula (which his clients say is unintelligible) while holding a bouquet of *san cap* over the lamb, but without touching the animal either with the plant or his hands. He then gives the bouquet to the client with instructions to return the lamb to its fold and to suspend the bouquet there. The healer also advises the client to forget about the bouquet after hanging it up. This advice, verging on taboo, is a way of saying that one must have confidence in the remedy and give it time to work. The healer notes that just one of his 'sacred' bouquets suffices, no matter what the size of the building or the flock within (see below).

As with *marcioré*, the collection of *san cap* is not sacralized; the plant can be picked by the healer or brought by the client. According to both parties, what matters is that it be whole and fresh. However, the presence of the most afflicted lamb from each fold is imperative. This lamb plays the role of 'substitute' (Mauss and Hubert 1950:58–9). If the contagion originated with this lamb, then in the same way that the animal transmitted the disease in the first place, with 'conjuration' it can transmit the cure. If the conjured lamb dies, another sick lamb must be brought to the healer so he can 'work it over' and give the shepherd a new *san cap* bouquet.

For the healer, each element in his conjuration is interconnected. The lamb without the plant, the plant without the lamb, or the incantation alone are all equally ineffective. In addition, the 'healing contagion' that is the aim of his efforts applies only to lambs that contracted *muguet* before the conjuration. If new-borns or lambs that were healthy at this time are later infected, then the healer must 'work over' another lamb (preferably the sickest one in the new group) because his treatment is '. . . good for the harm that exists, not for the harm to come'. In other words, it is a curative rather than a preventive measure.

The healer inherited the secret of *san cap* from his father, just as he inherited his family flock. While his father's clientele consisted of a close circle of neighbours, the son's practice extends to shepherds of other districts, whom he calls 'neighbours from afar'. Thus, proximity is now defined occupationally rather than residentially. Word of the healer circulates at fairs and weekly markets, where shepherds have the chance to meet and exchange professional, and especially veterinary, information.

The healer's clients are loyal, except, he says, for 'those over yonder', that is, shepherds from a group of villages some 30 km away. The healer is worried about reports that people there have started using 'his' plant but without 'his' formula and without consulting him. Worse still, they '. . . hang it [*san cap*] as a preventive', he says. This behaviour constitutes a direct challenge to the healer's professional integrity; it calls into question the plant's mode of functioning and hence the 'secret' handed down by his father.

Modern usages
Experiments with san cap *bouquets* G.—a man in his 30s at the time of research—is the individual responsible for the behaviour of 'those over yonder'. G. comes from a long line of Cévenol transhumants, but he also attended a technical school for shepherds. He thus controls both traditional and modern sheep-raising techniques.

Originally, G.'s knowledge of medicinal bouquets was limited to *marciouré*. However, a few years ago during a particularly virulent attack of what he diagnosed as *muguet*, G. consulted the healer of St M. After this first visit, however, G. never returned to the healer because he later identified *san cap* in his own pastures. And the next lambing season he 'dared' to hang up *san cap* bouquets without the healer's services. G. thus demonstrated his total disbelief in the power of what he calls the healer's *charabia* 'prayer'. However, G. does not question the effectiveness of the plant itself. He offers the familiar explanation that the bouquet aerially diffuses a beneficial constituent and that the *muguet* scabs dry up in parallel with the desiccating bouquets. During the following lambing season, G. also used *san cap* prophylactically. In this 'profane' usage, G. increased the number of bouquets suspended within the protective/curative space.

After these initial experiments, G. experienced two years of doubt about *san cap*. During this time, he vaccinated his ewes instead of hanging up bouquets. This period coincided with an epidemic of what G. terms *ecthyma*, the clinical signs of which are virtually identical to those of *muguet* (Table 1). He probably learned this technical term from the new veterinarian in the region. It is unclear whether G. adopted the term and the associated vaccine because he had lost confidence in the bouquets or because of the severity of the infection. In any case, he later decided that the veterinarian's 'shots' were ineffective and so he returned to hanging up preventive bouquets. Now, however, he alternates bouquets of *san cap* and *marciouré* in his folds. This innovation is designed to enhance the plants' effects and to minimize risks—not only the health risks to the lambs but also any potential supernatural risks to G., who in a sense has desecrated a plant inscribed in a sacred context.

G. found this strategy effective and he told others of his success in appropriating and administering the *san cap*. His confidants included the shepherds of his winter mutual-aid network, as well as other stockowners whose lambs he takes on the summer transhumance. His example has led still other shepherds in the region to incorporate his methods into their own technical repertoire. Functioning as a professional intermediary, G. desacrilized and modernized the healer's traditional technique, thereby making it available to many others.

Adoption of chancrée *bouquets* This case from southern Sologne concerns an ultra-modern, high-technology breeding farm for ewes. Its director is C., a young sheep breeder who is also president of the local butchers' cooperative. C., who comes from a family of cattle breeders, acquired his professional knowledge of sheep raising at a school for shepherds. For many years C. has combated a disease that he knows only as *ecthyma* by vaccinating pregnant ewes approximately one month before term. However, as evidenced by repeated outbreaks of the disease among the lambs on the farm, the vaccines did not seem wholly or consistently effective. One such outbreak occurred during the lambing season of 1981. When C. noticed the first signs of ecthyma in his bucket-fed lambs (the twins and orphans), he promptly called in a zootechnician from the Departmental Breeders Association.

This technician serves all the sheep farms in the region, traditional and modern alike. He first observed the use of bouquets in the folds of elderly shepherds in neighbouring Perche, near Vendôme. But for ten years he got no answers anywhere to his discreet queries about this practice. (The technician says veterinarians did not know of it because it was kept secret.) During the 1981 epidemic, local shepherds finally told him how they both cured and prevented ecthyma with bouquets of *Geranium robertianum* L., known locally as *herbe-à-Robert* or *chancrée* (from *chancre*, a term for ulcerations in humans). The shepherds instructed the technician in details of the plant's identification and biotope, as well as its curative and preventive applications.

The technician shared his information about the therapeutic use of *chancrée* with C. Because there was not enough time during the epidemic to vaccinate all the farm's sheep, they decided to try the traditional remedy. Fortunately, the herb is a common, anthropophilic species that is readily found along hedges and embankments. However, this plunge into folk veterinary medicine likely caused some misgivings on the part of both C. and the technician, both of whom were trained in the latest husbandry methods. But C.'s qualms were allayed by the technician's social and professional status and his reputation for seriousness and competence. Doubtless, too, the lack of alternatives in an urgent situation was a factor in their decision.

Unlike *marciouré* and *san cap*, the therapeutic use of *chancrée* requires a phase of contact between the diseased part of the body and the plant. Contact consists of rubbing the lambs' mouths (where the red spots of ecthyma first appear) with a handful of the herb before it is hung in the fold. C. carried out this treatment scrupulously and found it quite effective. But he also introduced a 'posology' of his own invention in which he treated his lambs in batches of five, changing the herbs for each batch. According to C., the phyto-therapeutic benefits lie in the juice of the crushed geraniums. He compares *chancrée*'s morphology and curative action to that of another local plant, *herbe aux verrues* (*Chelidonium majus* L.), which he knew is used on warts in humans.[6]

For the prophylactic use of *chancrée* bouquets, however, the technician failed to leave C. any specific instructions as to number and placement. The technician suggested only that the bouquets be renewed every two or three weeks to reinforce their effectiveness—which, as usual, C. ascribes to the plant's 'strong odour'. C. therefore decided to diminish the circulation of air in the folds and to hang the bouquets as low as possible. He was especially careful to do so over the enclosure for the bucket-fed lambs which, because they do not benefit from the antibodies in ewe's milk, are at greater risk. C. was so pleased with the bouquets' results that he has now totally abandoned the ecthyma vaccination.

Clearly, C. sought to rationalize his therapeutic use of *chancrée* by applying a 'scientific' posology. The same concern led him to advise a disbelieving trainee from Burgundy to conduct an experiment to verify the prophylactic efficacy of *chancrée*. C. suggested comparing three groups of lambs: one born of vaccinated ewes, another protected only by the bouquets, and a third group as a control. During his interview, C. repeatedly returned to the theme of 'After all, it's not magic!' as though he needed to convince not only his interlocutor (the author) but also himself. He displayed a certain uneasiness because of his inability to explain fully the effectiveness of the *chancrée* treatments. But he felt the method had many compelling arguments in its favour: its simplicity; the fact that it is free; and for prophylactic use, the ease of administering bouquets to the flock as a whole, in contrast to the tedious work of vaccinating each animal individually.

C.'s use of *chancrée* was somewhat serendipitous; but not so the technician's. The technician says he is always 'attentive to what can be learned in rural areas'. He now recommends this providential plant to all his clients, though for him, it is only a first response to certain problems in modern veterinary care—particularly the 'wrongful use of antibiotics', he says. Normally, the technician serves as a change agent to transfer modern technology to stockowners. But in this case, he has inverted the order of things to become a proponent of 'tradition', a label that is usually pejorative.

His is not an isolated case. The technician says some of the region's young veterinarians are also interested in local veterinary know-how. Field research by the author in Côtes-du-Nord and Mayenne has revealed that livestock technicians there also play the same mediating role between traditional and modern methods and stockraisers. Moreover, information about local plant treatments circulates among different parts of France via technicans' professional meetings, where the relative merits and methods of using bouquets and other traditional treatments in place of commercial pharmacueticals is often discussed.

Tradition and modernity

This overview of the uses of medicinal bouquets among traditional and modern sheep raisers in present-day France reveals that, in fact, tradition and modernity are not so far apart. Both groups use the same plants to treat and/or prevent the same diseases, i.e., dermatological problems. And all those men in both groups who employ the bouquets attest to their effectiveness. However, more traditionally inclined shepherds use bouquets in a 'routinized' way and with unquestioning confidence. As one of these men explains, 'My great-grandfather, my grandfather, and my father did it that way, and I am going to do the same. What's important is that it works!' In contrast, the more modern users of this centuries-old practice have modified and to some extent 'scientized' it by excluding the services of healers or priests, rejecting magico-religious reinforcements, adding posological details, and employing technical instead of local disease names. They desire a rational, 'scientific' explanation for the bouquets' healing and protective power.

Some veterinarians are alarmed by technicians' increasing adoption of traditional practices. One veterinary author brands this 'new empiricism' as '. . . legalized, regulated, codified, structured and bureaucratic obscurantism' (Villemin 1982:288–9). Yet such shifts are not without precedent. Mauss provides a parallel in the scientization of massage in France, which removed this skill from the hands of traditional healers. Emphasizing the historical bond between magic and the evolution of science and technology, he wrote:

> The techniques are like seeds that have germinated in the soil of magic but are then dispossessed of the latter. They are progressively stripped of all they have acquired from the mystical; the processes that remain are increasingly valued differently; where before they were attributed a mystical value, now they are only a mechanical action (Mauss and Hubert 1950: 135).

In the same fashion, by introducing quantification and causality into their thinking about medicinal bouquets, modern stockowners and zootechnicians have transferred this technique from magic to science, from credulity to experimentation and from tradition to modernity.

By way of epilogue, it is noteworthy that—after learning of the research described here—in March of 1989 France's professional association of sheep and goat producers disseminated a survey on the use and efficacy of medicinal bouquets to the 4800 subscribers to its *Bulletin de l'Alliance Pastorale* (Cornuau 1989). Although the results are not yet analysed, stockraisers are clearly eager to learn more about the mechanisms behind this technique, which so many of them use. It will be interesting to see whether the survey stimulates any serious, laboratory-based research on the properties of the plants in question and their possible effects on the dermatological conditions they are employed to treat. One can only wonder, too, what might be the reaction of the vast pharmaceutical industry to any suggestion of replacing its modern vaccines and drugs with simple, traditional bouquets . . .

Notes

1. Translated by Dan McConaughy, with many thanks from the author.
2. Venomous animals in particular are suspended thus. Their desiccation seems to be seen as medicinally more important than the odour they emit (see text).
3. For humans, the objects may be hung above the sick-bed or tucked under the patient's pillow. The remedy has a continuous effect if the patient remains in bed. If she/he is up and about during the day, the remedy takes effect at night while the patient sleeps. The use of bouquets is especially popular for childhood ills.
4. Fournier makes no reference to *lathrée clandestine*.
5. Some such transfers are not only symbolic but also semi-biological, at least in the sense that the transfer object may indeed have been contaminated with the disease agent or vector. For example, a common generalized therapy for both animal and human ills is to take biodegradable objects (like leaves and herbs or an apple, onion, egg, piece of lard, etc.) that have touched the diseased part of the anatomy and bury them underground or, so as to accelerate putrefaction, in manure or in anthills. As the items rot, the disease magically disappears (see Lévi-Strauss 1962).
6. In fact, Herb Robert is a well-known veterinary herbal medicine in Europe, where it is used as a wound powder, an insecticide, and a retardant for internal bleeding. Similarly, the use of the stem juice of Celandine is a common treatment for warts in both livestock and humans [editors' note].

8. The interpenetration of endogenous and exogenous in Saami reindeer raising

MYRDENE ANDERSON

THE SAAMI PEOPLE (formerly known as Lapps) inhabit the arctic regions of north-western Europe—specifically northern Fennoscandia, which is comprised of Finland, Norway, Sweden and the Kola peninsula of the former USSR. Although Saami are stereotyped as 'the reindeer people', in fact only some 10 per cent (approximately 6000) of all Saami engage in any form of reindeer production. However, in some of the northern hinterlands of Fennoscandia, as much as 35 per cent of the population (mostly Saami) may do so. All told, the Saami manage about 500000 head of reindeer (Aikio 1987), mainly on public-domain rangelands under an extensive stockraising regime involving seasonal migrations.

Both traditionally and today, Saami reindeer producers use their animals' products for home consumption—hides, blood, viscera, sinew, antlers, bones, hooves, milk and stomach contents, in roughly that order. However, cheap commercial alternatives to many reindeer products are increasingly available. Consequently, some traditional Saami food preferences and skills have changed and atrophied (Anderson 1981). Today, Saami reindeer production mainly focuses on the sale of meat to domestic, regional and international markets. There is also an active east Asian export market for antler velvet for medicinal and aphrodisiac uses. In Fennoscandia, however, new government regulations prohibiting the de-antlering of live animals have limited this market. Taken together, these shifts in consumption and marketing patterns constitute one, highly visible, example of the penetration of exogenous forces into the endogenous/traditional systems of Saami reindeer raising.

Indeed, for several centuries, Saami reindeer raising has been regulated in one fashion or another in every Fennoscandian country. But the regulation of endogenous practices of reindeer husbandry and healthcare and their penetration by exogenous political and scientific structures accelerated after World War II. Before then, few veterinarians practised among the Saami; and those who did typically also served as district agricultural agents. In the post-war period, however, government-sponsored schools were set up for Saami youth interested in formal training to supplement their traditional knowledge of reindeer management. At the same time, the Fennoscandian nations fostered increased research in reindeer demography, nutrition, husbandry practices and veterinary medicine. Today, there are government research stations that specialize in the study of reindeer; and a number of government-subsidized research and/or extension journals are devoted exclusively to reindeer production issues (see the reference list for examples). Livestock regulations, land-use laws, and other policies deriving from these new R&D thrusts and from the exigencies of the modern nation–state have increasingly affected traditional Saami reindeer raising. The most significant of such policies pertain to the timing and use of rangelands and to veterinary/public-health measures (Beach et al. 1991). The latter largely centre on quality control in slaughter and meat production. After the Soviet nuclear accident at Chernobyl in late April 1986, such policies understandably proliferated.

Below, the history of Saami/reindeer relationships is briefly overviewed. Then, the system of extensive livestock production pursued by most Saami today is described, drawing upon the author's field research among Saami of northern Norway and Sweden[1] and upon the literature documenting both traditional and modern husbandry and healthcare practices.[2] In the process, some of the exogenous impacts upon traditional husbandry and healthcare practices are noted. The chapter concludes with a discussion of how the Chernobyl catastrophe has accelerated and intensified the interpenetration of endogenous and exogenous systems in Saami reindeer production.

The Saami/reindeer relationship

Saami and reindeer have been a part of each other's history for as far back as the existence of Saami in Fennoscandia can be reconstructed, several thousand years ago (Vorren 1973). A migratory herd species, the reindeer[3] (*Rangifer tarandus*) was one of a number of important terrestrial and marine animals that, via hunting, made it possible for prehistoric Saami to survive in the frigid reaches of Fennoscandia. Saami hunting doubtless had an impact on the genetic history of the reindeer, too, by virtue of the hunters' selecting for (or in consequence of) individual animals' differential vitality, age, sex, colouration and antler size. This earliest, hunting stage of the Saami/reindeer relationship can be characterized as one of predation by the former species upon the latter.

Stage II of this interspecies relationship is defined by the first steps toward some management of the wild herds of reindeer plus the occasional taming of individual animals. This stage began at the prehistoric juncture, about 400 years ago (ibid.).[4] Captured wild reindeer (bulls as well as cows) were routinely used as decoys in hunting and to attract bulls in the fall rutting season. Possibly some of these captured animals were retained and, with castration, even tamed enough to be used as pack or draught animals. (Only a few Siberian peoples have ever used reindeer as mounts.) At this point, any such control over individual animals could have inspired the idea of veterinary care. Also, given that the domestic dog accompanied Saami in their move into Fennoscandia, canine ethnoveterinary practices may have been generalized to reindeer; and both may have been modelled after some of the more pragmatic aspects of ordinary human ethnomedicine.[5] This second stage of the Saami/reindeer relationship has been described as a sort of pastoralism, with humans following (or transhuming) along the seasonal migration routes of the reindeer. In certain areas and in more recent historical periods, this stage has been characterized as involving large herds with high reindeer-to-human ratios, minimal human surveillance of and interaction with the animals, and only incidental husbandry and healthcare interventions.

Stage III of the Saami/reindeer relationship begins with the maturation of the international fur trade in the seventeenth century. By then, most pelt-and-fur species in Saamiland had been driven to extinction or were greatly diminished in number or in value in competition with the North American supply. Only then did some Saami groups begin to concentrate their trading activities on reindeer. At that point, the over-hunted and increasingly scarce herds of reindeer became individually owned, although they were managed by corporate groups loosely organized bilaterally. At this point, too, owners understandably began to take more systematic herd husbandry and healthcare measures (Vorren 1973). For example, dogs were used to ward off predators and to contain the herds during their moves (Anderson 1986). And some reindeer were tamed enough to milk, pet and, with castration, use as draught and pack animals.

This history of the Saami/reindeer relationship is reflected today in three core types of reindeer economies. They pivot on the tensions between predation and protection, between sharing and accumulation, and between subsistence and market—roughly corresponding to hunting, pastoralism and ranching (after Ingold 1980). An alternative taxonomy is Paine's (1964) on hunting, herding and husbandry.

Within these two typologies, a minority of today's reindeer producers can be classed as ranchers or 'husbanders'. They manage herds ranging in size from fewer than 100 head up to several hundred head under fairly intensive conditions, with fairly limited herd movement (Anderson 1984a, 1986, Beach 1981). Such systems are mainly found in the more heavily populated, farmed and forested regions of southern Saamiland, especially in Finland. However, the majority of Saami reindeer producers in Norway and Sweden today fall into the category of pastoralists (or, in Paine's taxonomy, herder–husbanders). Operating on open tundra, their management systems can be characterized as extensive. Herd size ranges between several hundred and several thousand; seasonal migrations are usually long in both duration and distance (100 km and upwards); and direct husbandry and healthcare interventions are perforce more limited than in intensive stock operations, due both to herd mobility and dispersion and to the non-tameness of most of the animals. Indeed, these extensive reindeer production regimes are perhaps more akin to wildlife management than to pastoralism as it is normally defined. Indeed, in many respects they wisely mimic and build upon reindeer ethology and environmental aids (see below), reinforcing rather than combating natural processes.

Reindeer husbandry and healthcare

For the purposes of the present discussion, husbandry practices can be grouped into three broad categories: herding and range management; management of herd composition, including culling and breeding; and other husbandry operations, such as slaughter, castration, earmarking and velvet harvesting. Healthcare interventions traditionally were, and still are, fairly minimal. However, producers did and do monitor and manage aspects of herd health and nutrition generally; in addition, they attend to the condition of certain individual animals, especially geldings. The range of health concerns attended to includes: most notably, pests and parasites; a variety of diseases in individual animals; diet and nutrition; and since Chernobyl, radioactive contamination of forage, live animals and meat.

In each of the following sections, Saami husbandry and healthcare measures are described first in their endogenous form. Then, where relevant, exogenous impacts that have led to changes or modifications in traditional practice are discussed. It should also be noted that all these practices are reinforced by supernatural ones designed to protect the collective *sii'da*, that is, the herd together with its range, migration routes, owners, herders, infrastructure and pastoral paraphernalia (Anderson 1978). Still today, shamans (*noaidi*) and ordinary producers make general-purpose offerings on stoney promontories in order to ensure herd health and well-being. Magic in the form of the *juoigos* ('yoick' or 'chant') is also sometimes used to ward off predators and to calm reindeer as well as people (Anderson 1984b).

Husbandry

Herding and range management The hardy and indigenous reindeer browse and, to a lesser extent, graze freely on open range throughout the year. This management regime stands in sharp contrast to all other livestock in Fenno-scandia, which are sheltered and provisioned at least eight months of the year. The general annual pattern of herd movements can be described as follows. During the winter, a given herd remains together on the delicate lichen pastures of inland mountains and plateaux. These winter pastures contain barely enough lichens to supplement the few other palatable plants that survive under snow cover. As May approaches each spring, the herd disperses. Cows are the first to begin migrating to summer pastures, as they head for traditional calving grounds where there is little ice build-up and fewer predators; bulls begin their migration somewhat later. The summer pastures are rich in herbaceous plants; and the pastures are located in areas such as mountain slopes or shore lines, where breezes ward off insects. Thus summer pastures may be found either higher or lower in elevation than the herd's winter range, depending on the region. In the autumn, the animals range widely in search of mushrooms. But eventually the herd reunites at its traditional rutting grounds. This is the first stage in the return migration to winter pastures.

In certain seasons (such as the summer, when cows and calves move together in nursery groups) and locations (for example, natural cul-de-sacs), reindeer are left under little or no surveillance for long periods. Minimal oversight of herds is facilitated by certain aspects of *Rangifer* ethology. Reindeer will not range far afield in deep snow or on circumscribed land masses; and in the presence of some disruption, such as predators, they move allelomimetically (as a group) with their agitated fellows.

Traditionally, producer interference in herd movements and forage use was minimal. The migration routes taken entailed little producer decision-making, since they were equally familiar to herds and humans. Or as Saami often put it, 'People just followed the herd'. Indeed, it was arguable which species was herding which—humans or animals. Occasionally, however, herds would be manoeuvred according to longer-term migration plans or the presence of other herds nearby, in order to avoid herd mixing. Traditionally, such manoeuvres were executed by one or more persons, with or without dogs, on foot or on skis, or by reindeer-drawn sledge. Today, these methods may be supplemented by the use of snowmobiles, boats, trucks or even airplanes.

Reindeer–human contact was most intimate during two types of husbandry activities: during round-ups, when operations such as earmarking, castration and culling were performed; and during migration. Nowadays, the spring migration is the largest and most socially significant. At this time, the children of producers who follow this migratory system are even given a school holiday so they can accompany their families and learn the traditional routes and husbandry methods.

Today, however, traditional migration routes and the larger sweeps of seasonal migrations have been curtailed by government regulations on animal movements within each reindeer district. These districts in part follow the longstanding flows of herds across the landscape. But these flows have also been re-shaped by contemporary political boundaries. Saami herding and range management have been considerably complicated by these and other exogenous factors. Examples include the intrusion of sedentary farmers on traditional rangelands; modern resource-extraction activities such as mining, logging and the generation of hydro-electric power; transport and communications infrastructure, such as roads, snowmobile routes, power lines and stations; usurpation of traditional rangelands for recreational, tourist and military activities; and pollution, which now includes nuclear contamination. Contemporary herders must therefore exercise much greater control over migration routes so as to keep reindeer away from crop lands or from dangerous places such as roads, power lines, dams and the most severely contaminated patches in the landscape.

With dwindling range lands, producers also must take greater pains to protect and conserve the remaining forage resources, especially the fragile winter lichen pastures that are critical to herd survival. During the summer, the exposed and desiccated lichens are brittle and flammable, so producers make extra efforts to protect them from both livestock and human abuse (including the all-terrain vehicles popular among tourists). This concern over scarce winter pasturage has contributed to the proliferation of regulations designed to orchestrate the movement of herd segments: groups of bulls, pregnant cows or nursery groups composed of several cows and their calves. For example, bulls—who lag behind the pregnant cows in the spring migration—must be nudged off the winter grazing grounds by early summer. And after the autumn rutting season, the reassembled herd must be held back until conditions on the winter range can withstand renewed human and animal traffic and grazing.

Such strategies for controlling migration and range utilization make for added pastoral work, however. When herds or herd segments must be transported any distance by truck or ferry, calves and younger animals have no opportunity to learn the traditional migratory routes. This means that, unless such freighting is systematically instituted thereafter, the younger generation of animals will require much closer guidance and attention in herding.

Herd composition, culling and breeding When left to their own devices—as in the wild or under extensive management regimes—reindeer herds will vary in size and age/sex composition, depending upon a variety of factors. These include the season of the year, the weather, available pasturage, the proliferation of pests and predators, and anthropogenic disturbances on the range. Traditionally, Saami did little to control herd composition other than culling according to immediate enabling conditions (the number, type, condition or health of the animals at hand) and owners' short-term needs—usually for meat or for rituals like weddings, which require white hides for clothing. For meat, only sick, lame, old or infertile animals typically were culled.

Pressures on range resources backed by the urgings of reindeer researchers and extension workers have made for changes in herd composition and culling practices, however. For example, Saami are now advised to keep no more than 5 per cent of a herd as studs. Today, producers may slaughter most male calves not selected for breeding or for gelding and training as draft animals. Culling takes place at the end of the calves' first or second summer, at ages four and 16 months, respectively. Even though the calves still have several years of potential growth and weight gain at these ages, they would strain the carrying capacity of today's more limited rangelands. Since winter mortalities are highest among calves—with many not surviving their first year anyway—early culling makes good sense in terms of conserving scarce forage.

However, rationalizing herd composition through culling assumes implicitly that producers will select carefully for breeding stock. But in fact, some of the young male animals slated for culling still manage to breed before they are slaughtered. Indeed, few producers see selective breeding as a management priority, even though they have a good working knowledge of animal genetics. Nor are Saami always easily convinced of the value of systematic culling, because large and robust herds constitute a visible index of a family's wealth and prestige. Moreover, certain animals are culturally highly valued despite the fact that they may have genetic shortcomings. An example is white reindeer, whose hides are prized for ritual, aesthetic and social purposes; but white reindeer are born with poor hearing and often fail to thrive. Reflecting these differences between modern and traditional herd-management wisdom, people vary in their breeding and culling choices. Two siblings with reindeer in the same herd, for instance, commonly make independent (and sometimes contradictory) husbandry decisions. Even though both share the cultural value placed on white reindeer and both know that such animals tend to be less hardy, one sibling may prefer to keep this status marker on the hoof while the other decides to wear it on his/her back in the form a white hide tunic.

Other husbandry operations Traditionally, slaughter was performed with a knife stab to the nape of the neck, followed by another to the heart (or in some regions, only the latter). While this procedure is still followed, government regulations now stipulate that the animal must first be stunned by a bolt to the forehead. Also, producers who plan to market the meat are no longer free to slaughter animals when and where they please. Instead, slaughtering must be supervised by (typically non-Saami) meat inspectors/veterinarians at government-built district slaughterhouses, where certain promoted practices are subsidized.

Government mandates have also affected traditional methods of castration, earmarking and velvet harvesting. Castration was typically performed by the herder's crushing the testicles between his teeth—as sheep raisers around the world have long done and, in some areas, still do. Now, this operation must be done using tongs. Government regulations also prescribe the timing of traditional earmarking, when registered patterns are incised and excised along the edges of the ears to record ownership. This procedure is now restricted to the warmer months, when surgical complications are less likely. (When the temperature falls too low, for example, the wounds on the ears may freeze rather than heal.)

Another law prohibits the ancient practice of cutting antlers from live animals. Reindeer of both sexes grow antlers each spring, which is when the velvet stage occurs; the antlers are then shed later in the year. But Asian markets reject velvet harvested from shed antlers as having no medicinal or aphrodisiac value. The new government regulation means that for the velvet to be harvested, the entire animal must be sacrificed. Thus, velvet production is greatly depressed. Moreover, this restriction entails major wastage in meat production, because reindeer slaughtered in the spring are usually too emaciated from winter stress to yield much meat.

Healthcare

In general, producers rarely note the health of individual animals; or if they do, most animals are given no clinical or other attention. Eventually they die an accidental death or are slaughtered. The main exceptions to this rule are geldings used as draught animals. Their health is closely monitored, for several reasons. They represent a sizeable investment of time and training, and they are essential to seasonal transport. Furthermore, they may be the oldest and largest animals in a herd; and because of hormonal changes induced by castration, they do not shed their antlers during the winter. Thus, they literally 'stand out' in the herd. They are given pet names, and also thus become an enduring feature of the social landscape. With the exception of geldings, however, people usually make concerted efforts at healthcare only if a number of head are afflicted simultaneously.

Pests and parasites The main herd health problem of reindeer is pests and parasites, which can affect vitality without necessarily leading to death. Insect pests such as mosquitoes, midges and gnats all torment the reindeer and interfere with grazing. But the most noxious and economically destructive pests are two ectoparasites: the reindeer warble (*Oedemagena tarandi*) and the bot fly (*Cephenemyia trompe*). Warbles lay their eggs on the back and sides of the animal; when the eggs hatch, the larvae burrow beneath the skin, puncturing the hide and lowering its value. (Also see Shanklin, this volume.) Bot flies lay their eggs in the nostrils, and the larvae mature as far down as the throat passage, where they cause considerable respiratory distress. In both cases, the larvae leave the host in the spring and early summer, to become egg-laying flies by mid-July.

The natural inclination of the reindeer—and of their herders—is to avoid fly-infested areas as much as possible. Faced with plagues of insects, the animals will try to head into the wind or move to smoky areas; with the surcease of wind or smoke, they cluster together; or if they can find no relief, the herd scatters. To avoid or combat the pests, herders employ strategies mimicking reindeer ethology—such as herding the animals onto a breezy slope. Or they may light smudge fires. To forestall scattering, they may drive the herd into a cul-de-sac.

A wide variety of endoparasites also plagues reindeer. Often carried by dogs or snails, different species of parasites settle in the lungs (*Echinococcus granulosus*), liver (*Cysticercus* spp., *Dicrocoelium* spp.), brain (the nematode *Elaphostrongylus rangiferi*), intestines (tapeworms) and muscles (*Setaria tundru, Cysticercus tarandi, Sarcosporida* spp.). Calves and yearlings are the most apt to be seriously affected; but as much as 70 per cent of a herd may be infected by one or another endoparasite—most commonly, liverflukes. Factors identified by scientists as promoting endoparasitism generally reflect traditional understandings and include: over-population of reindeer; keeping herds in the same corrals two years in a row; the amount of infected scrap meat, especially lungs, scavenged by dogs; and mild summer weather, which provides favourable conditions for parasite proliferation. For ectoparasitism, avoidance of infested areas has always been the traditional, and best, method of control.

In contrast to traditional methods of pest and parasite control that take advantage of reindeer ethology and natural environmental phenomena, exogenous efforts have centred on treatment and vaccination campaigns. The case of warbles is illustrative. As early as 1958, campaigns were mounted to treat reindeer against this scourge. Although the drugs used (for example, the organo-phosphate Warbex) were effective, they were never applied on a large enough scale to make much difference. Later, in the 1980s, massive programmes of inoculation with ivermectin were instituted. However, they led to some controversy after over-optimistic expectations were disappointed (Haugerud 1990). The problems facing any such treatment or inoculation campaigns are daunting. Most notable are the practical difficulties and costs of treating many thousands of head of only semi-tame migratory animals, not to mention the dangers of overdosing and the threat of drug resistance.

Other diseases Aside from parasites, the most common diseases of reindeer are sores, bladder and eye infections, hoof problems and a nerve affliction that causes lameness in the hindquarters. With the exception of geldings, lame or lagging animals are usually simply slaughtered. But if a gelding is involved, herders may treat the animal with folk and/or modern remedies. Sores are treated topically with pine pitch, tar or juniper (*Juniperus communis*) or marsh-tea (*Ledum palustre*) infusion. Bladder infections call for feeding the animal reindeer hair, usually mixed with a fat, or for drenching with an infusion of juniper tea. For eye infections, a commercial antibiotic ointment may be applied.

Diet and nutrition Weak animals may be coaxed to eat lichens of certain genera (especially *Cladonia* and *Stereocaulon*), horsetail, or even the *Carex* sedge hay used as boot insulation. Sometimes people collect lichens and horsetail in advance, to be saved as emergency fodder. In particular, this is done for tethered draught animals. But these plants will also be offered to any weak or sick animal that has been sequestered for observation. Yearlings following their first winter are the most apt to need this extra attention. Today, mineral blocks may also be provided, at least for draught animals. However, these practices represent a luxury that the majority of Saami, who follow an extensive production regime, cannot afford.

When most of the herd is seen to be suffering from a presumed dietary problem, producers may seek veterinary advice. But often the only possible remedy is to remove the animals from the range and provide them better forages and supplements. However, this strategy is problematic because reindeer do not tolerate well sudden changes in feed. Nowadays, mineral blocks may be used to try to entice a group of ailing animals to accept 'artificial' feed. But even if the animals are given natural forages gathered by hand from their home ranges, this remedy may not suffice.

When only a few weak or ill animals require special feeding, adult women often take charge. They are less likely to migrate than are men, since women are charged with the care of children in school or with dealing with other exigencies of modern life that have made many husbandry tasks, and especially herding, a now-mainly-male role. If an entire herd or herd segment requires supplemental feeding—as has been recommended since Chernobyl—feed must be freighted to the herd. In this case, men are primarily responsible.

Radioactivity The Chernobyl disaster dumped significant amounts of radioactive fall-out in patches over Fennoscandia, with some of the northern hinterlands experiencing the greatest contamination. This is precisely where substantial reindeer production takes place, as well as many other primary subsistence activities such as elk hunting, freshwater fishing and mushroom- and berry-picking. Along with tourists, all residents of the hinterlands engage in all these other activities. However, radioactive contamination of reindeer meat was an especial concern. In large part, this concern related to the reindeer's heavy dependence on lichens, which were perceived as harbouring especially high levels of radioactivity. The question for Saami producers and their consumer markets was: How safe was it to eat reindeer meat?

The answer to this seemingly simple question was not clear, however. For one thing, as migratory animals, reindeer visit many sites across the course of a year, all with potentially different levels of contamination. Moreover, during the first years after Chernobyl, radioactivity could not be, or was not, tested in live animals in Fennoscandia; this could be done only upon slaughter. Reindeer carcasses that showed high readings of radioactivity based on the technology available at the time were simply buried or, insofar as possible, diverted to pelt farms as feed. Governments instituted systems to compensate people whose animals or other products were condemned. Meanwhile, researchers set about investigating ways to make contaminated food products 'safe' for human consumption. For reindeer, the strategies devised included feeding pellets designed to absorb the radiation or providing a special diet prior to slaughter. After several years of experience, the latter strategy came to be preferred.

Before the Chernobyl incident, Fennoscandian regulations concerning radioactivity in foodstuffs were in part shaped by the European export market, where a common limit was 600 becquerels of caesium-137[6] per kilogram of food (hereafter, bq/kg). Depending on the region, some of the reindeer meat tested during the first year after Chernobyl registered 10000bq/kg or more of radiation.[7] By way of contrast, for some of the fish tested during the same period, this figure exceeded 20000.

Within weeks of the Chernobyl disaster, however, governments began revising their food-safety regulations. To take one example, in Sweden the National Institute of Radiation Protection and the National Food Administration lowered the safety limit for milk to 300bq/kg. This new figure was calculated based on the risks to the main consumers of milk: babies (Jones 1989). Subsequently, this 300bq/kg limit was extended to *all* human foodstuffs in Sweden. Among some Saami, these shifting regulations and figures were interpreted as a government ploy to justify ending compensation for condemned reindeer.

A year after Chernobyl, however, Sweden set a new and much higher limit of 1500bq/kg specifically for 'wild' products such as reindeer, game, fish, mushrooms and berries (Beach 1990). Of course, few non-Saami proportionally consume as much reindeer meat as a baby would milk. But with public fears depressing reindeer-meat markets, many Saami (and especially Saami reindeer producers) increased their consumption of reindeer meat to much greater levels than non-Saami populations. There was some speculation about a lack of government concern for Saami health and well-being, with the implication that this lack bordered on passive ethnocide. Subsequently, expert discussion claimed that occasional doses of up to 10000bq/kg of contaminated foodstuffs would not endanger consumers so long as the annual maximum dose of one millisievert was not exceeded.

Like Sweden, other countries of Fennoscandia promulgated new and rapidly changing regulations, with little congruency among them.[8] Both producers and consumers of reindeer products have been subjected to seemingly arbitrary and inconsistent modifications in the policies thus established (Beach 1990, Paine 1987, 1988b). Further complicating the meat production picture are the many different food-safety standards and laws that have proliferated in distant internal and external markets in the wake of Chernobyl. As research continues, food safety and exposure levels are still being revised, with perhaps the most common measure now in use being the acceptable total lifetime dosage [editors' note]. But informed choices are still difficult to make about products that derive from animals that frequent a number of different locales and habitats.

In summary, as a result of Chernobyl, Saami and non-Saami alike have had to cope with the stress of living with levels of pollution that can soar far above the scientifically established and nationally sanctioned thresholds for safe food consumption. But the Chernobyl incident struck a particularly hard blow at Saami reindeer production, as well as at the producers themselves, who may be at greatest risk from contaminated reindeer products. Although the media have widely touted the threat to Saami reindeer production, there are signs that production will endure,[9] albeit probably with modification as a result of increasing interpenetration.

Accelerated interpenetration

The interpenetration of endogenous and exogenous systems in Saami reindeer production is a longstanding process. Although it began to accelerate after World War II, ever broader yet more tightly integrated international markets (now including the former USSR republics as well as the nascent EC) and inescapable transnational events like the Chernobyl catastrophe have added fresh impetus to this process. As a result, interaction between Saami reindeer producers and government and scientific agencies has increased markedly, with both positive and negative consequences.

On the positive side, Saami are tasking such agencies in new and more demanding ways, and they now scrutinize government policy and animal husbandry and veterinary advice much more critically. For example, reindeer producers would like to understand better the changing regulations and the units of analysis on which they are based. They are asking questions like the following. Will the meat of animals that are penned and fed special diets to bring them within food safety limits before slaughter actually be as safe to eat as that of stock that never exceeded the contamination threshold? And, what is this threshold, really? How should risks to humans from consumption of contaminated reindeer meat best be calculated? And what can governments and scientists do to reassure consumers about the healthfulness of reindeer meat?

Conversely, greater interaction has stimulated government and R&D professionals (e.g. in veterinary science, animal genetics, forage agronomy and range science) to learn to accommodate the pragmatics and traditions of Saami reindeer management. This has led them in the direction of devising husbandry and healthcare interventions that are tenable at the grassroots level. For example, many researchers have come to appreciate that certain techniques may not fit well with the extensive reindeer production regimes of most Saami. Examples include the establishment of blood lines and the use of artificial insemination. On the other hand, scientists and developers now understand better the kinds of measures that many Saami producers would welcome—for instance, parasite control strategies, cost-effective mineral and feed supplements, and local ensilage methods to offset critical forage bottle-necks. Researchers and extensionists are also learning to work more closely alongside producers, and to draw on Saami's local-level knowledge—not only in matters of food safety but also in coordinating stocking levels on range lands and determining optimal herd size and composition for cultural needs as well as for profit.

On the negative side, not a few Saami and even some researchers have felt a sense of conspiracy in the post-Chernobyl contamination rhetoric of the press and officialdom. They suspect that governments and/or dominant ethnic factions are weary of accommodating the to-their-eyes exotic livelihood of a stubborn Fourth World people and so are seeking ways to use Chernobyl against Saami (see Beach 1990, Edelstein 1988, Paine 1987, 1988b). If this discourse of suspicion spreads, Saami could become a textbook case for ethnic extinction. Alternatively, a nativistic movement could ensue, including revitalization of endogenous husbandry and healthcare practices. Perhaps not such a negative outcome after all . . .

Notes

1. Intensive field research was conducted during 1972–6 and 1979–80, with additional periods of fieldwork between and after these dates. Unless otherwise noted, the discussion throughout this chapter applies mainly to Saami of northern Norway and Sweden.
2. This literature derives from three types of sources: Saami authors themselves (e.g., Aikio 1987, Ruong 1968, Turi 1931, 1965, Utsi 1948), documents produced from and for Saami reindeer producers (e.g., Skjenneberg 1965, Skjenneberg and Slagsvold 1968), and studies and reports by contemporary ethnographers and linguists (e.g., Anderson 1978, Beach 1981, Ingold 1976, 1980, Nesheim 1966, Nielsen 1928, Paine 1964, 1971, 1972, 1988a, Vorren 1973, Wiklund 1916).
3. English 'reindeer' and 'caribou' refer to the same species, with the former term applying to the tame or somewhat more domesticated animals mostly in the old world and the latter to wild ones in the new world (Zeuner 1963). Interestingly, today the only Saami term regularly used to refer to reindeer is the opaque and irregular lexeme *boazo* (pl. *boc'cut*), specifying 'domesticated reindeer'. While the Saami language retains a regular lexeme *god'di* (pl. *goddit*) for 'wild reindeer', in fact this term is transparent, deriving from *god'dit* 'to kill, to murder', harking back to hunting times.
4. The change from hunting to herd management in Fennoscandia may have been a local-level transition, a local-level transformation, or a cultural borrowing from the Siberian east, where reindeer management can be documented for several thousand years (as versus only several hundred years in Fennoscandia). In other words, for Fennoscandia this shift is difficult to pinpoint not only temporally and spatially but also in terms of transitory evolution versus transformative development. The former is more non-predictable, open-ended and creative, while the latter is somewhat determinate, progressive and phased (Salthe and Anderson 1989).
5. History is moot on this point. However, contemporary Saami ethnomedicine includes a number of shamanistic elements that do not seem to transfer to either dogs or reindeer. Only human medicine commonly entails trance, laying on of hands, stanching of blood, suction, cautery and charms fashioned of sinew or leather.
6. Although caesium-137 is only one of the contaminants, it is of special concern because of its long half-life (about 30 years). In contrast, elements like iodine-131, with a half-life of eight days, are no longer an issue.
7. It should be noted that radioactive contamination had visited Saamiland before, from atomic testing in Siberia in the 1950s and 1960s. The accumulated dosages of radiation in humans, livestock and especially lichens were regularly monitored and found alarming. At the time, even though Saami were warned about the danger of eating reindeer meat, few took the warning seriously or were able to do anything about it. The current situation appears more real, perhaps because of the enormous effort to educate the public, but also because Chernobyl was a major media event. Some people who had reindeer meat in their freezers at the time of Chernobyl later had it tested for radioactivity, out of curiosity. They sometimes found that they had routinely eaten meat with over 300, 1 500, or more bq/kg.
8. For Norway, for example, the limit was 300bq/kg of food in May 1986, 370 in June 1986 for children's food but 600 for other foods; and for reindeer meat as of November 1986, 6000.
9. In fact, in certain regions spared serious fall-out (including northern Norway), the reindeer industry is thriving, perhaps even to the point of straining forage resources.

9. Ethno-agroveterinary perspectives on poultry production in rural Nigeria

MAMMAN AMINU IBRAHIM AND PAUL AYUBA ABDU

Nigeria's poultry population has been established at 10 million exotic and 124 million 'local' chickens, 45 million guineafowl, and one million each of ducks, pigeons and turkeys (Nawathe and Lamorde 1982). At the height of the exotic chicken industry, in Nigeria as in many developing nations, the numerous local breeds were viewed as a barrier to poultry development because of their comparatively lower productivity and their presumed status as carriers of disease (ibid.). Several developing countries in Africa have therefore sought to upgrade small farmers' stock via programmes that substitute exotic cocks for local ones.

In Nigeria, one such scheme known as Operation Coq was instituted (Taran 1974). It endeavoured to replace all local cocks in co-operating villages within one to two years. In such operations, all village cocks must be removed because the exotics cannot compete with them (AERLS 1976). However, this scheme—like most others involving importing 'improved' breeds into Africa—did not live up to its promise of greater productivity (CTA 1987, Wilson 1979). To attain efficient levels of production with imported stock in the tropics, poultry management and dietary systems must equal or exceed those practised in climates more favourable to the exotics (Bushman 1974). In Nigeria, this has not been achieved due, among other things, to the ongoing economic crisis that began about 1984 and caused a severe slump in all import-dependent sectors. As a result, the present population of exotic chickens in Nigeria is probably far fewer than the 1982 figure cited above. Not only did Operation Coq fail; it also absorbed almost all of the nation's poultry research and veterinary resources while at the same time branding the 124 million local chickens a health menace to the exotics.

As McCorkle (1989) has observed, the litmus test for the sustainability of a development package is a crumbling economy. Nigeria's current economic crisis has at long last kindled some interest among national scientists in the country's local poultry breeds and husbandry systems. Unfortunately, in their efforts to develop a poultry industry based on local stock and materials, Nigerian scientists continue to rely on research objectives and production criteria appropriate to exotic birds under intensive management. Thus they risk producing breeds and management recommendations that are just as ill-suited to the biophysical and human environment of rural Nigeria as those imported from abroad. Poor understanding of local management objectives, knowledge, beliefs and practices has been recognized as one of the major factors constraining the poultry industry in developing countries (McArdle 1972). Before successful poultry improvement schemes can be mounted, an in-depth appreciation of indigenous poultry husbandry systems is imperative.

This chapter describes selected aspects of ethno-agro-veterinary belief and practice pertaining to poultry varieties and production systems among Hausa and settled Fulani in rural Nigeria. In addition, the authors analyse how local ideas and techniques—even seemingly mistaken ones—often serve useful stockraising purposes and offer some tantalizing clues for appropriate research and development. The focus here is on chickens and guinea-fowl, but other species are also mentioned. The chapter draws on a spectrum of sources: reviews of relevant literature; informal interviews and discussions with adult Hausa and Fulani men and, especially, women[1] over a period of more than 10 years; and the authors' firsthand experience and observation of poultry raising in rural Nigeria—both as scientists and as members of the two ethnic groups discussed.

Farmers' poultry production objectives and criteria

Hausa and Fulani women traditionally manage the household poultry (Ibrahim 1986, Ibrahim *et al.* 1983). Almost every family in rural Hausaland keeps some poultry. These animals are used for both home consumption and sale, with sales being somewhat more important for settled Fulani (Waters-Bayer 1988). Like commerical poultry raisers, rural people keep some birds mainly for eggs (layers) and others for meat (broilers). Guineafowl are raised primarily for eggs while chickens, ducks and pigeons are kept mainly for meat.

Thus, for farmers in Hausaland, layers and broilers are comprised of different species. There are good reasons why this is the case. Among the domestic birds of Nigeria, the guineafowl is by far the best egg producer. A local chicken lays only 50 to 60 eggs per year in four clutches.[2] In contrast, under the same environmental and managerial conditions and with the regular egg collection that farmers practise, a guinea-fowl gives 100 to 150 eggs annually (AERLS 1976). Even with intensive management, under Nigerian environmental conditions the layers of exotic chicken breeds average no more than 159 eggs per year (Nwosu 1987). This slight advantage of exotics is more than offset by the guinea-fowl's much greater hardiness and more consistent laying.

Although traditional guineafowl husbandry is practised only in the northern parts of the country, it accounts for up to 53 per cent of all eggs consumed in Nigeria (Akinwumi *et al.* 1979 cited in Ayeni and Ayanda 1982, Ayorinde 1988). For taste and quality (including, for example, a larger yolk) Nigerian consumers prefer guineafowl eggs to all others (Ayeni and Ayanda 1982). Guineafowl eggs therefore fetch a relatively higher price in the market-place.[3] Equally important, they more often survive transport on the nation's poor roads because they have harder, thicker shells than chicken eggs (Ayorinde 1988).[4] They may also store better insofar as the thicker shells may retard evaporation. Certainly, along with more conventional considerations—such as market price and reliability and the quantity and quality of egg production—farmers consider shell strength crucial for a successful egg operation. Yet this is a criterion that scientists often overlook.

Aside from eggs and meat, there are other reasons why rural Nigerians keep poultry. Along with small ruminants, poultry play a unique savings and investment role in rural household economies. Small stock in general are referred to as *quarkuwar qarke* 'shield of the herd'[5] because they protect the reproductive integrity of the family herd of cattle. When domestic needs or social obligations arise, small stock can be slaughtered instead of large stock. They are also seen as a good investment towards eventual or additional cattle ownership. As one folk proverb admonishes:

If you lack the resources to establish a herd of cattle, then buy a hen; you can be sure that the neighbour's cock will find her. With the proceeds from the sale of her chicks, buy a ewe. The neighbour's ram will find her, too. From sales of the resulting ram lambs, buy a heifer.

Such wisdom generates verifiable economic propositions. For example, the authors purchased a local female chick of the *wake-wake* variety for about 10 naira. The chick cost virtually nothing to raise in terms of feed or veterinary care. But within a year, it generated between 200 and 300 naira (US $20.00 to $30.00)—enough to buy two young ewes!

In addition to their nutritional and economic roles, poultry are seen as fulfilling other, predictive and protective functions for humans. It is customary to assign or give a hen to the new-born child of a relative or friend in order to test the child's 'hand' at poultry raising. As in many other cultures around the world (McCorkle, pers. comm.), the fate of these first animals is believed to predict the child's future expertise and success (or lack thereof) at stockraising. In addition, all members of a family usually have an animal nominally assigned to them as a protective totem. People believe that ill health or other misfortunes intended for humans will often strike their animal alternates instead. The latter belief directly influences people's attitudes towards animal illness. For example, if a chick displays neurological symptoms typical of Newcastle disease, people may assume it has been attacked by a malevolent spirit that was aimed at its owner.

Varieties and qualities of local poultry

Poultry science in Nigeria recognizes only one type of non-exotic chicken, which it labels merely 'local'.[6] In contrast, Hausa and Fulani name and distinguish at least 15 different types of local chicken based on such considerations as productivity, colouring, feathering, body size and conformation, and ideological association with certain spirits (Table 1). Along with other parameters, the last factor figures in the cost and availability of different varieties. For example, only members of the *bori* cult of the spirit-possessed raise certain varieties of chickens. These are used to invoke the birds' associated spirits to heal a patient, harm an enemy, and so forth (Callaway 1984, Ibrahim this volume). Such birds are more costly and difficult to obtain than other varieties because many people do not keep them out of fear of the evil or dangerous spirits with which they are linked.

The beliefs associated with these special varieties are suggestive for geneticists and breeders. For example, might the *durgu* 'dwarf' chicken be associated with the luck-spirit because of its excellent performance under harsh conditions? Rural people rank the *durgu* as the 'best' of their local chickens; poultry scientists would agree with this ranking. Along with the *kwaye* (naked neck) and the *burtsa* or *fingi* (frizzled feather) varieties, the *durgu* is thermodynamically best adapted for hot environments; the *kwaye* additionally shows an advantage on a suboptimal protein diet (Merat 1986). While the authors know of no genetic studies on the *burtsa*, unselected genes for dwarfism and naked neck have been documented in the local poultry population of several other countries in the subtropical, tropical and equatorial zones (ibid). Indeed, several dwarf (the Vedette) and naked-neck (the Transylvanian) breeds are highly recommended for tropical Africa (Bushman 1974, CTA 1987, Merat 1986).

Table 1. Varieties of local chickens in Hausaland

Hausa name	Description and associated spirits (if any)
Bacam	A small but well-proportioned chicken.
Ba'ka	Pure black. Such birds are associated with *Kunnau*, one of the most malevolent of the evil spirits. Its name literally means 'the ignitor' and suggests lack of caution. Children and pregnant and nursing women keep well away from *bori* festivals featuring this spirit and the *ba'ka* chicken.
Ba'kar shirwa	Colour of the African black kite, *Milvus migrans parasiticus*.
Burtsa, birci, fingi, or 'kudugu	Birds with sparse and permanently ruffled or 'frizzled' feathers. These chickens are kept almost exclusively by *bori* cultists and are associated with *Kuturu* ('the leper' spirit) and *Abba*. *Kuturu* is an aggressive, short-tempered and malevolent entity.
Durgu	Short-legged or dwarf chicken. The associated spirit is *Gajere* 'the short one'. This spirit is consulted mainly by hunters since it dispenses good luck.
Fara	Pure white. Such birds are linked to a royal spirit known as *Dan galadima*. People possessed by it affect 'royal' attributes such as extravagance.
Jar shirwa	Colour of Ricour's kite, *Chelictinea ricourii*. Such birds are associated with *Yar mairo*, the wife of *Abba*; she is greedy, envious, sugar-loving and miserly.
'Kurar fatake or toka	Ash (*toka*) coloured. The first term refers to the dust ('*kura*) raised by foot or mounted merchants (*fatake*).
Kwaye or jimina	Naked-neck chickens. The second name refers to the neck of an ostrich.
Mai sirdi	Cocks with an arrangement of feather colours and a certain shape of the back that resemble a saddled horse.
Mai tukku	A chicken with a crest of feathers on its head.
Maiwa	Colour of the *maiwa* variety of pearl millet.
Sha zumami or ja	Light red, like the colour of the sugar ant.
Wake-wake	Black with white spots.
Zabuwa	Grey spotted with black (the colour of the most common type of guinea-fowl).

Similarly, the *jar shirwa* chicken is linked with the fierce and possessive *'yar mairo* spirit because of this bird's aggressive behaviour. Unlike Nigerian geneticists, rural producers judge a variety not only by its qualities as a layer or a broiler but also by its hens' overall ability as mothers. In addition to more conventional considerations such as broodiness and the number of fertile eggs laid per clutch, rural people value aggressiveness in a mother hen. They see this trait as an important factor in chick survival. This makes good sense, given that under indigenous poultry management, a hen often must fight off other birds to secure sufficient feed for her offspring and must protect her chicks against predators. Indeed, the authors have witnessed prize local hens chase off dogs!

Thus it is no surprise that Hausa actively select for aggressiveness, as well as broodiness, in their hens. The value people place on both these traits is evidenced in local aphorisms, proverbs and customs. For example, a common saying, *Dan tsako samu ka'ki dangi*, makes reference to a chick's (*dan tsako*) aggressiveness in claiming its share of food from its clutch mates. And Hausa say a person who perseveres at something despite immense obstacles 'has the heart of a chicken', paralleling a hen's great patience and perseverance in brooding.[7] The dried and powdered heart of a chicken also figures in a local love philtre used to keep a lover or spouse from straying, just as chickens cannot be driven away from their home foraging grounds. These examples illustrate how, again, geneticists and breeders can take a cue from rural producers, proverbs and customs in identifying important traits to be selected for under indigenous management systems, plus possible genetic sources for such traits among local poultry varieties.

Poultry management practices and beliefs

To label all styles of poultry management that are not intensive or semi-intensive as 'free range' is misleading. Such non-discriminate labelling implies strong cross-cultural similarities where few in fact exist. Hausa and Fulani husbandry differs from that reported for neighbouring Sudan (Wilson 1979) or even for other parts of Nigera (Nwosu 1987). The following sections exemplify specific poultry management techniques based on Hausa and Fulani concepts of the biological requirements of their birds, especially chickens and guineafowl. Building upon these concepts and their management correlates, the authors also offer suggestions as to how such indigenous practices and perspectives actually or potentially promote healthy and productive poultry raising.

Flock size, composition and culling
Several factors determine the distribution, size and composition of flocks. Ducks are kept mainly in towns because of the availability of borrow-pits, which serve as handy ponds. Almost every ward has its own, named pond (*tafki* or *kududdufi*). Guineafowl are easily alarmed, so they are mainly kept in villages or on the outskirts of towns.[8] Despite the preference for guineafowl eggs, this species is always kept in smaller numbers than chickens, for several reasons. Guinea-fowl can be serious agricultural pests; they are especially destructive of fields during the planting season. Also, as a mainly arboreal species, they are more difficult to manage. Furthermore, the guineafowl's habit of communal egg-laying may cause quarrels between neighbours as to who owns which eggs.

Chickens are kept in flocks of about fifteen. Farmers say that when the flock surpasses this number, the hens begin to lay eggs communally, just as guinea-fowl do. This leads to fights among birds and disrupts the incubation process. As soon as women notice communal laying, they sell or slaughter some of the chickens, retaining only the offspring of the best birds. Ageing cocks are also culled and replaced with young ones whenever women find tiny, yolkless 'pigeon eggs' in the nest. Farmers believe such eggs are due to old, impotent cocks,[9] although Western science indicates they are caused by foreign material in the oviduct (Ensminger 1980). Any sick adult birds with poor ethno-prognoses are promptly sold or consumed locally. Young birds, however, are virtually never culled or consumed.

All the foregoing practices have beneficial implications for flock health and productivity. Culling unproductive, aged or sick animals improves the flock generally. And culling sick adults helps limit the spread of disease. For the often small flocks of rural Nigerians, not slaughtering young animals also makes good sense, if the flock is to reproduce itself.

Housing, watering and feeding
Although guineafowl are sometimes allowed to roost outside in trees or on huts, poultry usually are housed in well-ventilated wicker coops (*akurki*) ideally made

from young, split stems of *geza* (*Combretum micranthum*). The coops are placed under shade trees or grain bins (*rahoniya, rumbu*), with the bottom 5cm or so firmly buried in the earth to withstand buffeting by small ruminants (Plate 1). Chickens are never cooped with ducks, because ducks often attack and kill chicks. In contrast, guineafowl keets are often placed with foster hens (see below).

Water is provided *ad libitum* in large earthenware basins (*kwatarniya*) specially crafted or purchased for this purpose. For chicks and keets, a much smaller bowl-shaped pottery vessel (*kasko*) is used. There is very little spillage or faecal contamination. In the case of pigeons, sugar is added to the drinking-water to encourage them to stay close to the house. And for all poultry species, prophylactic botanicals are regularly administered in the drinking-water (see Prevention and Control of Mortality, below).

As a feed supplement for guineafowl, occasionally poultry owners excavate a termite-hill (*suri*), bring it home and crush it for the birds to pick through. By and large, however, Nigerian farmers do not collect and feed insects to their poultry; it is more practical to let the birds forage for themselves.[10] For chickens, the main feed supplements are kitchen scraps and the coarse part of floured grains that remains after sieving (*tsaki*). Ducks receive a paste or slurry of water and bran (*tsaki* or *dussa*). Turkeys are fed onion leaves and a mineral-rich aquatic

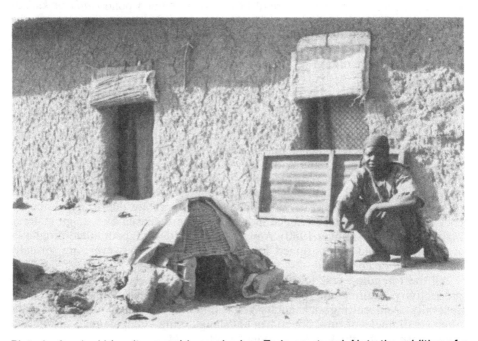

Plate 1. *An akurki (poultry coop) in a suburban Zaria courtyard. Note the addition of a polythene covering. Normally this would not be necessary if the coop were properly located in the shade and if the wicker were plastered with cowdung and mud. Although the coop is firmly planted in the ground, the stone wedges provide extra protection against dislodgement.*

lettuce (*Pistia stratiotes*, Hausa *kainuwa*) that grows wild in ponds; Hausa reportedly also feed this lettuce to ostriches (Dalziel 1937).

Whole grains such as guineacorn (sorghum) and millet are usually given only to hens and newly hatched chicks. According to rural Hausa and Fulani, the choice of whole-grain supplements determines the sexual differentiation of chicks, which they believe begins only after hatching. People say that if a hen and her chicks are fed guineacorn, most of the chicks will become females; if fed only millet, males. Since a flock needs both sexes, people usually give hens both grains during the first few weeks of brooding. This emic rationale for feeding mixed grains serves a useful etic purpose. A diet of only guinea-corn would prejudice young chicks' growth and development because the relatively large grains are difficult for chicks to pick up and swallow. Conversely, while an all-millet diet would ensure good chick nutrition, millet grains are too small for the mother hen, and she would thus tend to lead the chicks off to forage elsewhere. But the mixed diet allows both chicks and hens to benefit from supplemental feeding, while also enjoying a more balanced diet. Moreover, the combination may be beneficial in that it reduces the total consumption of guineacorn, which some studies have found to be toxic in chickens (McClymont and Duncan 1952).

Egg and chick production
Rural Nigerian poultry raisers know that a young hen is approaching maturity when she begins calling a mate (*kyarkyara*); likewise for the cock when he begins to crow (*cara*). They also believe that the male selects the location where the hen will nest—an observation confirmed by the authors in many instances. Hausa and Fulani say that frequent *kyarkyara* calls and an enlarged crop (*bali koto*) are sure signs that the hen will lay within a few days. Perhaps not unreasonably, people believe the crop is the site of initial egg formation because they observe that the crop distends just a few days before laying. (In fact, distension results from increased food intake, a dietary change, or both). In any case, an enlarged crop tells the poultry owner that it is time to make or purchase a new coop.

Women are generally familiar with each of their birds' egg-laying patterns, especially if a hen commonly skips a day or so between clutches (*fashi*). They also know that most hens will lay an extra egg a day or two after brooding commences—an observation that the authors have confirmed. While guineafowl are recognized as superior layers vis-à-vis chickens, they are considered poor mothers (Ayeni and Ayanda 1982, Ayorinde *et al.* 1988). Typically, five or so guineafowl lay their eggs together in a single, secluded nest outside the home. Called *gamaiya*, this communal behaviour is good from the point of view of gathering up the eggs for sale or consumption. But it is bad in terms of natural incubation, in that one bird cannot cover all the eggs in the communal nest. This presents a technical problem. How to produce an adequate supply of future guinea-fowl layers in the absence of artificial incubators?

Hausa confront this problem in a rather ingenious way. They know that the incubation periods for chickens, guineafowl and ducks are 21, 28 and 31 days, respectively. Producers therefore allow a chicken to finish laying her clutch of, say, 10 eggs. On the day she begins to brood (*kwanci*), all her eggs are removed. Some may be sold or consumed; others may be temporarily placed with a hen in-lay or on the point of brooding; or they may be stored in a cool, dark place until they can be returned to the original hen or given to another. Meanwhile, the hen's clutch is replaced with five guineafowl eggs. At the end of seven days, five of her own eggs are returned, making a total of 10. Rural producers feel that more than 10 eggs would over-tax the hen (see below). The five chicks and five keets hatch 21 days later, and the hen mothers both satisfactorily. In fact, using chickens as foster mothers for keets appears to improve keet survival (Ayeni and Ayanda 1982).[11]

A similar method is used for hatching ducks, which are also considered poor mothers. In this instance, the chicken sits on the duck eggs for 10 days before her own eggs are reintroduced. Farmers do not use chickens as foster mothers for ducklings, though. Poultry raisers correctly note that the foster hen will reject or wean ducklings prematurely because they grow much faster than chicks or keets. Ducklings' non-chick-like behaviour (swimming and sieving the mud for worms instead of pecking) may also be a factor here.

Unlike poultry scientists, rural Hausa believe that the hen is entirely responsible for the process of hatching. People think the brooding hen gradually abrades the shells of the eggs on which she sits. This belief in turn provides the emic explanation for the varying incubation periods of poultry species: the thicker and tougher the shell, the longer the hen must brood. In evidence of this explanation, people also point out that a hen that has just finished brooding feels lighter and looks fatigued. Although farmers know that a hen eats much less when brooding, they feel this does not adequately account for all the weight loss.

Because of such beliefs, it is considered cruel to add to the hen's work by replacing all her eggs with those of guineafowl. Moreover, women try to ease the hen's work of hatching the guineafowl eggs by carefully but thoroughly rubbing the eggs with ash (*toka*) or dried bran before introducing them into the nest. This practice in fact serves a useful purpose, albeit not the one that people think. During the rainy season, guineafowl usually lay their eggs outside; rubbing the damp eggs dry with absorbents may help reduce embryo and even hen mortality. Moisture encourages the multiplication of micro-organisms on the shell, thereby increasing the chances of their gaining entry into the egg, where they would kill the embryo. Drying off damp eggs may also decrease heat loss during the incubation process and prevent illness among brooders.

Sometimes hens abandon their nests before all the eggs have hatched. This results in a high proportion of *dakwaye* 'dead-in-shell'. To encourage hens to continue brooding, towards the end of the incubation period a few seeds of *geza* are placed on the eggs. The seeds seem to serve as a simple lure. Research has suggested that this practice may somehow also enhance communication between the hen and the unhatched chicks or among the embryos, thus synchronizing the hatching of eggs laid at slightly different times (Nesheim *et al.* 1979).

Rural Hausa believe local hens have invisible mammary glands that emerge only when chicks suckle their also-invisible milk. (This explains why the glands cannot be detected on slaughtered hens.) Certain behaviours are cited supporting this belief. First, flock owners observe that chicks do not seem to eat during the first few days after hatching. Instead, they stay in the nest with the hen. In fact, a chick retains enough yolk to nourish it for several days after hatching, so it does not need to forage for food (ibid). Second, people point out that chicks often huddle under a hen's breast, with their heads raised and their beaks open as if they were nursing. But in fact, chicks assume this posture in order to dissipate excess heat and possibly in order to peck at parasites on the underside of the hen's wings and body.[12] Ectoparasitism is the most prevalent health problem among chickens in Hausaland (Abdu *et al.* 1985b). Hens that have just finished brooding can be expected to be more heavily infested than others, since incubation requires them to remain in the nest during most of the 21-day period. Chicks are known to recognize and peck at small ectoparasites and insects such as ticks and termites. Thus, the 'suckling posture' may be linked to two useful functions: decreasing hens' parasite loads and increasing chicks' protein intake.[13]

Traditional Hausa and Fulani husbandry takes advantage of any such potential benefits, plus many others, in that it makes taboo the taking of young chicks away from their mother. Separating them is seen as the height of cruelty since, according to farmers, it would deprive the chicks of life-giving milk and maternal care. Such an act carries the supernatural threat of insanity or death. Only a person who possesses magical powers and follows a careful supernatural protocol to ward against these dangers can safely separate young chicks from their mother. The strength of these beliefs is illustrated in a Zaria poultry scientist's year-long but fruitless efforts to purchase day-old chicks from villagers for his experiments. People could not fathom how he could make such a heartless and risky request—although they were quite willing to give him adult birds free.

Under indigenous 'free-range' poultry production, such beliefs have real husbandry value, however. Chicks weaned prematurely hardly ever survive. It is exceedingly rare to see orphan chicks, unless by chance or design they have been adopted by another hen. Orphaned chicks are denied the many vital survival services that only a mother hen can provide. These include: protection from predators; provision of night-time warmth during the cold dry season; guidance to safe shelter and appropriate food; and via exposure to low levels of pathogens that the hen has experienced, resistance to certain ills. As a local saying notes, out of compassion 'God never takes the life of a mother hen without first taking those of her chicks'.

Taboos and beliefs such as those described above have direct implications for poultry development and extension efforts. For example, even at the peak of Nigeria's Operation Coq campaign to replace local stock with exotic chickens, very few Hausa or Fulani dared to buy day-old-chicks from the hatcheries (Waters-Bayer 1988). Even the most vigorous encouragement from extension workers could not overcome farmers' fears of supernatural reprisals for being party to separating young chicks from their mothers. Equally if not more important were producers' essentially accurate assessment that such orphan chicks would not long survive the rigours of indigenous husbandry without the care of a mother hen. Realistically, in most of rural Nigeria, there are few or no alternatives to the hen's life-giving warmth, protection against predation and disease, and provision of nutritious foodstuffs. Veterinary services and commercial feeds, for example, are either unavailable or far too costly for the average poultry raiser. The campaign might have met with better success if the time and trouble had first been taken to understand and respect rural people's poultry-raising beliefs and practices. For example, if fertilized eggs or weanlings had been offered instead of 'motherless chicks', producers might have been more responsive.[14]

Prevention and control of mortality
Flock mortalities can result from accident, predation or disease. Drowning and trampling of chicks are common accidents, especially wherever sheep are also

raised. The most common predators are dogs, cats, snakes, and other birds, mainly hawks (*shaho*). Hausa rarely keep dogs, and any stray is usually killed on sight. While cats are well-liked, any cat implicated in killing a fowl is immediately destroyed.

To ward off snakes, poultry owners grow certain repellent plants or place sliced garlic (*Allium sativum*, Hausa *tafarnuwa*) around hen houses (Ibrahim, this volume). On occasion, they may employ a snake charmer to locate and remove especially destructive reptiles. Cobras and night adders, for example, can decimate a flock in a single night.

To 'immunize' chicks and keets against hawk attacks, the spiny fruits of *tsuwawun zaki* (*Cucumis pustulatus*) are placed in their drinking-water. More important, however, is the growth pattern of local chickens and guinea-fowl. In comparison to exotic poultry, they develop much faster initially, with growth slowing later on (Ayorinde *et al.* 1986, Nwosu 1987). Thus they more rapidly reach a size that may deter hawks. Growth then slows before it can produce serious nutritional deficiencies. As noted earlier, there is both deliberate and natural selection for aggressiveness in local poultry and this, too, may help reduce losses to hawks and other predators. However, Hausa recognize the limitations of this trait in young birds, as evidenced in the proverb 'Whatever a chick can know, a hawk has long known'.

Local chickens suffer from diseases such as Gumboro and Newcastle disease, salmonellosis, coccidiosis and helminthosis (Abdu *et al.* 1985b, Aire and Ojo 1974, Umoh *et al.* 1982). Studies of unvaccinated but apparently healthy chickens in rural Fulani flocks showed that 69 per cent were seropositive for Gumboro (Abdu *et al.* 1985a), 99 per cent for *Mycoplasma gallisepticum*, 99 per cent for *M. synoviae*, 52 per cent for *Salmonella pullorum*, 47 per cent for *Coxiella burnetti* and 5 per cent for *Brucella abortus* (Abdu *et al.* 1984). Similarly, high antibody titers to *M. gallisepticum* have been demonstrated in apparently healthy local guineafowl, ducks, pigeons and turkeys (Adesiyun and Abdu 1985). But local stock succumb to these clinical diseases much less often than exotic breeds. Since 1981, only one case of coccidiosis and two cases of helminthosis have been diagnosed in local chickens at the Ahmadu Bello University Veterinary Teaching Hospital. This contrasts with 48 and 16 outbreaks of these diseases, respectively, recorded among exotic breeds at the same clinic between 1981 and 1984 (Abdu *et al.* 1985b).

It is difficult to interpret the significance of such contrasts because of confounding variables and practical research difficulties. For example, local birds raised in towns are likely to be exposed to vaccine virus, thus complicating the results of serological surveys for Gumboro disease (Abdu *et al.* 1985a). Further confounding comparisons between local and exotic stock is the fact that rural people have little access to veterinary clinics; and the few ambulatory services treat only cattle and small ruminants. Moreover, definitive diagnostic data on diseases among local poultry are difficult to obtain due to the practice of promptly selling or consuming adult birds that fall sick. Comprehensive simulation studies of local poultry management would be necessary to ascertain the true prevalence of disease among flocks in rural Nigeria.

Pending such research, however, the usual explanation scientists give for the lower incidence of clinical disease in local birds is genetic resistance acquired through natural selection. Given producers' practice of promptly culling sick adult birds, this explanation makes sense. In essence, this practice makes for generalized selection for disease resistance. Farmer opinion and belief reinforce this assessment, and even suggest some specific links between local poultry varieties and resistance to certain diseases. An example is some Hausa's claim that *burtsa* chickens survive Newcastle disease better than other local varieties— although the affected animals reportedly show neurological signs resembling spirit possession for a long time thereafter. Such signs are part of what cause people to associate certain varieties with the spirit world (see above) and to employ the birds in magico-religious contexts. Again, such empirical observations offer tantalizing clues for geneticists and breeders. It may be worthwhile to evaluate all chicken varieties used in *bori* rituals for genetic resistance to Newcastle disease.

Other reasons for the lower incidence of clinical diseases in local breeds may include the beneficial culling, feeding and watering strategies described earlier. In fact, like poultry raisers elsewhere in the world (Vondal, this volume), rural Nigerians generally take a prophylactic rather than therapeutic approach to poultry disease, and their measures are aimed at the whole flock rather than individual birds. As noted earlier, both Hausa and Fulani continuously administer prophylactic botanicals in birds' drinking-water. Some of the plants used to control poultry diseases in Nigeria have been reported in Nwude and Ibrahim (1980). Although the therapeutic efficacy of most such botanicals has not yet been determined, information about their pharmacological properties is often available. To take just one example, farmers use the fruits of *Solanum incanum* (a bitter variety of garden egg) to control bacterial infections and gastrointestinal disorders in Nigerian poultry. This vegetable is known to contain solanine (ibid., Dalziel 1937), an alkaloid that inhibits a variety of micro-organisms, including *Staphylococcus aureus, Candida albicans*, and *Trichophyton mentagrophytes* (Etkin and Ross 1982; also see Roepke, this volume).

Conclusions

Hausa and Fulani beliefs about poultry biology are not always scientifically correct. But as McCorkle (1989) emphasizes, the issue is not how closely folk knowledge and practice parallel Western veterinary medicine or whether indigenous beliefs and practices are 'right' or 'wrong'. Rather, what is important is '. . . the extent to which they promote productive animal management given the resources actually or potentially and realistically available to stockowners' (McCorkle 1989:160; also see Schillhorn van Veen, this volume). Indeed, many Hausa and Fulani management practices *are* of scientifically demonstrable benefit in promoting poultry health and productivity. Were they not, how could rural Nigerians maintain approximately two poultry units for each of the country's 100 million people—and do so at no cost to the nation in terms of expensive imported birds, equipment, feeds or drugs?

In the indigenous husbandry system, valuable techniques include active selection for productive and pro-survival traits, good housing and watering habits, strategic culling, well-formulated supplemental feeding for hens and newly hatched chicks, the astute manipulation of natural incubation and mothering processes, and the regular administration of natural drugs to prevent disease. While the efficacy and significance of other practices or beliefs may be less clear, they should nevertheless be explored for any possible benefits they may provide within the local poultry-raising system. A case in point is the practical value, under free-range conditions, of the taboo on separating young chicks from their mothers. Thorough investigation of all aspects of indigenous agroveterinary knowledge and praxis might suggest some realistic, new directions for improving poultry production in Nigeria and other countries in the tropics.

Unfortunately, current, Western-derived criteria and research goals for genetically improving local poultry do not fit Nigerian needs, nor those of other developing nations. Indeed, sometimes it almost seems as though scientists' goal is to breed out all the characteristics that make for a desirable animal from the point of view of rural producers. Research by national agricultural institutions that ignores farmers' own production objectives and criteria, their indigenous genetic resources, and their local management savvy can yield only breeds and husbandry recommendations that are just as alien and unworkable as those elaborated abroad. Unless all the components in local production systems are understood and incorporated into experimentation and extension, farmers are not likely to adopt new breeds and techniques.

The potentials of ethnoveterinary R&D for agricultural development have been reviewed by McCorkle (1986), who also hints at useful interactions with other fields of human endeavour. The present authors would like to add their observation that there are many potential advantages to combining such investigations with educational curricula. Across more than a decade of research, it has become clear to us that Nigeria's agro-educational system has no roots in the nation's own cultures. Hence the educational system has made little headway in dispelling unfounded beliefs, validating useful ones, or extending new information about agricultural production processes among rural people.

But attempting to change local poultry management or any other agricultural practices without first understanding their place and meaning in farmers' current production system, economy, society and culture is foolish. Accordingly, we urge the systematic study of indigenous knowledge not only for guiding agro-veterinary research, development, extension and policymaking, but also for grounding educational curricula in more relevant and realistic contexts. The result will be more appropriate agrilcultural development schemes that rural people can put to active use.

Notes

1. Both because they are the flock managers and because of Islamic religious and cultural mores, women in Hausaland are in a better position than men to observe the flock in and around the house. They are therefore a richer source of information on poultry matters than men.
2. However, the production potential of local birds may be much higher; see, e.g., Wilson (1986).
3. Although guineafowl eggs cost 0.67 naira each compared to 0.80 for local chicken eggs (1992 prices), they are in reality more expensive than chicken eggs because of their smaller size.
4. Because of this characteristic, boiled guineafowl eggs are preferred for the Hausa gambling game called *fashe* 'to break', wherein the owner of the strongest boiled egg wins the other players' eggs.
5. All non-English terms glossed in this chapter are from the Hausa.
6. Needless to say, this makes it virtually impossible to obtain and analyse comparative scientific data on indigenous varieties of chickens. However, significant differences in mortality and in feed intake and conversion that can be attributed to genotype have been reported for four varieties of helmeted guineafowl in Nigera (Ayorinde *et al.* 1988).
7. For more such aphorisms concerning the behaviour of local chickens, consult Abraham (1958).

8. Due to their loud, cackling call, however, guineafowl are increasingly being kept in towns for use as burglar alarms!

9. The notion that cocks lay eggs may be fairly widespread in West Africa. Zeitlyn (1991) has also documented it for the Mambila of the Cameroons.

10. Interestingly, though, during the 1988 grasshopper plague, in parts of Hausaland insects were collected and marketed as a dietary supplement for local chickens and ducks. In a personal communication, McCorkle notes that farmers in other parts of Africa 'farm' termites for poultry feeds.

11. Such findings have led some experts to recommend that *all* chicken eggs be routinely replaced with those of guineafowl. Yet if this recommendation were taken, there soon would be no chickens left to act as incubators in rural areas!

12. This posture can also signal gapeworm infection (syngamiasis). However, this disease can be ruled out here for several reasons. First, its prepatency is about three weeks; yet even younger chicks display this behaviour. Second, animals with gapeworms would assume this posture under any variety of circumstances; but chicks typically do so only when they are underneath a hen. Finally, this disease is most common during the dry season when birds concentrate around the few moist areas to compete for earthworms; but chicks manifest this behaviour year round.

13. On the other hand, this behaviour might also facilitate the transmission of parasites from hens to chicks. This hypothesis cannot be tested in Hausa villages, however, because in order to obtain parasite counts, chicks and hens would have to be separated. But such separation is strongly tabooed (see text).

14. In the Operation Coq, however, this is not certain because local people astutely associate high mortality rates (*wabi*) in chicks with exotic breeds. Thus they see purchase of such breeds as a waste of money.

10. *Madosha*:
traditional castration of bulls in Ethiopia[1]

MAURO GHIROTTI AND MULATU WOUDYALEW

CASTRATION IS ONE of the most ancient techniques for improving livestock performance. It is documented in the Bible (Leviticus 22:24–5) about 1250 BC, but it was certainly well known before then. It was performed by the ancient civilizations of the Fertile Crescent, the cradle of livestock domestication, where cattle played fundamental socio-cultural and productive roles. Cattle were probably first domesticated for religious purposes, and only secondarily for agricultural use (Mason 1976). The oldest remains of domesticated cattle date back to 7000 BC, while evidence for the use of oxen as draught animals dates from about 3200 BC.

For ancient pastoral societies, cows were symbols of abundance and fertility, and bulls of virility and strength. The male's power and aggressiveness were believed to lie in the testicles (see also Schwabe, this volume). Removing an animal's testicles meant eliminating these characterisitics. Castrated animals were indeed found to grow more docile and fatter than bulls.

In Africa, different traditional methods of castration are currently used. Most involve surgery with a knife or spear, as among the Fulani of Mali, the Somali, various Nilotic or Nilo-Hamitic peoples of East Africa and the Tonga of central and southern Zambia (for example, Elmi 1984, Evans-Pritchard 1940, Ligers 1958, Schwabe and Kuojok 1981). Today, many of these methods are slowly being replaced by the use of Burdizzo pincers, which crush the spermatic cord without cutting the scrotum. This stops the flow of blood to the testicles, which then atrophy. A bloodless and relatively simple operation, this method is safer than open surgery because it minimizes the risk of infection.

This chapter reports on another bloodless castration method long used and still widely popular in highland Ethiopia. As part of a study on livestock grazing and the role of the male in herd fertility (Ghirotti and Woudyalew 1990), an appraisal of animal health, husbandry, and production was conducted in the Ghibe valley of highland Ethiopia in September 1985. Most cattle in this area are small East African Zebu. The study included an investigation of traditional castration methods among the main ethnic groups in the region: the mostly Christian Oromo and the mainly Muslim Amhara. Information on castration practices and related beliefs was obtained from key informants through semi-structured interviews, and from four clusters of 33 farmers through questionnaires. In addition, castration ceremonies were photographed.

The *madosha* castration technique

In Ethiopia, male animals have traditionally been used for draught (ILCA 1981). Without oxen, many farm families would be hard-pressed to do their cropping.[2] The more land a family cultivates, the more oxen it owns. Up to four hectares of land can be cultivated for each pair of oxen (Brumby and Scholtens 1986). As a result, one-third of a typical highland family herd are oxen. The great importance of oxen is further suggested by the *thmad*, the traditional unit of land measurement in the highlands. One *thmad* equals the amount of land that a pair of oxen can plough in one day. This amounts to about 0.20ha in hilly regions or 0.25ha in flat areas (Ghirotti 1988).

Given the tremendous importance of oxen, it is no surprise that Abyssinian farmers have developed methods of bull castration that are both effective and safe. The farmers interviewed said they castrate bulls to make them stronger and more tractable for ploughing, to forestall fights among males, and to obtain a better fat cover. All male cattle are castrated when they are four to six years old, regardless of their conformation or performance. The *madosha* (Amharic 'hammer') is the tool used. The operation, which is bloodless, involves crushing the spermatic cord.

The castration ceremony takes place on *Maskal* day, on 27 September each year. Castrating bulls at *Maskal* is part of a long-standing highland tradition (next section). Animals are free from work at this time, and their recovery is less problematic because there is plenty of good pasturage and because, as farmers put it, 'the river waters are clear'. Moreover, flies—which can infect the cuts made in the scrotum—are fewer during this season. Finally, since *Maskal* falls during the dry season, the risk of infection is less (see also Evans-Pritchard 1940).

A community elder experienced in animal husbandry performs the castration procedure at dawn. The bulls are first gathered in the *kraal* of one of the village headmen who is responsible for the operation that year. After a bull has been tied and cast, its testicles are pulled backwards from the perineum and a pole is driven into the ground behind the scrotum. Two sticks are then fixed just above the testicles. The front stick stretches the spermatic cord, while the other prevents the testicles from being accidentally hit during the operation (Plate 1). The

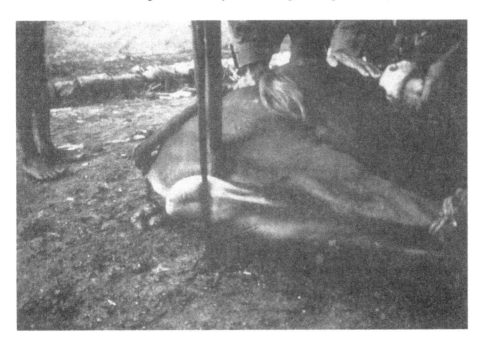

Plate 1. *After the bull has been tied and cast, a pole is driven in the ground between the scrotum and the perineum, and two sticks are placed just above the testicles.*

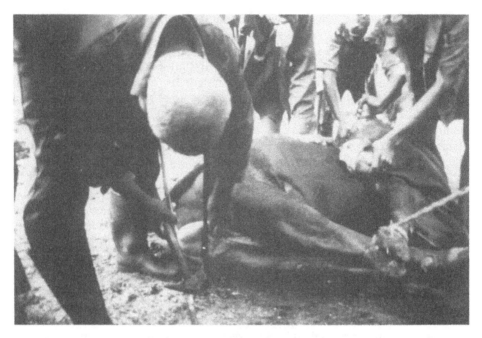

Plate 2. *The spermatic cords are struck with the* madosha, *thereby crushing them in a bloodless operation.*

cords are crushed by striking the front stick with a hammer (Plate 2). In this way, the effect of the trauma is distributed.

If the animal is well restrained, the operation lasts only three to five minutes, during which time the elder palpates the cord to evaluate progress. Finally, he makes a few cuts on the scrotum with a razor or other blade and applies *fetho*, a traditional medicament made of ground seeds (possibly *Linum* spp.) that have been soaked in water. According to experienced informants, the incisions 'release the bad blood that eventually forms under the sac'. The medicament, which is also used in human ethnomedicine, is said to reduce inflammation and local congestion.

Immediately after the operation, the bullock is freed and made to run. Its quick return to activity signals that it will soon recover. If all seems to be in order, the animal is sent to graze with the rest of the herd while the farmers castrate another bull or turn to the rest of the *Maskal* celebrations. Farmers check that the castration was successful by watching for the testicles to atrophy some two months later. If this has not occurred, the procedure is repeated during Ethiopian Christmas, at the beginning of January.

The cultural context of bull castration

Highlanders of Ghibe prefer their traditional castration method to Western alternatives for a variety of reasons. First, as noted above, it is quite safe. Second, they have great confidence in it. Third, however, the operation forms an integral part of community ceremonies on *Maskal* day, which is one of the most important religious and political festivities in the central highlands of Ethiopia. *Maskal* is not only an occasion to have a good time; it is also an age-old Ethiopian religious and historical tradition (Sottochiesa 1936). It dates back to AD 1400 when King David IV of Ethiopia was battling the forces of Islam that sought to conquer the Abyssinian Highlands (Pollera 1926). *Maskal* commemorates the arrival of St Michael in Ethiopia, bearing the Holy Cross from Jerusalem after a dangerous and eventful journey. The cross ended a long period of starvation, drought and disease; many miracles occurred; and a time of faith and plenty began (Sottochiesa 1936). *Maskal* falls at the end of the rainy season, which signals a propitious period of change. The crops are nearly ripe, and there is great rejoicing in every village (Pollera 1926, Walker 1933). Also, *Maskal* day constitutes one of the rare occasions during the year when both farmers and their animals have a break from work and when livestock are slaughtered for feasts.

Conclusions

Interviews with farmers in other parts of Ethiopia (specifically, the areas around Debre Brahan and Debre Zeit) indicate that bloodless castration methods are widely used throughout the central highlands. For many reasons, stockowners prefer such methods despite livestock agents' efforts to promote the use of Burdizzo pincers. Even though these instruments are now available at every veterinary field station, in the countryside the pincers are employed in only about 2 to 3 per cent of all castrations (Ghirotti and Woudyalew 1990). Significantly, most Burdizzo castrations are also done on *Maskal* day.

Other bloodless methods of castration have been described among African pastoralists. To the Western eye, they might seem crueler than open surgical techniques (Mathias-Mundy and McCorkle 1989). However, bloodless methods greatly reduce the risk of tetanus (notably in horses), screw-worm infestation, fly-borne infection, and the post-operative diseases that are so frequent in hot environments. Traditional African techniques of bloodless castration are based on the same principles as the Burdizzo. Further, they are more familiar and acceptable to many peoples. And in many traditional societies, castration is not merely an operation; it is also a social and cultural event.

Still, relatively little is known of the benefits and efficacy of traditional methods. The reputedly positive effect of *madosha* castration on carcass composition is doubtful, since the operation has little effect on fat deposition in zebu cattle (McFarlane 1966). And where cattle breeding is uncontrolled (as in the Ethiopian highlands), incompletely castrated oxen may still compete in mating, thus reducing herd fertility. They may also fight with younger uncastrated males. Yet Ethiopian stockowners consider behaviour modification and reduced fertility in castrated bulls very important. In order to record and compare changes in behaviour, hormone levels and degree of testicular atrophy in bulls castrated traditionally versus with the Burdizzo, the authors began a study in Ghibe. Unfortunately, due to civil unrest in Ethiopia and other problems, it was not possible to complete the study.

Nevertheless, we strongly recommend conducting comparative investigations of traditional and modern veterinary methods, under varying husbandry conditions and with stockowners participating as co-researchers, as a way to improve rural people's farming, and the stockraising upon which it so often depends. In the case of *madosha*, for example, comparative research could point the way to increasing the reliability and safety of this traditional technique. Investigation of the plants used locally to treat castration wounds and other problems is another promising area of research. Moreover, developers and livestock agents should consider extending basic veterinary assistance (for example, vaccination against clostridial diseases, treatment of complicated traumas) at strategic times of the year when castrations or other husbandry operations are typically performed. Rather than struggling to introduce exotic and often expensive new techniques, equipment, and time-tables, it makes far more sense to build upon useful local equivalents that are already widely accepted and culturally valued.

Notes

1. The authors are indebted to the many farmers who shared their knowledge with us. Special thanks are due to Ato's Bekele M., Markos K., Abafagi A., and W.ro Ghifty A. for their wonderful co-operation. Likewise for the field staff of the Veterinary Services of the Ethiopian Government and the Trypanotolerance Network of the International Livestock Centre for Africa (ILCA). Field research was conducted under the auspices of ILCA. Dr R. B. Griffiths provided helpful editorial comments on this chapter, and Ms S. Z. Babsa typed earlier drafts.
2. If a farmer does not have enough male cattle, however, he may yoke together an ox and a horse to pull the plough, as is also commonly done in Gojam Province.

11. Aspects of animal healthcare among Samburu pastoralists

CLAIRE HEFFERNAN, ELLEN HEFFERNAN AND CHIP STEM

BASED ON FIELD research in 1987 and 1988, this chapter reviews concepts of livestock disease and healing among Samburu pastoralists of northern Kenya.[1] This effort explored four major topics: traditional and current management practices and productivity problems (see also Heffernan 1987, 1990); pastoralists' views on the etiology, symptomology, prevalence, zoonotic properties, and economic importance of different livestock diseases; herders' recourse to traditional versus modern treatments for their major livestock healthcare problems; and Samburu knowledge of and access to commercial pharmaceuticals and formal-sector veterinary services. Attention was also given to herd size and composition, the socio-economic characteristics of Samburu healthcare practitioners, and both past and present veterinary interventions in the region.

After summarizing the research findings, the chapter offers suggestions for improving government delivery of veterinary services in the context of Samburu's changing social, cultural, and economic realities. The larger aim here is—by defining ethnoetiologies, therapies, attitudes, and roles and responsibilities concerning livestock disease among one pastoral people—to contribute to the growing literature on culturally appropriate and cost-effective veterinary interventions for pastoralists and other stockraisers in the developing world.

Study site, methods and subjects

The study site
The Samburu are a Nilo-Hamitic pastoral people who speak a Maa-related language. In 1984, they numbered 99 200 (Ominde 1988). They inhabit Samburu District, an area of 20 808 km^2 in north-central Kenya (Ojang and Ogendo 1973). With less than 500 mm of rain annually, most of the district is semi-arid scrubland that is suitable only for livestock production (Fumagalli 1977). Cattle are everywhere the mainstay of the Samburu economy, although smallstock and camels play a greater role in livestock production in the lowlands (Lamprey and Yussef 1981). The research reported here was conducted principally among Samburu of the Leroghi Plateau, where rainfall is slightly higher than the average for the district as a whole and where pastoralists are increasingly adopting small-scale agriculture.

Samburu society is organized in a segmentary descent system, with males divided into age sets: the *morani* or warriors, junior elders, and firestick elders (Spencer 1965). Although the latter two groups are generally the 'owners' of animals, the extended family is the labour unit responsible for livestock management. In the rainy season, when good pasture and water are abundant, herds are grazed around the *manyatta*, a semi-permanent settlement. During the dry season, the family cattle are moved to temporary camps in higher parts of the district where pasture and water are still available. Small stock and several cows in milk are left behind at the *manyatta*, to provide food for family members remaining there. These animals are tended by younger boys and girls while *morani* take primary responsibility for dry-season herding.

Methods and subjects

Qualitative data were gathered on the topics outlined above, using an open-ended but structured questionnaire developed during field consultations with anthropologists and economists. This instrument was administered verbally in Samburu and KiSwahili, with a Samburu interpreter translating from the former to the latter when necessary. The objective of the questionnaire was not to gather statistical data regarding livestock and veterinary care. Rather, interviews focused on herders' perceptions of animal diseases—how to identify, treat or prevent them—along with other parameters of livestock healthcare and husbandry. Questionnaire data were supplemented with a literature review. Additional information regarding cultural and socio-economic processes was gathered through participant observation in the daily life of the Samburu. Daily interaction with pastoralists also permitted visual confirmation of questionnaire responses.

Herders were usually interviewed while they were with their herds. During the interview, notes were made as to the specific number and condition of the animals. This strategy allowed researchers to ask detailed questions about the illnesses or demeanours of specific animals and to observe healthcare techniques directly. All interviewees were eager to discuss their animals' ills, the possible causes, and the treatments they employed. People were less inclined to discuss the size and composition of their herds; this is tantamount to Westerners' revealing their salaries and personal net worth. Nevertheless, interviewees answered all of the questions in at least some form; and many volunteered considerable additional information, well beyond the confines of the questionnaire.

Each respondent was identified as to sex, age, clan affiliation and other social indicators. The majority of interviewees were junior elders. Few *morani* were available for interviewing because many had left the pastoral lifestyle for urban areas. Whenever the researcher learned of other individuals with particular livestock management or healthcare powers, follow-up interviews were sought with that individual as well, or with clan members of similar repute. Ultimately, the study sample (29 males, five females) ranged all the way from tribal elders to young boys and girls responsible for herding small stock. Women interviewees provided informative perspectives on their traditional and present-day roles in animal healthcare, while the youngsters furnished a tangible view of herding techniques and of family and clan approaches to educating future herders. This sample allowed researchers to assess animal healthcare knowledge and practice across genders, ages and generations in terms of both past and changing social, cultural and economic norms among Samburu.

Samburu animal healthcare

Social roles and responsibilities

Veterinary care among Samburu is largely the job of men in the junior-elder and firestick-elder age sets. However, *morani* may assist with treatments and deal with minor ills that arise during dry season herding. In difficult clinical cases, collective consultations, diagnoses, and treatment decisions are often conducted among all the male members of the *manyatta*.

For certain types of animal health problems or for ailments that do not to respond to conventional therapies, extra-familial elders with specialized knowledge or powers may be called upon. Interviewees explain that these men's expert knowledge is passed down through generations from father to eldest son. They also note that different clans have special skills in treating certain illnesses. For example, the Lmasula Clan is reputed to be particularly good at curing eye ailments. Other clans are noted for totemic relationships or supernatural powers that aid in finding lost animals or inducing a cow to accept its calf (Fumagalli 1977). In addition to the foregoing specialists, Samburu recognize some individuals as having a particular knack or affinity for animal healthcare that is not ancestrally derived (Heffernan 1987).

While men typically deal with diagnosis and choice of treatment, women have traditionally played an integral role in healthcare, too—albeit one largely ignored in the literature to date (Beaman 1983, Sollod *et al.* 1984, Stem, this volume). Interviewees indicate that because women do the milking, women are frequently the first to notice behavioural changes or other early signs of disease in cows. Respondents further note that women prepare and often collect the various herbs and plants used in traditional treatments. However, women generally do not administer medicines or other treatments, except when male members of the *manyatta* are unavailable or when ills are minor ones. For example, women may treat calves with mange with a wash of rock-salt from the riverbank or an unguent of motor oil.

Ethno-etiology and diagnosis
Samburu livestock are subject to a number of debilitating diseases—principally East Coast fever (ECF), trypanosomosis, anthrax, rinderpest, contagious bovine pleuro-pneumonia (CBPP) and foot-and-mouth disease (FMD). As in ethnoveterinary systems worldwide (McCorkle 1986), Samburu name and classify many livestock diseases according to their most prominent clinical signs. For example, herders call Nairobi sheep disease *nadomanyita* 'red intestines' because of the bloody diarrhoea that is its principal clinical sign. The etiological agent is a tick-borne bunya virus, which can cause fatal gastroenteric haemorrhage.[2]

Relying upon far more subtle clinical signs, however, Samburu can often accurately diagnose diseases with very similar symptoms. For example, ECF and trypanosomosis are often difficult to distinguish between clinically. Even modern veterinary science cannot confirm a presumptive diagnosis without a blood test. But Samburu note that in ECF, lymphadenopathy (swelling of the lymph glands) begins with the parotid lymph node and spreads caudally, whereas trypanosomosis is usually characterized by generalized lymphadenopathy accompanied by localized swelling in the region of the fly bite. This same kind of attention to clinical detail is evidenced in the way Samburu classify diseases. For example, they distinguish between peracute and acute forms of anthrax (*mporoto* versus *lokushum* 'running blood'). Indeed, Samburu consider these to be two distinct diseases. Although interviewees do not identify either as contagious, they describe *lokushum* as zoonotic and note that it can be passed to humans through contact with the blood in an open cut on an infected animal.

Samburu may also use post-mortem lesions to characterize a disease. An example is rinderpest, a usually fatal gastro-enteric disease of cattle caused by a paramyxo virus and characterized by necrosis of the intestinal and upper respiratory tracts and an enlarged gallbladder. Significantly, the Samburu name for rinderpest is *lodua* 'gall bladder'. In fact, necropsies are performed on all dead animals and form part of the Samburu's regular diagnostic regime.

Recognizing that different diseases can share similar symptoms, Samburu sometimes use *both* clinical signs and post-mortem lesions to classify livestock disease and make a definitive diagnosis. For example, they distinguish explicitly the moist, foamy cough of CBPP (*ikipei*) from the dry, hacking cough (*lboliboli*) of other respiratory ailments. However, the Samburu name for CBPP translates as 'lung against the ribs'—a descriptive term based on post-mortem observation. In fact, in Western veterinary parlance, CBPP produces a severe, acute, fibrinous pneumonia with consolidation of the lung lobes; and upon post-mortem examination, the lungs are firm, enlarged, and often appear to adhere to the ribs.

Samburu also recognize the role of insects as disease vectors. Interviewees note that *ltikana* 'trypanosomosis' is transmitted by the tsetse fly. Herders indicate that they therefore avoid grazing animals in areas heavily infested with this pest. Samburu also practise controlled burning of range lands during years of high rainfall in order to destroy ticks and other carriers of disease. Burning promotes the growth of more nutritious grasses, too—a further factor in the maintenance of herd health.

When no other etiological information is available, Samburu may identify diseases according to their suspected place of origin. For example, ECF is called *lipis*—the Samburu rendering of Levi, the name of the European farmer whose cattle were the first in the district to contract ECF.

Unlike many other stockraising peoples discussed in this volume, Samburu generally do not view disease as a punishment for wrongdoing. Rather, they see both animal and human illness as linked to one's fate. While they do acknowledge that some animals are weaker and more prone to illness than others, they nevertheless believe that morbidity and mortality are determined from birth. Hence, they seldom separate sick animals from the rest of the herd.

ECF constitutes an exception to the foregoing ethnoetiological rule, however. This tick-borne protozoan (*Theileria parva*) disease is new to Samburu District. Herders recount that the first clinical cases of ECF appeared only in 1977. Pastoralists are therefore understandably unclear as to the etiology of this disease. It initially struck in the highlands, where higher rainfall makes for larger tick populations. However, some interviewees hypothesize that *Nkai* 'God' visited ECF upon the highlands in retribution for the elders' refusal to extend watering rights to lowland herders during the severe droughts of the 1970s. This was an unprecedented decision and one that is antithetical to Samburu ideals of co-operation and sharing. The elders' decision was primarily motivated by the droughts; however, the increasing scarcity of resources due to pastoralists' expulsion from their traditional grazing grounds by encroaching farmers was also a factor (Halderman 1985).

Ethnotherapies

Venipuncture is one of the most widely prescribed Samburu therapies. A rawhide tourniquet is used to occlude the jugular vein, which is then punctured with a small, sharp arrow. Performed primarily on cattle, venipuncture is usually done at the first sign of almost any illness. According to Samburu, most diseases affect the blood. Venipuncture is designed to reduce the amount of 'bad' blood in the animal's body and thus expedite recovery. Venipuncture is also performed on cows believed to be dangerously overweight and hence prone to abortion. Herders believe that too much fat increases the cow's body temperature to a point where the embryo cannot survive. Finally, venipuncture is also used for ceremonial purposes.

The blood collected through venipuncture is consumed as a dietary supplement mixed with milk. Blood drawn from sick animals is almost invariably consumed because Samburu recognize few livestock diseases as zoonotic. Aside from anthrax, herders identify only FMD (*lkulup*) as possibly zoonotic. They say that pregnant women who drink the milk or blood of an animal with FMD will abort. FMD is also one of the few diseases that Samburu correctly recognize as contagious and for which they quarantine affected animals. But because of FMD's low mortality rates, few herders consider it an economically important problem. In any case, interviewees know of no effective traditional therapy for FMD.

Another widespread traditional therapy is branding with a hot piece of metal. Always performed by elders, branding is prescribed for recalcitrant cases of any disease, and specifically for arthritis, swollen joints or down cows. It is especially popular for treating paralysis. In such cases, branding is done around the spine, which Samburu believe is the site of the problem. In all other cases, however, heat is applied only to tissue that is close to a bone because Samburu believe the skeleton is inert and plays no role in disease processes. Neighbouring Rendille pastoralists often place hot stones on the bellies of animals suspected to have worms (Spencer 1973). When queried about this difference in technique, Samburu say that applying heat so close to organs would likely cause internal ruptures and haemorrhaging.

Interviewees explain that branding draws illness away from the surrounding tissue and into the bone, thereby disseminating and 'diluting' the harmful effects of the ailment. Respondents add that there is a specific time-frame for therapeutic branding within a treatment regime and that moribund animals will not benefit from the procedure. In fact, branding can be beneficial for many ailments insofar as it produces localized stimulation of the haematopoietic and immunogenic systems.

Most herders are adept at basic perinatal procedures such as performing episiotomies and assisting in normal deliveries. Elders with specialized knowledge of obstetrics are called upon to attend to more complex needs such as dystocia (abnormal or difficult birth). These elders can reputedly assess the size and position of the foetus, and accordingly they perform a foetotomy or, if the dam dies, a Caesarean section. For a foetotomy, the specialist uses small knives that can be cupped in the palm of the hand, thus avoiding injury to the vagina and uterus. In addition to such obstetrical skills, some elders are recognized experts at setting complex fractures.

For many significant animal illnesses, Samburu have developed herbal medications. For example, the plant *seketet* (*Kyllinga flava*, a Myrsinaceae) is used as a multipurpose cure-all for both human and livestock ills. Animals with ECF may be drenched with an aqueous suspension of the powdered seeds of this plant. A decoction of this same preparation is given hot, as an anthelmintic. However, the most popular Samburu treatment for intestinal parasites employs a preparation of the plant *lmokotan* (*Albizia anthelmentica*). For conjunctivitis, Samburu use a decoction of crushed tea leaves, sugar, and water as an effective eyewash. For mastitis, herders boil sheep fat in water and rub the warm mixture over the affected parts of the udder. To prevent louse infestations in new-born calves, the animals are bathed with a mixture of milk, water and *labai* leaves (*Psiadia punctulata*, a Compositae).[3]

Changing dynamics of animal healthcare

Samburu livestock treatments today are a mix of old and new. Traditional medicines and techniques are often supplemented or substituted by modern veterinary drugs and vaccines. To take just one example, interviewees say they prefer tetracycline to their multipurpose tonic of *seketet* for treating ECF. All interviewees indicate that ECF is the most economically devastating disease, both in terms of livestock mortalities and treatment costs. There has been little time to elaborate ethnoveterinary solutions to this newly introduced disease. Hence Samburu welcome modern drugs to combat it.

At a broader level, as Western medicines and techniques become available and as herders discover them to be effective, Samburu may drop traditional therapies in favour of the new ones. In fact, most of the pastoralists interviewed participate in vaccination campaigns and/or use Western drugs. Although such treatments are very expensive and difficult to obtain in the district, demand for them is growing.

Shifting from traditional to modern treatments and techniques has contributed to several significant problems in Samburu systems of animal healthcare and husbandry, however. For example, in order to earn cash with which to purchase Western veterinary products, more and more *morani* are entering the wage economy. In response to the loss of their pastoral labour, women and young boys and girls are assuming greater herding responsibilities; indeed, stockraisers often now must 'borrow' children of kin for this purpose (Sperling 1984).

The growing demand for and use of Western pharmaceuticals has also eroded traditional authority structures and social roles in animal healthcare. The principal consumers of Western veterinary medicines are men of the warrior and junior-elder age sets, since they are the ones working in the wage economy. They can thus afford to buy expensive Western drugs when their elders cannot. Moreover, these younger men are typically better informed about the use of such drugs. In short, much of the power and knowledge to heal no longer rests with the senior elders. As a result, even elders with extensive diagnostic and therapeutic skills are now consulted only infrequently and, according to interviewees, usually only for obstetrical and bone-setting needs. Similarly, with the growing use of Western pharmaceuticals, women are less often called upon to prepare traditional medicines.

A more generalized problem is herders' imperfect knowledge of the use and specificity of modern pharmaco-therapies. Word-of-mouth is the primary method for acquiring such information, and dosages are often calculated by trial and error. This has occasioned serious difficulties with modern veterinary drugs. Many interviewees recount how animals have died from overdosing or have been literally 'dipped to death'. Although respondents report that most herders are somewhat familiar with giving injections, they confess that often the same needle and syringe are used to administer all medications. Also, although some herders are aware that many medications should be administered in specific sites (intravenous, intramuscular, subcutaneous), in practice they give most injections intramuscularly in the neck.

A further factor in the widespread misunderstanding of modern pharmaco-therapies in the district has been the paucity of government veterinary attention to the region (Meck 1971, Raikes 1981).[4] Since independence, however, the number of government veterinarians in Samburu District has increased substantially. Yet, given the very nature of pastoralism—the constant movement and dispersion of herds and people across vast distances—the livestock service's limited budget makes it difficult to deliver veterinary assistance to pastoralists except at population centres (Heffernan 1987, Stem, this volume).

Most interviewees share this assessment, indicating that their access to veterinarians is limited and that formal-sector livestock services are generally inadequate. In evidence, respondents cite the many government-run tick dips that are inoperable due to disrepair. They add that the few dips that are functional are often ineffective because they have been diluted so as to divert acaracides to the black market. In fact, pastoralists usually must buy their veterinary pharmaceuticals on the black market, with all the attendant problems of questionable quality and appropriateness.

Government veterinarians do run twice-yearly vaccination campaigns, however; and they hire Samburu herders to assist them in animal restraint and inoculation. Most interviewees had participated in such campaigns. Nevertheless, they express uncertainty about how the vaccinations worked or exactly which diseases were being immunized against. Researchers, too, have observed that the livestock service does little to increase herders' information about veterinary drugs and treatments. For example, pastoralists understand (correctly) that recent vaccination campaigns have been primarily aimed at FMD. Because Samburu do not consider FMD economically important, they have not bothered to participate in such campaigns. But they did not realize that rinderpest—a disease for which they *do* value Western vaccines—was also being vaccinated against in the FMD campaign. Such misunderstandings obviously have immediate consequences for animal health.

Conclusions and recommendations

Livestock healthcare in Samburu District could be greatly improved by expanding herders' roles as veterinary auxiliaries and redefining their duties to include healthcare education. Programmes that have taken this approach have been successful in other pastoral areas (Grandin and Young, this volume, Halpin 1981, Schwabe 1981, this volume, Sollod and Stem 1991, Stem 1983 and this volume). Trained veterinary auxiliaries would provide a substantial and more comprehensive network to instruct other pastoralists in the etiologies of important diseases, in preventive measures, and in the proper selection and posology of commercial drugs. Auxiliaries could also alert herders to upcoming vaccination campaigns and their purpose, and inform stockraisers of the availability of other veterinary services. Furthermore, auxiliaries could collect much-needed epidemiological intelligence and relay it to the veterinary department to aid in national livestock disease monitoring. In short, a corps of herder–auxiliaries can provide a vital two-way link between pastoralists and government veterinary services.

Such paravet programmes furnish minimum-cost disease control at the same time that they extend the range and application of veterinary services within a cultural context. In additional to paravet training for pastoralist men, for example, women's traditional role in milking could be taken advantage of in designing an auxiliary programme. Women are in the vanguard in noting changes in animal health as signalled by milk production (Sollod *et al.* 1984). As the processors of milk and milk products, women are also in a good position to monitor for certain kinds of zoonoses. Training women in disease recognition could therefore form the framework of an early warning system for outbreaks of contagious diseases that are most readily detectible in milch animals.

Like other pastoralists, Samburu persist in the face of overwhelming change (Rigby 1985). In part, their success can be attributed to their empirical veterinary knowledge. Today, however, the Samburu world is changing rapidly. Tourism, the exploding population of Kenya and the concomitant invasion of grazing grounds, the assimilation of young warriors into the wage-labour market and the national culture—all affect traditional Samburu ways of life. Western pharmaceuticals also play a role in the changing patterns of Samburu life. Knowledge of commercial drugs is largely restricted to younger, cash-wealthy, and typically better educated people. Other herders' information is sketchy, leading to dangerous and counterproductive misuse of alien pharmaceuticals. To improve livestock healthcare for the majority of pastoralists, development projects must address these emergent socio-economic dynamics. Formation of a veterinary auxiliary corp of herders would be a useful first step.

Notes

1. Research among the Samburu was jointly funded by the Department of International Programs at Tufts University School of Veterinary Medicine and the Tufts University School of Veterinary Medicine Summer Research Fellowships. The authors are indebted to Drs Albert Sollod and Sheila Moffet of Tufts School of Veterinary Medicine, without whose guidance and support much of this work would not have been possible. Special thanks are due the Samburu of Seketet, whose hospitality and patience were heart-warming and inspiring.
2. Throughout the chapter, etic-scientific descriptions of diseases are taken from Blood and Radostits (1989) or Losos (1986). Information and classification of plants used in Samburu veterinary medicine are from IPAL.
3. For greater detail on the Samburu veterinary pharmacopoeia, consult Heffernan (1990).
4. Historically, the Northern Frontier (of which present-day Samburu District was a part) was administered as a 'special area' and the movement of both livestock and people in and out of the area was restricted (Hogg 1986). Restrictions were designed to protect European settlers' imported, exotic cattle (which were to form the foundation for a national beef industry) from the presumably disease-ridden native cattle. Pastoralists' participation in the national beef market was thus blocked (Jacobs 1973) and the veterinary needs of the Northern Frontier were virtually ignored. By the 1950s, however, the government finally recognized that the livestock industry could not survive on exotic cattle alone. Despite all the laws and restrictions, the exotics were being decimated by disease. During the 1950s, therefore, massive vaccination campaigns were mounted against anthrax, rinderpest, CBPP, FMD and blackquarter (after Fumagalli 1977).

12. Traditional management of camel health and disease in North Africa and India[1]

ILSE KÖHLER-ROLLEFSON

As a SPECIES native to the subtropics, the dromedary camel did not become a subject of Western veterinary research until the turn of this century. Colonial officers and veterinarians from France, Great Britain and Italy wrote the first manuals on camel health and husbandry during the early decades of the twentieth century (for example, Cauvet 1925, Cross 1917, Curasson 1947, Droandi 1936, Leese 1927). These comprehensive works make frequent reference to traditional ways of managing camel diseases, and their authors note that such practices are often as effective as Western ones.

An extensive tradition of familiarity with camel diseases and their treatment in North Africa and adjoining areas is hardly surprising. The dromedary has played a central role in Arab and Islamic culture for millennia. The species is immortalized in the Koran, the Hadith, and the writings of many Arab scholars; by the twelfth century AD, 12 general treatises on the camel had been written. Although there appears to have been no work on camel medicine *per se*, many references in these early documents attest to a detailed inventory of camel diseases and treatments (Froehner 1936). Early veterinary procedures included not only relatively simple remedies such as bleeding and the use of plant-based ointments to treat skin diseases, but also such complicated manipulations as vaginal suturing of prolapsed uteri and inducing abortions in females impregnated by stray bulls. A high standard of animal care and attention to detail can be inferred from references to leather shoes for protecting camels' feet and leather blinkers for shielding camels' eyes during sandstorms (ibid.).

A similar level of sophistication about the maintenance of camel health and productivity is found among many camel-keeping peoples of Africa and India today. Twareg of the African Sahel, for example, distinguish among some 30 diseases of camels; and they resort to a wide variety of procedures to treat these ailments, including, for example, cauterization and the application of wooden splints to broken limbs. They even know how to remove a persistent *corpus luteum* by rectal manipulation (Nicolaisen 1963:121).

Twareg also have detailed knowledge of the pharmaceutical properties of most of the plants in their habitat, and they use them in remedies against an array of animal diseases such as constipation, stomach upsets, worm infestations and congestion. Camels that are not acquainted with the poisonous plants of an area are systematically sensitized against them. For instance, Twareg force camels unfamiliar with *Nerium oleander* to inhale the smoke from burning oleander leaves; alternatively, an oleander leaf may be inserted into the camels' nostrils, thereby inculcating a strong dislike of this toxic plant and training the animals to avoid it from then on (Nicolaisen 1963:120–5).

Twareg knowledge of camel health and husbandry is matched or even surpassed in elaborateness and sophistication by Somali and other camel-keeping tribes of Africa and the Levant. One index of the extent of such knowledge systems is the number of terms in a language for describing the characteristics and conditions of individual animals. Twareg use 43 terms to denote the exterior body parts of a camel (Apoggi 1933, cited in Nicolaisen 1963:125). The vocabulary of Arab camel raisers in the Butana region of eastern Sudan includes over 17 terms for camel age classes, along with 36 expressions for different defects and diseases (for example, 'dry on one teat', 'dry on four teats', 'cow-hocked', 'narrow-chested') (Acland 1932). In studying the semantic systems of camel pastoralists in the western Sahara, Monteil (1952:107) compiled a list of 600 terms for body parts and diseases, of which 180 related to reproduction and 300 concerned husbandry practices.

It would take an entire volume to do justice to the vast storehouse of indigenous knowledge about camel health and husbandry that is alluded to in the colonial, travel and ethnographic literature of the nineteenth and early twentieth centuries. Hence this chapter limits itself to a discussion of indigenous methods for combating three of the most common and serious camel diseases: mange, camel pox and trypanosomosis. Together, these illustrate of the depth, breadth and astuteness of ethnoveterinary knowledge among camel-keeping peoples.

Ethnoveterinary knowledge and practice for three major camel diseases

Mange
Although infection with the sarcoptes mange mite (*Sarcoptes scabiei*) is not usually lethal, it does have a great impact on camel productivity. This ectoparasite leads to loss of condition and weight, reduced milk output, and a predisposition to other diseases. Mange occurs throughout the distribution range of the camel. But because it is more difficult to control in animals with long shaggy hair, it is economically more significant in areas like North Africa and the Levant, where the winters are relatively cold.

A wide variety of plant tars and oils are used as topical applications to treat and prevent mange. In regions where this affliction represents a severe problem, prophylactic applications may be made seasonally. Among Arab camel raisers, one of the most widespread and successful preparations is a tar distilled from the Phoenician juniper (*Juniperus phoenicea*) or from *Thuja articulata*. These tars are very practical, since they can be easily stored in goat skins, and thus were once universally available (Cauvet 1925: 490). The tar is applied in a solution of one to two parts of warm water. Cauvet calculated that 4 to 6 litres of this mixture would be required for each animal. Algerian Arabs often treat their camels with such preparations at least once a year, preferably after shearing. With the exception of nursing females, all animals over two years of age are included. The procedure leaves the animals indisposed for two weeks, during which time they must be rested.

An alternative treatment is a mixture of oil or sheep fat with powdered sulphur (although Cauvet considers the tar preparations superior). Certain mineral springs and sea water are also ascribed therapeutic benefits against mange. However, water has to be applied with caution, since during the hot season camels are very susceptible to chilling.

Twareg camel herders prepare yet another mange remedy from animal bones that have been crushed in a large mortar and then heated over the fire; the marrow that oozes out is rubbed into the skin of the affected animal (Nicolaisen 1963: 121). The fruits of the *aborak* tree (*Balanites aegyptiaca*) may be similarly processed and applied. Ahaggar Twareg also use the pounded leaves of *Cleome arabica* and *Capparis spinosa* mixed with sour milk. Other Twareg preparations are based on: the ashes of *Chrozophora brocchiana* or charcoal of *Calotropis procera*; tar from *Tamarix gallica*; Colocynthis vulgaris seeds (ibid.); *Calligonum comosum*, *Diplotaxus Duveyriana*, or *Eruca sativa* (Cauvet 1925: 493); and a mixture of *Cleome arabica* and *Colocynthis vulgaris* with the urine of healthy camels (Monteil 1952:42).

Some of these plant genera also figure in the anti-mange treatments of other camel-raising peoples. In Eritrea, a tar is extracted from *Tamarix aphylla* and *Acacia loeta*. In Sudan's Butana region, herders cut away the hair in the infected areas and then apply a dressing of colocynth or sesame (*Sesamum indicum*) oil (Acland 1932: 138). Other Sudanese pastoralists, including Rashaida of the Kassala area, use *goudran*, a home-made topical treatment prepared by grinding the seeds of *Colocynthis vulgaris* and then heating the paste until it liquifies (Köhler-Rollefson *et al.* 1991; see also Nayel and Abu-Samra 1986).

Nigerian Hausa use a complex tar preparation called *alkibri*. It is mixed using gourd seeds, castor-oil beans (*Ricinus communis*), the epiphyseal parts of long bones and the fruits of *Balanites aegyptiaca*. These ingredients are placed in a special jar with a very small opening. The jar is inverted and aligned over the mouth of a second such container that has been buried in the ground. A fire is lit around the surface jar and kept burning for one night; the carbonized material that accumulates in the buried jar represents the end-product (Curasson 1947: 384; see also Bernus 1981:191).

An effective treatment for mange used by Indian camel owners is the following.

> In the Northern Punjab, in April, camelmen make a routine of oiling their camels as well as clipping them . . . The oil used by Punjabis is Taramira oil (made from *Brassica eruca*), and it is applied all over the body with a rag. The camel must be kept in the shade while the oil is on its body, because exposure to the sun's rays will cause it to blister. The oiling causes the camel's temperature to rise 1 to 2 degrees and may give rise to oedema under the belly. When Taramira oil is not available, oil from [*Sesamum indicum*] can be used. When the oil has been applied 48 hours the camel is taken to the bank of a stream and covered all over with mud, which is left on for three days, and then removed with the fingers. This practice I can strongly recommend as a sound one wherever the cold season has been severe enough to give the camel a long winter coat which gets infested with all kinds of parasites (Leese 1927:132)

Although the contemporary Western pharmacopoeia provides a much wider selection of treatments for mange, such commercial drugs are hardly more efficient than traditional concoctions. 'Oil is replaced by "hog's lard" and lanoline by vaseline, but the principle remains the same' (Cauvet 1925:492).

Camel pox

Camel pox is the most important viral disease of camels. It is manifested by vesicles and pustules that subsequently form crusts or scabs. It generally causes fatalities only among young animals, and during the rainy season. A number of herding groups therefore inoculate their camels to ensure that the animals contract the disease only during the dry season.

Leese (1927:64) describes how herders in south-eastern Punjab and Rajputana vaccinate young animals before the onset of the monsoon in order to bring on a mild attack of camel pox. They do this while good grazing is available

(May–June). The herders take crusts from an infected animal and keep them dry until needed. To prepare the vaccine, they break up the crusts and mix them with a little milk. Then the stockowner pricks the lip of the young camel several times with a needle and rubs the mixture into the punctures. The incubation period is about four days. Only one or two calves need be inoculated because the disease soon spreads to the others in the herd. Most of the camels to be inoculated are about four months old, but animals of up to 16 months of age may be included. Arabs employ a similar preparation, using an acacia thorn for the inoculation (Curasson 1947:57, Higgins 1983:1 094).

Trypanosomosis

Trypanosomosis is arguably the disease of greatest economic significance in camels. Widely known in North Africa as 'surra' (a Western term), it is caused by infection with the protozoan *Trypanosoma evansi*, or more rarely *T. brucei* or *T. congolense*. The disease is vectored by biting flies, mostly tabanids. Manifested by intermittent fever, anaemia and progressive unthriftiness, surra can take either an acute or chronic course, frequently ending in death. It also causes abortions and reduces milk yields. The occurrence of this disease and its insect vectors effectively define the southern limits within which camel husbandry can be safely practised in Africa. The safety line follows the 15°N latitude in West Africa, and the 13°N latitude in Chad and Sudan. In the Horn of Africa, however, camels thrive as far south as 2°S latitude.

Especially during drought—when lack of forage in the safe zone forces herders to take their animals into fly-infested areas—trypanosomosis will almost certainly strike. This scenario prevailed in Sudan during the 1984–5 drought, for example. Then, camel herders from northern Kordofan were forced to drive their animals into southern Kordofan (Abdalla and Akasha 1988)—an area regarded as distinctly unsafe for camels.

Camel herders are very much aware of the mode of transmission of trypanosomosis. They have therefore developed a wide variety of strategies to avoid exposing their animals to flies (also see Schillhorn van Veen, this volume). Vegetation that is known to host breeding populations of insects is burned or chopped down. Watering is scheduled so that it does not overlap with the activity periods of tabanids. For example, during the hot season when flies are active in the morning and afternoon, camels are watered at noon; but during the cooler season when tabanids swarm during the day, watering is done at night. When herds are trailed into fly-infested areas, marching is done only at night; during the day, flies are kept away with smoke and fire.

During camel raisers' temporary forays into southern Kordofan, extensive precautions must be taken if camels are to survive even brief visits. The animals are kept in straw huts with smoldering smudge fires; they are fed exclusively on dry feed; and they are not used for work (Schinkel 1970:255, 258). If daytime travel is necessary, topical ointments (often plant tars) are applied to ward off flies. This is apparently a very ancient practice. Pliny (cited in Cauvet 1925:479) makes reference to dugong fat being sold along the Red Sea coast for use as a camel grease against insect bites.

Diagnosing surra is not easy. The only sure method is to examine blood smears under a microscope. However, the trypanosomes occur in the peripheral blood system only during the paroxysmal stage of the disease. During the other stages, even microscopic analysis may not give accurate results. In consequence, more than 80 per cent of infected animals may not be identified by this procedure.

It is noteworthy that certain camel pastoralists have developed diagnostic tests of at least equal accuracy. For example, Rebaris of the south-eastern Punjab and Bedouin of Arabia take a handful of earth, let the camel in question urinate on it, then shape the mud into a ball. After drying for half an hour, the ball is broken apart and smelled by the herder or healer. In camels with many trypanosomes in the peripheral blood, a characteristic sweet, pungent, 'sickly' smell can be detected. According to Leese (1927:240), this method has the same level of accuracy as examining blood under the microscope—although he understandably prefers his microscope to the indigenous procedure. In India, the Rebaris are the only ones with knowledge of this traditional diagnostic procedure. Accordingly, camel owners seek them out avidly to have their herds examined during the months before the monsoon season so as to weed out animals infected in the previous year. Another traditional diagnostic test used in India consists of pulling out tail hairs from a suspect animal and applying the roots of the hair to the down-turned palm of one's hand. An animal is diagnosed as healthy if the tail hairs stick to the palm. The basis of this test—considered by Leese to be of some value (ibid.)—is that in healthy camels a bit of flesh is yanked out with the hair, and this is what then adheres to the hand. Both these tests were also known and used by camel pastoralists of the western Sahara (Monteil 1952:44).

In North Africa, trypanosomosis is diagnosed by a bone-marrow-like flavour in the milk of affected female camels (Curasson 1947:134). Also, if upon pinching the skin of a camel's thigh between thumb and index finger, the fold does not even out, this is regarded as an infallible indication of trypanosomosis. (In Western veterinary medicine, this is a generic test for dehydration.)

Traditional cures appear to be non-specific. They are aimed mostly at enhancing natural resistance. Examples include drenching or feeding with preparations such as the following: an infusion of henna; a broth of mutton, jackal meat or fish; salted, scalded milk; *Tragama nudatum*, a plant rich in certain salts; or other plants such as *Nucularia perrini* and *Cornulaca monocantha* (Curasson 1947: 155, Monteil 1952:44). Twareg make a special concoction of sheep urine, jackal meat and *Boscia senegalensis* leaves that is administered intranasally (Bernus 1981: 192). Sudanese camel herders are reported to take especially elaborate measures. They 'transform the ruminant into a carnivore' (Cauvet 1925:482) and feed it boluses of boiled and minced meat alternating with balls of crushed millet.

Western researchers have noted that different breeds of camels display varying levels of resistance to trypanosomosis (Schillinger and Rottcher 1984). Camel pastoralists recognize that some infected animals may develop lifelong resistance to the disease. In Sudan's White Nile Province, camels diagnosed as having surra are frequently handed over to an expert for a special treatment that lasts more than three years. Fewer than 50 per cent of the creatures survive long enough to complete the treatment regime; but those that do are considered immune and hence are extremely valuable—especially in the fly-infested southern regions (after Reid 1930:167). Such animals are called *afiq* 'salted'. Similarly, in the El Arish and Katieh regions of Egypt, certain camels regarded as 'immunized' are much sought-after (Cauvet 1925:479).[2] Furthermore, in Sudan and in the central region of the Niger River, some camels are able to remain in the river valleys throughout the year without contracting trypanosomosis, whereas this would mean certain death for the others. However, these 'immune' animals reportedly do not have as much endurance as their Saharan cousins. In Senegal such survivors are called *onoloff* and in Mauritania *zaguer* (ibid.).

Since early in this century, when colonial camel corps were often afflicted with trypanosomosis, Western veterinary medicine has endeavoured to eradicate this scourge. Control of this protozoal disease, however, presents almost insurmountable obstacles. Because of the great variety of insect vectors and the huge area they inhabit, control can be practically ruled out as a measure of containment. Attempts to develop a vaccine have been unsuccessful because of the immense antigenic variation within the trypanosomes. A number of trypanocides of varying efficiency exist. For example, Naganol (also known as Suramin) has been used since the 1920s; but now, many strains of trypanosomes are resistant to it.

Another substance, Anthrycide, was highly successful. But it has not been produced or marketed since 1974 (Mahmoud and Osman 1984, Schillinger and Rottcher 1984). It seems that the manufacturer, ICI, considered it unprofitable. Overall, pharmaceutical companies have shown a remarkable lack of interest in developing trypanocides for camels, because such drugs are not considered commercially viable (Mahmoud and Osman 1984). Thus, Western approaches to combating this disease have stagnated. Here, the large body of traditional knowledge regarding the prophylaxis, diagnosis and treatment of trypanosomosis offers promising alternative approaches.

Implications for development

A great many traditional methods of managing camel diseases qualify as rational and efficient by even the most rigid standards of Western veterinary science (see also Schillhorn van Veen, this volume). The information presented in this chapter—almost all of it culled from books by colonial officers and veterinarians in the early part of this century—illustrates the value of systematically recording and analysing ethnoveterinary techniques for deriving workable solutions to camel health problems. Ideally, such research should be conducted by scientists or scientific teams who have both anthropological and veterinary training. That way, the potentials of traditional healthcare knowledge and practice can be realistically assessed, in both socio-economic and technical terms, for their usefulness as cheap, accessible, effective and environmentally sound alternatives for improving camel health and productivity.

The wide variety of traditional ointments for treating mange is a case in point. There is certainly no shortage of commercially produced acaricides that are effective against the sarcoptes mange mite. These products are, however, generally based on highly toxic organophosphorus or chlorinated hydrocarbon compounds. These substances can lead to accidental poisoning of both animals and people and to the accumulation of chemical residues in the environment. From an ecological standpoint, there is no question but that a locally produced, plant-based ointment stored in a goat skin is preferable to a toxic chemical imported from overseas and marketed in a plastic container. It would thus make sense to support cottage industries that manufacture effective traditional preparations, whether for mange or other ailments (see also Anjaria, this volume, and for commercial possibilities for homemade feedstuffs, Vondal, this volume).

The Indian and Arab method of vaccinating against camel pox speaks for itself. Knowledge of this simple procedure requires dissemination to other camel-keeping peoples and countries.

In the fight against trypanosomosis, neither indigenous nor Western efforts offer an immediate solution. However, the elaborate precautions that camel herders take to prevent this disease are noteworthy. In recent years, though, pastoralists have had no alternative but to move their animals into areas known to be infested with insects that transmit trypanosomosis are vectors. This fact suggests that the low productivity and the high losses currently besetting camel husbandry may be fairly recent phenomena. Such setbacks may be common now because many traditional mechanisms for maintaining herd health and productivity are no longer feasible in the face of cultivators' encroachment on prime grazing grounds or the deterioration of the remaining pastures due to the overgrazing attendant upon human overpopulation and/or climatic shifts.

One possible avenue for attacking trypanosomosis would be to combine pastoral and Western know-how. As noted earlier, some camels appear to be naturally resistant to this disease. Pastoral knowledge regarding such animals' pedigrees and peculiarities is phenomenal, as evidenced in the reports of many early travellers and colonial officials. A telling anecdote related by Davies (1957:32) concerns a Sudanese Arab whose female camel had been stolen. The owner searched for her unsuccessfully for many years. Finally, he came across the track of a young camel with a peculiarity of gait that he was certain had been inherited from his missing animal. By pursuing this clue, he was ultimately able to trace his camel. While Davies tells this story to illustrate camel pastoralists' tracking skills, it also speaks volumes about their knowledge of applied genetics and their intimate familiarity with practical aspects of animal breeding. With pastoralists' participation, it should be possible to identify particular camel blood lines with an inherited resistance to trypanosomosis. Such individuals could then be selectively bred—where helpful, with the assistance of artificial insemination or even embryo transfer.

It is appropriate to conclude with a quote from Cauvet, who compiled an incredible amount of information on camel lore and all aspects of traditional camel husbandry. His commentary on Arab camel keepers holds for many camel pastoralists: they profess '. . . with a certain arrogance that only the one who has been raised on it will ever get to know camel medicine well' (Cauvet 1925:514). He emphasizes that camel pastoralists have adopted prophylactic measures of great efficiency: they flee regions with stinging insects; avoid areas and oases where camels can contract microbial diseases and parasites; change their encampments as frequently as possible; and make certain that their camels receive a varied diet according to the seasons. Cauvet's observations underscore the fact that camel-herding peoples have developed astute and elaborate management methods to keep their animals healthy and productive. Indeed, they have adapted their whole lifestyle to this end. They need relatively little outside assistance to instil greater efficiency into their camel husbandry. Rather, Western veterinarians and animal experts could learn from them how better to rear these useful and unique animals within the constraints of their natural environment. This would lay the groundwork for expanding camel husbandry as a much-needed yet sustainable means of food production in arid and semi-arid areas.

Notes

1. Preparation of this chapter would not have been possible without the monumental compilations of camel knowledge by two colonial experts in particular—Commandant

Cauvet and A. S. Leese—both of whom were obvious sticklers for detail. Also, the monograph by H. G. Schinkel provided many useful references.

2. Although Cauvet uses the term 'immunized', I suspect the more appropriate description would be 'tolerant'.

13. Ethnoveterinary pharmacology in India: past, present and future

JAYVIR ANJARIA

IN MANY ASIAN countries, traditional medicine exists side by side with modern Western medicine. Recently, both scientific and commercial interest in ethno pharmaceuticals and their applications has grown appreciably. Scientists and developers have increasingly come to recognize that many local remedies work, are readily available and provide cost-effective alternatives to Western drugs. At the same time, Western medicine is being examined more critically. Many synthetic drugs have side-effects and sometimes environmental implications; there is a risk of iatrogenic (doctor-inflicted) illness with powerful Western drugs and highly invasive procedures; and patients complain that Western-style medical professionals are cold and uninterested. Moreover, according to the World Health Organization (WHO 1976), 85 per cent of people in developing countries still rely on traditional medicine as their first choice in human health-care. WHO emphasizes that, if its goal of 'Health for All by the Year 2000' is to be achieved, traditional medicine perforce must play an important role in primary healthcare (ibid.).

Traditional medicine is experiencing a revival in the veterinary sector, too. Beginning more than a decade ago, the Asian Office of the Food and Agricultural Organization (FAO) recognized the importance of ethnoveterinary medicine and commissioned a number of reports on its status in six Asian countries (FAO 1984a, 1984b, 1984c, 1986, 1991a, 1991b). All these studies found that ethno-veterinary practices could be usefully incorporated in animal health services. And in 1986/7, the Livestock Development Programme of the Asian Development Bank launched a project in Sri Lanka to institutionalize the use of traditional veterinary medicine at the national level (Anjaria 1986a).

Most of the foregoing efforts have focused on ethnoveterinary botanicals. India is particularly rich in medicinal plants. An estimated 20000 plant species are found across India's highly varied topography and climate. Of these, about 2500 are used medicinally, and nearly 1300 have aromatic properties (Arora 1965). Considerable research has been devoted to India's medicinal plants and other indigenous drugs. So far, however, very little attention has been paid to their possible applications to livestock. Yet with concerted interdisciplinary research and systematic testing under field conditions, many traditional botanicals offer promise for the development of a thriving industry in veterinary drugs that often derive from age-old practice. This chapter describes the past, present and possible future of such developments in India.

The past: traditional medical systems in India

India has three major traditional medical systems: Ayurveda, Siddha and Unani-Tibb. Although they are most commonly thought of in association with human medicine, all three also apply to animals.

Ayurveda or 'the science of life' defines life as a constant and continuous union of five basic elements: earth, water, fire, air and ether. Together, these elements constitute the body, organs, mind and soul. The origins of Ayurveda date back to the Vedic period, *c.* 1500 to 600 BC. Ayurvedic belief holds that Lord Brahma defined this medical science when he created the universe. He taught Ayurveda to Daksha Prajapati who in turn passed it on to the twin Ashwinikumar brothers and through them to Lord Indra. To combat earthly diseases, Sage Bhardwaj learned Ayurveda from Indra. Bhardwaj then taught it to other sages who transferred the knowledge to other disciples. In this fashion, Ayurvedic knowledge was traditionally transmitted orally.

In the first century AD, this knowledge was committed to writing in the Charaka and Shusruta Samhitas (Anonymous 1941a, 1941b). These two Sanskrit works on medicine and surgery form the theoretical foundation of classical Ayurvedic medicine. However, still earlier Vedic scriptures such as the Atharvaveda, Rugveda and Yajurveda (Anonymous 1958a, 1958b, 1958c) also mentioned therapeutic measures and numerous medicinal plants, along with many incantations, charms and spells. It seems that in its earliest form, Ayurveda practice was dominated by religious and magical elements. Diseases were thought to be caused by demons and were often cured with charms and rituals.

The Vedas also make reference to early veterinary arts. The Rugveda shows *ashvini* healers ('divine physicians') replacing the severed leg of a prize mare with an iron prosthesis (Anonymous 1958b:1.116.15). A hymn in the Yajurveda (Anonymous 1958c:1221) prays for medicinal plants for cattle health and production. Veterinary skills and practices are also referenced in Indian mythological scriptures. The Mahabharata epic (Anonymous 1958d), dating from the fifth century BC, speaks of Nala as a great animal trainer and caretaker and mentions the animal physicians Raj and Bij. Other early scriptures that contain information on animal management, feeding and veterinary care are the Puranas, including the Agni, Brahma, Devi, Garuda, Linga, Matsaya and Skanda (Anonymous 1954a, 1954g).

The first Sanskrit book devoted solely to veterinary medicine is the Shalihotra. Shalihotra was a famous authority on equine medicine during the late Vedic period. Another well-known veterinarian from that period was Palakapya, a specialist in elephants. The first animal hospitals in India were erected by order of King Ashoka in the third century BC; he also formulated rules for their operation. These early Ayurveda clinics used a wide spectrum of herbal remedies. They also stimulated many written works on veterinary treatments that employed herbal and other indigenous drugs. Examples of such Sanskrit documents from that period include the Aswa Chikitsa and the Gaja Chikitsa on equine and elephant medicine, respectively. (For greater detail on ancient Ayurvedic veterinary medicine, see Lodrick 1981 and Shirlaw 1940.)

Some authorities consider Siddha merely a local variant of Ayurveda. However, its followers believe that Siddha is quite distinct and perhaps even more ancient (Satyavati, 1982). Siddha medicine is practised in the Tamil Nadu region of south India. Despite the limited geographic and linguistic (Tamil and some Telugu) extension of Siddha, there is a great quantity and variety of literature about it. This literature spans medicinal plants, non-herbal drugs, alchemy, disease syndromes, diagnoses and therapies, plus treatments for animals.

The third medical tradition, Unani-Tibb, originated in Greece and is based on the teachings of Hippocrates (born *c.* 460 BC) and Galen (*c.* 130–200 AD) on the humoural theory of pathology. The Arabs further developed this system, which came to India along with Islamization. (*Unani* is an Arab corruption of the Greek word for 'Ionian'.) Experimentation and clinical tests in India added many local drugs to the original pharmacopoeia. Unani-Tibb shares with Ayurvedic medicine a recognition of four basic elements (earth, water, air, fire) that are in turn linked with four 'humours' (blood, phlegm, black bile and yellow bile) (Foster and Anderson 1978). Also like Ayurveda, Unani employs a wealth of plant, animal, and mineral *materia medica*. However, Unani disease concepts and diagnostic techniques have much in common with early allopathic medicine (Zysk Keni 1979), and they emphasize treating the patient as a whole. Unani also recognizes that constitutional differences influence the action of drugs (Satyavati 1982). Unani is applied to animals as well as people, and research within the Unani system has contributed to the development of veterinary treatments in India (Razak 1982).

The present: research on ethno-pharmaceuticals

Clearly, veterinary medicine has a long tradition in India, and many ancient skills and practices are still widely used in rural areas today. Along with stock-owners' and healers' own innovations, the medical traditions outlined above have given rise to a great variety of local veterinary treatments and techniques. Among them are: cauterization, fumigation, surgery, obstetrical procedures, inoculation and various ritual and magical operations.[1] But medicinal plants form the cornerstone of Indian veterinary medicine. And while some ethnoveterinary practices are harmful, many others—especially those using medicinal plants—appear to be generally safe and effective.

Use and potentials of ethno-botanicals
Although little scientific research has focused on the use of herbal remedies in animal healthcare and production, many of the plants used in ethnoveterinary practice are also applied in human medicine and have been intensively studied in this context. The combined efforts of numerous projects launched by national laboratories and universities and by veterinary, medical and pharmacology colleges in India have resulted in considerable (though still incomplete) experimental data on many of the nation's indigenous medicinal plants. A bibliography of studies between 1950 and 1975 on Indian botanicals lists some 2500 plants and 400 references (Iyengar 1976). Vohora's (1989) analysis of the entries in this bibliography found that phytochemical studies predominated (60 per cent of the plants investigated). Next in order were pharmacological studies (about 16 per cent), pharmacognostic and botanical reports (13 per cent), and investigations of plant cultivation or of other, general topics (8.5 per cent).

Again, these studies have focused primarily on applications in human health-care. Yet many of the plants employed in human ethnomedicine have potential veterinary applications as well, if dosages and modes of administration are tested and adjusted for each animal species. Drawing upon recent research findings reviewed in Anjaria (1986a, 1986b, 1986c) plus the author's own decades of experience in Indian ethnopharmacology, the potentials of some of these traditional botanicals for improving animal health and productivity are outlined below.

Milk and egg production Many traditional plant remedies of varying efficacy exist for agalactia, or failure to produce milk. For example, feeding cows tinctures of jaborandi (*Pilocarpus* spp.) and *Nux vomica* (Ghokale 1926), sometimes in combination with powdered tubers of *Euphorbia nana* (Raju 1932), has been shown to increase milk yields. Likewise for the roots of *Asparagus racemosus* fed to buffalo cows (Patel and Kanitkar 1969).

For centuries, Indian stockraisers have also used *Leptadenia reticulata* (LR) as a galactagogue, as well as a remedy for a number of other ailments (see later sections). Its medicinal use is described in both the Atharvaveda and the Charaka Samhita (Bagayitkar 1959). LR is a creeper that grows year round near thorny trees in forests and gardens in certain regions of India and some other Asian countries (Anjaria and Gupta 1969b). LR has been studied for its chemical composition (Anjaria and Gupta 1970a, 1970b), the pharmacological activity of aqueous and alcoholic extracts (Anjaria and Gupta 1970b, Shrivastava *et al.* 1970, 1974), and the effects of stigmasterol and lipoid fractions (Anjaria *et al.* 1975a, 1975b). Controlled pharmaco-dynamic experiments have confirmed the lactogenic action of LR in cattle, water buffalo, sheep and goats (Anjaria and Gupta 1967).

For these studies, experimental animals were selected that were similar in age, number of lactations, date of calving and body weight. Lactating female cattle and buffalo fed crude LR powder at a dose of 1 340mg per cow twice a day for 12 days with six days each of pre- and post-drug periods showed significantly increased milk yields—12.5 per cent in cattle and 9.8 per cent in buffalo (Anjaria and Gupta 1967, 1969a). In another study with cattle, oral administration twice daily of 2.5g of LR per cow for 15 days resulted in a net gain of 10.5 per cent in milk production (Anjaria *et al.* 1974). LR powder fed to sheep and goats at a dose of 536mg per animal twice daily for 12 days produced significant net gains (14.2 per cent and 10.8 per cent, respectively) in milk production as measured by pre- and post-suckling weight of offspring (Anjaria and Gupta 1967). Quantitative and qualitative analyses of milk constituents and blood during the experiment showed no changes. In all experiments, milk yields were maintained even after the drug was stopped. Moreover, in all species treated, hard-milking animals became soft-milking with smoother milk let-down. Also, milk yield began to increase about five days after treatment began, with an overall rise of 11.8 per cent. (For details of these and other LR investigations, consult Anjaria and Gupta 1967, 1969a, 1969b, 1970a, 1970b, 1972.)

LR has also been used in combination with other medicinal plants known to Indian stockraisers. Galog™—which contains LR, *Asparagus racemosus, Tinospora cordifolia* and some other plant extracts—increases milk yields in cattle and buffalo after five to 10 days (Chaddha *et al.* 1977; Gahlot 1982; Kulkarni 1976; Pande and Rai 1982). The lactogenic effect of Leptaden™ tablets—which contain a mixture of LR and *Breynia patens*—has been tested in various species by a number of researchers (Anjaria and Gupta 1967, 1970b, Azmi 1970, Dash *et al.* 1972, Dave 1969, Harkawat and Singhvi 1977, Johari and Singh 1970, Kaikini *et al.* 1968, Kaikini and Pargaonkar 1969, Kulkarni 1970, Moulvi 1963, Narasimhamurthy 1969, Pal *et al.* 1979, Prasad 1970, Raghavan Nambiar 1980, 1981, Rajagopalan *et al.* 1972, Vaishnav and Buch 1965). With few exceptions, they report encouraging results with varying doses given over 15 to 20 days. However, the cost of treating an animal with Leptaden tablets is higher and the tablets are less effective than LR alone (Anjaria and Gupta 1967).

LR powder, stigmasterol isolated from LR, and Leptaden™ also significantly increase egg production in hens (Anjaria *et al.* 1970, 1975c). The effect of Leptaden™ on various other parameters in poultry production has also been studied (Ishwar 1980, Ishwar and Mohsin 1981a, 1981b, 1981d, 1981e, Natrajan 1968, Samal 1974). Other plant preparations that increase egg yields are a mixture of *Asparagus racemosus, Nigella sativa*, and *Withania somnifera* (Kumarasamy *et al.* 1986 cited in Anjaria 1986a), and Livol™ (Pradhan and Misra 1988), which contains *Boerhaavia diffusa, Solanum nigrum*, and *Terminalia arjuna* (Pandey *et al.* 1984).

Reproductive disorders Reproductive disorders in farm animals can result in infertility, sterility, or abortion. These conditions cause great economic losses in terms of milk and progeny. Many herbal preparations are available for controlling habitual abortion, inducing heat, and promoting conception. (For reviews of such preparations, see Anjaria 1981a, 1981b, 1986d).

One example is Prajana™, which has been used with encouraging results for post-partum anoestrus in farm animals. Elaborated on the basis of traditional pharmaceuticals, Prajana™ is a mixture of nutmeg (*Myristica fragrans*) and other herbs. It is commonly given orally in the form of capsules, but an injectable solution has also been developed. Several studies of the efficacy of Prajana™ in up to 110 anoestrous cattle and buffalo cows have reported the induction of heat in 50 to 86 per cent of the animals treated; following artificial insemination, conception rates ranged between 50 and 88 per cent (Galhotra *et al.* 1970, Kodagali *et al.* 1973, Kulkarni 1973, Patil *et al.* 1983). Some of these authors recommend a dosage of two capsules every 24 hours until the animal comes into heat. (For additional information and the results of laboratory trials with mice, see Deshpande 1976 and Naresh Chand 1974, respectively.)

Other plant-based preparations derived from ethnoveterinary practice to induce heat in cows include Heatrone™, which contains *Argyreia speciosa,* and Aloes Compound™, which is based on *Aloe barbadensis*. Of 30 heifers treated with Aloes Compound™ for 10 days, 18 came into oestrus within a month and were inseminated; of these, 13 conceived (Dutta *et al.* 1988). Aloes Compound™ and another plant-based pharmaceutical, Myron™, have been tried for reproductive disorders in female bovines, with encouraging results. These disorders include irregular oestrus, anoestrous, atonic reproductive tract, endometritis and metritis (Dange 1977, Rathore and Pattabhi Raman 1977). Leptaden™ is effective in cases of retained placenta and habitual abortion (Raghavan Nambiar 1980).

Plant-based remedies have long been used to treat reproductive disorders in male animals, too. Saxom™ is a mixture of three plants traditionally used for such problems (*Mucuna pruriens, Pedalium murex* and *Sida cordifolia*). It has shown promise for improving semen quality and libido in rams and for increasing libido and mounting aggressiveness in bulls (Jai and Joshi 1979, 1981). In tests on laboratory mice, *S. cordifolia* alone had a significant positive effect on testes weight, prostate, epididymis and seminal vesicles; and it significantly improved spermatogenesis. It also increased testis weight and comb size in 65- to 79-day-old chicks (Jai 1977). Given orally, Fortege™—a mixture of powdered *Anacyalus pyrethrum* compound, *Argyreia speciosa, Mucuna pruriens* and *Withania somnifera*—has been shown to improve semen quality in bulls (Sharma 1969).

Urinary disorders Bulls and rams are prone to urinary calculosis (Anjaria 1969). A number of Indian plants have proven helpful in treating diuresis, calculosis, and other urinary disorders in cattle. These plants include *Crateva nurvala, Tribulus terrestris, Boerhaavia diffusa, Saxifraga ligulata*, and *Hyoscyamus niger* (Anjaria 1986c, 1986e, FAO 1984a; for further detail on the use of *Crateva nurvala* and still other herbal drugs for urinary disorders, consult Chopra 1970 and Mukherjee *et al.* 1984). Cystone™ contains the plants just listed. Although *in vitro* pharmacological evidence is lacking (Anjaria and Kamboya 1970), Cystone™ and a decoction of *Dolichos biflorus* are reportedly effective *in vivo* (Angelo and Lavania 1976, Das 1956).

Respiratory disorders In many regions in India, farmers and local veterinarians alike treat cold symptoms in cattle with inhalations of *Eucalyptus*, turpentine, or benzoin. Indians also have a panoply of traditional herbal expectorants. Scientists have screened many of these in search of remedies or reliefs for nonspecific coughs and colds. Aulakh and Mahadevan (1989) review 22 single-component herbal drugs used against asthma, and they discuss the expectorant effects found in animal trials. Most remedies use plants such as *Alpinia galanga*, *Adhatoda vasica*, *Curcuma longa*, *Glycyrrhiza glabra*, *Ocimum basilicum*, *O. sanctum*, *Piper longum*, *Terminalia belerica* and *Urginea indica*, plus other ingredients such as camphor and ammonium chloride (Anjaria 1986e, FAO 1984a). Some of these plants have been studied quite extensively, such as *A. vasica* (Jain *et al.* 1984) and *G. glabra* (Tyler *et al.* 1988). Several commercial preparations containing mixtures of the plants just cited are available under different trade names. For instance, Caflon™ is effective for coryza in camels (Vashishtha and Singh 1975).

Digestive disorders Traditionally, a large number of herbal mixtures containing bitter tonics, carminatives, appetizers, alkalizers, and purgatives have been used to treat digestive disorders in livestock (Anjaria 1982, 1986a, 1986f, FAO 1984a). Many of these preparations are also used in allopathic prescriptions and have been much studied. Examples include *Nux vomica* tincture, and extracts of *Atropa belladonna* and *Digitalis purpurea*. Since considerable information on these plants has been published elsewhere (for example, Budavari *et al.* 1989, Tyler *et al.* 1988), they are not discussed here.

For digestive disorders, commercial formulae containing large numbers of herbs are abundant. An example is Himalayan Batisa™. Made of 32 different herbs, it is effective in alleviating indigestion in large animals (Basak and Nandi 1982, Gowal 1987, Nooruddin 1983, Singh *et al.* 1980). It has also proved beneficial in overcoming stress in sheep (Gowal 1987) and in increasing feed intake and conversion ratios in broiler chicks (Basak 1986). One of its ingredients is *Swertia chirata*, a bitter tonic also used as an appetizer. (For a review of pharmacological studies of this traditional medicinal plant, consult Edwin and Chungath 1988.)

Indian veterinarians prescribe various commercial herbal mixtures for bloat in large animals. These mixtures are compounded of species such as *Embelia ribes*, *Ferula assa-foetida*, *Gardenia gummifera*, mustard, *Trachyspermum ammi*, *Piper longum* and *Zingiber officinale* (Anjaria 1981a, 1982, 1986b, FAO 1984a). Tympol™, for example, has proven beneficial in relieving bloat in ruminants (Ehsham *et al.* 1977, Pal 1976, Tripathy and Pradhan 1977).

A number of herbal mixtures containing *Aegle marmelos*, *Areca catechu*, *Creta preperata*, *Embelia ribes* and *Holarrhena antidysenterica* have been used as antidiarrheals in large animals (Anjaria 1981a, 1982, 1986c, FAO 1984a). Although the chemistry and possible antimicrobial efficacy of *A. marmelos* have been thoroughly studied (Banerjee *et al.* 1984), its antidysenteric activity could not be demonstrated (Bhutani *et al.* 1984). However, the antidiarrhoeal efficacy of Neblon™—one of the many trade formulations based on the plants just mentioned—has been scientifically confirmed (Pillai *et al.* 1971, Rahman and Nooruddin 1981, Soni *et al.* 1980). Out of 35 plant extracts screened for activity against dysentery-producing bacteria and amoebae (Bhutani *et al.* 1987), an extract of *Terminalia belerica* fruit showed a wide range of antibacterial activity. *Parthenium hysterophoros* and *Ervatamia heyneana* also seem promising as antiamoebics. *Holarrhena antidysenterica* tested along with common adulterants such as *Wrightia* spp. had antiamoebic fractions in its extracts, although the plant's alkaloidal content varies regionally and seasonally (ibid.).

Hepatic benefits have been experimentally demonstrated for *Achillea millefolium*, *Capparis spinosa*, *Cassia occidentalis*, *Chicorium intybus*, *Solanum nigrum*, *Tamarix gallica* and *Terminalia arjuna* (Patel *et al.* 1988, Rathore and Rawat 1989). Various mixtures of these species are given both to animals and people. Livol™, described earlier, can reduce liverfluke damage in bovines and ovines (Mahanta *et al.* 1983, Pandit 1986). It is also used as a feed additive for kids (Arora and Mohini 1984), has a positive impact on broiler performance (Devegowda and Ramappa 1988), and reduces liver damage in dogs given carbon tetrachlorides (Pandey *et al.* 1984).

Helminth infections Helminths are a serious problem in Indian livestock, as they reduce both the quality and quantity of all animal products. Plants like *Alangium lamarckii*, *Areca catechu*, *Butea frondosa*, *B. monosperma*, *Holarrhena antidysenterica*, *Vernonia anthelmintica* and *Zanthoxylum alatum* are common ingredients of indigenous vermifuges available under various trade names (Anjaria 1982, 1986f, FAO 1984a). Laboratory studies on mice show good effects against oxyurids for *B. frondosa* and *V. anthelmintica* without being toxic to the host animals (Mehta and Parashar 1966). Singh *et al.* (1985) critically review the anthelmintic activity of *V. anthelmintica*. A single 0.25 g/kg oral dose of powdered root bark of *A. lamarckii* kills poultry ascarids (Dubey and Gupta 1969). Both *in vitro* and *in vivo* studies indicate that *Z. alatum* is ascaricidal (Singh 1969). The extract of *Piper nigrum* fruit kills tapeworms *in vivo* (Ali and Mehta 1986).

In dogs, an oral dose of 2 to 6 g of Wopell™—a mixture of *B. frondosa*, *Embelia ribes*, areca nut and male fern—reduced *Toxocara* spp. by 60 per cent, *Ancylostoma* spp. by 22 per cent and *Spirocerca* spp. by 7 per cent, all without toxic side-effects (Raghavan *et al.* 1976). The same mixture was also effective against hookworms in dogs, stomach worms in goats (Kumar *et al.* 1973) and *T. canis* and *Dipylidium caninum* in pups (Misra 1983). Preparations of *B. frondosa*, *Carica papaya*, *Momordica charantia*, and *Sapindus trifoliatus* have been found effective *in vitro* against *Ascaridia galli*, a poultry helminth (Lal *et al.* 1976). Anjaria (1986f) reports further indigenous anthelmintics that have been tested in India and in Sri Lanka.

Ectoparasitism A number of drug formulations based on indigenous plant extracts are reportedly effective against mange and other ectoparasitoses in livestock, including Himax™ (Sharma *et al.* 1982, Tripathy *et al.* 1986), Teeburb™ (Raghavan *et al.* 1983, Singh 1980), Pestoban™ (Ahmed 1986, Narang 1981, Sinha *et al.* 1987) and Blaze™ (Shrivastava *et al.* 1988, Supekar and Mehta 1986, Tripathy *et al.* 1987). Oil extracted from *Annona squamosa* kills lice (Anjaria 1986a). Furthermore, trials have shown that *A. squamosa* preparations can control flies by killing their larvae (Desai 1985).

Skin infections The antifungal, antiviral and antibacterial activity of some 100 plants in India (George *et al.* 1946) and about 50 plants in Sri Lanka (Vinayagamoorthy 1982) is well documented. Preparations from a number of plants used in traditional medicine have been well studied. Examples include *Enterolobium saman* leaves (Annapurna *et al.* 1989), *Senecio quinquelobus* leaves (Chaturvedi and Saxena 1983), *Phyllanthus fraternus* (Ramchandani and Chugath 1987) and

Parthenium hysterophorus (Rai and Upadhyaya 1988). The latter plant also shows antiamoebic activity (see above). *Juniperus communis*, *Euphorbia thymifòlia* and *Wedelia calendulacea* have demonstrated effective antifungal activity *in vitro* and in clinical trials with goats and buffalo calves (Gupta 1974).

Annona squamosa, *Azadirachta indica*, *Ocimum sanctum* and *Bergia odorata* all have promising antimicrobial properties (Anjaria 1986b, 1986c, 1986g, 1986h). Several of these also show anti-ectoparasite effects [editors' note]. *In vitro*, several bacteria (*Streptococcus*, *Staphylococcus*, *Escherichia coli*, *Corynebacterium*, *Pseudomonas*) that are resistant to many antibiotics and sulfonamides proved sensitive to chloroform extracts of the leaves of these first three plants. Ointments containing these extracts were tested on surgically induced wounds in mice that were infected with a mixture of these bacterial strains collected from animal wounds in the field. Treated daily with the ointments, the wounds healed within 12 days. In control experiments, the plant-based formulations were as effective as a commercial nitrofurazone ointment and better than a commercial antiseptic cream containing propamidine (Thaker and Anjaria 1986).

Antibacterial activity has been reported in *Cyperus rotundus*, *Holarrhena antidysenterica* and many other plants (George *et al.* 1946). The indigenous drug Himax™, which contains many such herbal agents, is effective in treating wounds, septic wounds, and skin mycosis in both large and small animals (Sharma *et al.* 1981, Thakur 1975). A dressing powder containing *Annona squamosa* and *Azadirachta indica* leaves, plus some other ingredients, was effective against septic wounds in field animals (Anjaria 1986b, 1986c, also see Malik *et al.*, this volume). Specifically, it promoted healing of wounds and ulcers caused by foot-and-mouth disease virus and other contaminated purulent wounds and indolent ulcers. Using these ingredients, Anjaria (1985, 1986g, 1986h) developed a cheap and effective wound powder for livestock that smallholder farmers can prepare and use themselves.

Inflammations Sharma (1978) obtained good results in testing topical applications of G32™—a mixture of 23 herbs—in 85 animals of different species with stomatitis, gingivitis, glossitis and pharyngitis. Fruit extracts of *Vitex negundo* and *Valeriana wallichii* (Shrivastava and Sissodia 1970) and *Cissus quadrangularis* (Singh *et al.* 1984) also exhibited significant analgesic activity in animal experiments.

Tumours According to Ambaye *et al.* (1984), many researchers have screened *Abrus precatorius*, *Saraca indica*, *Tylophora crebifera*, *Vinca rosea*, *Wedelia calendulacea* and *Xanthium strumarium* for anticancer activity, with varying results. *Semecarpus anacardium* was tried on cases of horn cancer in animals, but the results were inconclusive (Pachauri 1965).

The future: an enhanced ethnoveterinary drug industry

Currently, perhaps some 85 to 90 per cent of Indian stockraisers' veterinary budget is spent on commercially manufactured drugs, with perhaps a half of this going to life-saving drugs like antibiotics, and a quarter to supportive medicines.[2] As many of the chapters in the present volume argue, if small farmers were systematically taught the use of selected traditional home remedies, it would improve the routine healthcare of their animals and considerably reduce their veterinary expenses. To the extent that proven traditional botanicals can be cultivated, packaged and marketed commercially, there is also considerable scope for the growth of a national industry in indigenous-based veterinary pharmaceuticals. In fact, about 60 to 80 small industrial units in India presently produce trademarked herbal veterinary medicines. There are both problems and prospects in this industry.

On the problem side of this equation is the question of quality control. Although the industry claims that its pharmaceutical formulations are based on research, likely many preparations are derived empirically, with physicians and veterinarians collecting the prescriptions from stockraisers and then reporting them to the enterprises. Many such remedies contain a large number of different plants, and the dosages have not been scientifically verified. Only recently has a progressive trend toward organized research emerged in this respect.

Cost is another problem. Manufacturers' profit margins are high. Small farmers have to pay more for these ready-made drugs than it would cost them if they used crude plant materials as prescribed by local healers and veterinarians. For example, proprietary galactagogues containing LR with *Asparagus racemosus* or *Breynia patens* and some other ingredients cost about 60 to 80 Indian rupees (approximately US$2.00 to $2.60) per animal to treat agalactia.[3] The same treatment would cost only 5 to 10 rupees ($0.16 to $0.33) if crude, dried LR powder were used. Compared to the commercial preparation, the crude LR treatment gives the same or even better results; likewise for some commercial, botanically-based antidiarrhoeals.

On the other hand, proprietary herbal remedies do provide cheaper alternatives to many kinds of costly Western drugs. For example, in Sri Lanka, 18 such remedies for miscellaneous livestock ills were tested and found effective. Illustrating from just one of these 18—a herbal wound powder found to be as effective as Hoechst's Negusant™ powder—the local formulation cost 80 to 90 per cent less than the Western equivalent (Anjaria 1986a). If all 18 of these medicines were substituted for their Western equivalents, treatment costs to stockraisers would be cut by an estimated 60 to 75 per cent (Anjaria 1986a).

The optimal solution may lie in a combined approach. Stockraisers could be taught to prepare or improve upon simple home remedies themselves (also see Grandin and Young, this volume, Roepke, this volume). At the same time dairy co-operatives[4] and/or government agencies could oversee quality control in the production of proprietary herbal drugs and ensure that profits and prices are fair to the manufacturers and their customers, respectively. Another possibility is for co-operatives or states to manufacture traditional drugs themselves. In the author's opinion, such a move would furnish 40 to 60 per cent more drugs for the same amount of money. Any of these strategies would also help guarantee farmers a more ready supply of basic veterinary pharmaceuticals than the present, heavy reliance on imported drugs. These considerations of cost and availability are of great concern to stockraisers and local veterinary practitioners alike.

The growth of a national industry in indigenous drugs could also provide jobs, stimulate local economies and protect natural resources. Currently, the ethnopharmaceutical industry either gathers its raw materials directly from the forests and fields or purchases them from middlemen and traders. Recently, however, a few cooperatives have formed to regulate the harvesting and sale of medicinal plants. The author has visited one such co-op organized by inhabitants of the Gir forest of Gujarat State. Another area for national growth and development lies in the establishment of private clinics within the traditional veterinary service sector. An example is provided by a traditional healer in a village of Madhya

Pradesh. For over 50 years, this individual has run an animal clinic using only traditional remedies. According to reports during the author's fieldwork in the area, this clinic has successfully met virtually all of the villages' healthcare needs for their cattle.

At the international level, medicinal plants also have great export potential. Although synthetic organics have captured a substantial share of the global pharmaceutical market, plant-derived substances are still a vital part of modern medicine. For example, in 1973 community pharmacies in the United States dispensed 1 532 billion new and refilled prescriptions, some 25 per cent of which contained at least one active constituent from higher (seed) plants (Quimby 1977). If microbial and other natural products are included, prescriptions derived from natural sources accounted for almost 50 per cent of all drugs sold. Moreover, the Western market for natural medicines for humans is growing. It would not be surprising if the veterinary sector followed this trend.

It has been estimated that more than 75 per cent of the plants known in the Indian, UK and US pharmacopoeia grow in one or another part of India. Over the last 30 years, India has developed an industry of medicinal plants and phytochemicals with an annual volume of trade of more than one billion Indian rupees (INR). The total export of medicinal plants (including opium) increased from INR310.44 million in 1974/5 to INR450.99 million in 1977/8 (Chemexil 1986, GEC 1987, World Drug Market Manual 1982–3, cited in UNCTAD/GATT 1982). These figures include various items traditionally used in veterinary treatments.

Exports of veterinary herbal remedies may have a promising future, provided manufacturers declare the formulation and do quality-control testing as required by the registration regulations of many countries worldwide. Even now, some Indian manufacturers export trademarked veterinary drugs to the tune of INR4–6 million per annum through approved export agents (GEC 1987, UNCTAD/ GATT 1982). Laws to regulate and standardize manufacturing quality and processes in traditional formulations would give added impetus to the export of veterinary pharmaceuticals. At the national level, a more active export market would earn the country more foreign currency while simultaneously saving on exchange reserves for imports of drugs that cannot feasibly be produced in India. Appropriate laws might also facilitate collaboration and interchange of traditional veterinary remedies, resources, and information among Asian nations generally. Still, much more scientific work is needed to identify, and confirm the validity of, traditional botanicals. Of the 2 500 plants covered in Iyengar's bibliography, only 1.9 per cent reached the clinical trial stage; most were not investigated beyond the preliminary screening stage (Vohora 1989). More than 50 per cent of the plants studied were mentioned in only one paper; about 90 per cent had five or fewer entries, and only 37 (2.2 per cent) of 1 691 plants were studied for four to five pharmacological aspects. More, and more complete, scientific research would help to bolster the continued development of both national and international industries in ethnoveterinary pharmaceuticals. The ultimate result would be increased productivity, security, and income not only for nations but also for small farmers throughout Asia.

Notes

In the references for this chapter, the author was sometimes unable to cite page numbers because reprints of several Indian journals (for example, *Pashudhan,* published by the drug company Indian Herbs) do not reflect the actual page numbers of a publication. The same applies to early volume and issue numbers of articles from *Indian Drugs* (published by the Indian Drug Manufacturers Organization), copies of which show only the month of publication.

1. Examples and descriptions of such practices in different regions of India are found in FAO 1984a and in the first four volumes of the *Bulletin of Medico-EthnoBotanical Research* published by the Central Council of Research in Ayurveda and Siddha. Others are discussed in Malik *et al.*, this volume.
2. These are rough estimates based on the author's years of experience in the Indian pharmacological industry and fieldwork with farmers.
3. At the time of writing (late 1992), US$1.00 equalled 30 Indian rupees.
4. India has the largest co-operative dairy industry in Asia.

14. Ethnoveterinary medicine in western India

JITENDRA K. MALIK, ASWIN M. THAKER
AND ALLAUDDIN AHMAD

IN INDIA, LIVESTOCK farming forms an integral part of a diversified agricultural regime. Besides providing food (milk, meat, eggs) and raw materials such as fibre, skins, hides and manure, livestock constitute one of the main sources of traction. Agricultural productivity itself depends largely upon draught animals, which are critical for land preparation and cultivation. Indian farmers are becoming increasingly concerned about animal health because they see veterinary care as one of the most cost-effective ways to increase farm profitability.

However, modern veterinary assistance is not available in many of the more remote parts of India. There, people instead have recourse to home remedies derived from centuries of experience. Stockowners also consult local healers who possess diagnostic and therapeutic skills for many animal health problems that have clear clinical signs. The healers employ herbal and other medicines as well as drug-free treatments. Indeed, wherever indigenous veterinary medications and practitioners are to be found, farmers throughout India consider them cheap, safe and effective. Local people usually turn to these traditional veterinary resources first. Some stockowners further believe that traditional veterinary remedies can often succeed where modern ones fail.

Of course, not all traditional animal remedies can be or have been validated on scientific grounds. But certainly there are many indigenous drugs of great utility. And as indicated in Table 14.1 (displayed at the end of this chapter and in the preceeding chapter), there is a large and growing body of scientific literature on the practical veterinary potentials of medicinal plants in India. Based on this literature and on the authors' own research, this chapter describes selected ethnoveterinary practices still used today in western India.

Particular emphasis is given here to ethno-botanicals, because plants to treat and prevent animal illness and to promote livestock health and reproduction are perhaps the most prominent weapon in India's ethnoveterinary armoury. Stockowners believe that such plants, which are usually native to the local area, help an animal to recover on its own and/or correct functional abnormalities. Depending upon the disorder, a single plant or a combination of plants may be used, along with other, non-botanical, ingredients. Often, more than one remedy is available to treat or prevent a given disease.

As in human ethnomedicine, the use of the whole plant material is generally considered more satisfactory because various substances present in different parts of the plant may enhance absorption, add to the biochemical action of other ingredients or reduce undesirable side-effects. However, biological activity may be greater in certain parts of the plant—the leaf, flower, fruit, herb (that is, the finer stems, leaves and flowers), young wood or bark of the shoots, and roots or root bark. Bark, wood and roots are normally harvested in the autumn. Other plant materials are gathered in the morning, after the dew has dried. The timing of collection is important if the items are to be dried or further processed. Before drying, bark and wood are cut into small pieces; roots are cleaned, washed and chopped. All such material is best dried at room temperature in a shaded place with good ventilation. Botanicals are administered to animals in both fresh and dried form or in infusions and decoctions. In general, decoctions are more appropriate for bark, wood and roots.

The following sections describe just a few of the many therapeutic and prophylactic uses of botanical and other materials in farm-animal healthcare in western India. Insofar as possible, these are grouped by the problems they are intended to combat. But general and supernatural aspects of animal healthcare are also mentioned.

Traditional livestock practices

External injuries

There are numerous and often very effective home remedies to treat and relieve the pain of external injuries such as burns, abscesses and wounds. *Cyamopsis tetragonoloba* leaves and tea granules are commonly used for all such problems. Especially popular is a finely sieved ash of peacock feathers mixed with coconut oil. This preparation is used on many kinds of injuries because it repels flies. Specifically for burns, this peacock preparation is applied three times daily. But burns can instead be treated with a mixture of two parts honey to one part red lead, or with honey followed by red lead. Alternatively, the lesions may be dressed with a paste of fresh *Zizyphus jujuba* leaves mixed with groundnut oil (Patel 1967).

Abscesses are treated with various poultices and other preparations, for example: a warm mixture of one part turmeric and salt to two parts soap and groundnut oil; two parts wheat flour, one part salt, six pinches of turmeric, and four parts milk of giant swallow-wort (*Calotropis gigantea*); a mixture of groundnut oil, giant swallow-wort milk and red lead; or simply the milk of the common hedge cactus. A paste of 500g of granulated sugar in 500ml of polyethylene glycol and 0.5 per cent volume/weight (v/w) of hydrogen peroxide is reportedly particularly effective for large abscess cavities in domestic animals. It results in complete debridement, a significant reduction in the microbial population, and healing of the wound cavity within 18 to 25 days (Varshney *et al.* 1989).

Fresh human urine is poured on accidental wounds. And a bullock's urine may be applied to its hump to prevent yoke gall. Ewes' milk is massaged over fractures. Hoof wounds are dressed with a bandage containing a paste of calcium hydroxide and fresh custard apple leaves (*Annona squamosa*); the treated animal is then withdrawn from work in order to avoid complications. Alternatively, the wound cavity can be filled with oil from the seeds of the marking-nut tree (*Semecarpus anacardium*) and then cauterized.

The long horns of Zebu cattle and buffalo frequently sustain injuries. Horn wounds infested with maggots are thoroughly washed with a lukewarm aqueous decoction of neem leaves (*Azadirachta indica*) and then plugged with cotton soaked in turpentine (Gupt 1961). To arrest bleeding, a piece of gauze moistened with an aqueous solution of alum is applied to the wound. In cases of horn cancer, the horn is surgically removed and the cavity is washed as per the foregoing procedure; the wound is then packed with red lead containing a pinch of mercury and is bandaged. Another remedy is daily feeding a kilogram each of powdered *Trigonella foenum graeceum* and *Cassia tora* seeds after suspending them in four litres of water for about eight hours. Alternatively, 10g of powdered rabbit excreta mixed with jaggery (a crude, dark sugar) can be fed to the afflicted animal.

Ophthalmic disorders

Ophthalmic filariasis may be treated by applying a decoction of tobacco leaves to the eyes or, alternatively, a lukewarm, filtered aqueous decoction of neem leaves and salt. Salt and jowar millet (*Sorghum vulgare*) are sprinkled into the eyes of animals with conjunctivitis. To treat cataracts, the following may be applied to the affected eyes: finely crushed alum and fresh yellow turmeric in onion juice; a mixture or a decoction of tobacco, calcium hydroxide and salt; or ghee and salt. In yet another cataract treatment, part of the eyebrow is surgically removed using a sharp earthen instrument or a knife, and oil from the seeds of the marking-nut tree is applied to the eye with a bit of cotton; the animal is then kept out of the sunlight until it recovers—reportedly within about eight days (Patel 1967). An alternative treatment is cauterization (ibid.).

Ectoparasitism

For mange and other skin diseases, the essential oil of *Cedrus deodara* wood is applied externally. Ectoparasites can also be combated by thoroughly washing the afflicted animal with a lukewarm aqueous decoction of neem leaves and then massaging castor oil or neem-seed oil into the infested areas. An aqueous extract of *Ipomoea carnea* leaves in concentrations ranging from 0.25 per cent to 2 per cent is used against mites and lice on buffalo (Tirkey *et al.* 1988). Two other indigenous washes are: a lukewarm decoction of 1 kg of the bark of the bottle-guard shrub in five l of water; and 10 l of boiled water with 200g of tobacco, 100g of washing soda, 20g of calcium hydroxide, and 20g of salt or 10g of morphine. Finally, as a preventive measure, small smoke fires (usually of neem) are lit in animal quarters to drive off flies and mosquitoes during the evening.

Gastrointestinal disorders

Farm animals poisoned by consuming potatoes or potato leaves experience tympany and impaction. Treatment consists of drenching with 2.5 parts henna leaves (*Lawsonia alba*) and 10 parts coriander leaves, finely crushed and mixed in 80 parts water and then stored in a new earthen pot for 12 hours. This mixture is given twice daily until the animal recovers. It may be accompanied by 12 drops of lemon juice in both eyes twice daily. In addition, water is sprinkled on the poisoned animal. Alternatively, the patient may be covered with a wet gunny sack or cloth. For tympany suspected to result from excessive consumption of green fodder, castor oil or asafoetida (a carminative) are given as a drench. For tympany in general, ruminants can also be cauterized on the left flank. Alternatively, a 5cm incision may be made in the ear. Camels suffering from colic are purged with dried fish or a decoction of custard apple leaves.

Livestock owners take a systematic approach to countering diarrhoea in large ruminants. First, any fodder suspected of causing the diarrhoea is withdrawn. Second, a laxative/purgative consisting of 150ml of castor oil and 50g of powdered rock salt is given orally. Third, the animal is drenched with one of several preparations: 10g of finely crushed *Cannabis sativa* in about 1.5kg of curd, given twice daily; a sieved infusion of crushed *Ailanthus excelsa* bark in whey; 10g of henna leaves and 200g of fresh coriander leaves kept overnight in an earthen pot with 500ml of water and then administered twice daily for the first two days, and once daily thereafter; approximately 200g of crushed *Dalbergia sissoo* leaves in 800ml of water, given twice daily; or about 250ml of rice gruel containing a triturated mixture of 20g of bishop's weed (*Carum copticum*) seeds,

20g of catechu (an astringent obtained from acacias), and 30g of *Foeniculum vulgare* (Gupt 1961). For treating ascariasis in calves, *Canscora diffusa* is given orally. To prevent these and other intestinal worms, young calves are not allowed to suckle colostrum.

Reproductive and related disorders

For uterine prolapse, an extract of *Dudhiyo vachhanag* gathered during the monsoon season is mixed with colostrum from a buffalo's first lactation. After steeping for approximately 15 days, this preparation is topically applied to the prolapsed part of the genital tract, which has first been cleaned with onion water. Then the prolapsed part is corrected manually and, if necessary, trussed. For prepartum prolapse, the animal is drenched with a decoction of henna leaves in water. For recurrent prolapse, the animal is fed black gram, ghee, morphine and jowar millet, and the prolapsed part is topically treated with an extract of onion combined with morphine. Applying salt to the prolapsed part of the genitalia is another traditional remedy—as is cauterization, which has been successfully used as a styptic in such cases (Mathew 1990).

For expulsion of the placenta, 800g of *Urginea indica* bark and 20g of bishop's-weed seeds are crushed and combined with 20 g of jaggery. All these ingredients are boiled in 2.5 l of water until the volume is reduced to about 1 litre. After being filtered, the liquid is given twice daily. An alternative drench is crushed seeds of bishop's weed that have been boiled in linseed oil. Other practices include: drenching with a decoction of bamboo strips and leaves in water; feeding millet mixed with wood ash or sugar-cane leaves; and washing the external genitalia and expelled placenta with an aqueous decoction of neem leaves.

Garlic is sometimes used to treat nonspecific uterine infections in dairy cattle. Research reveals that the intrauterine administration of 20ml of garlic extract in water (1:5w/v) at 24-hour intervals is effective in controlling microbial infections of the reproductive tract in repeat breeding cows (Garg *et al.* 1983). Topical applications of alum or its aqueous solution are used to control uterine bleeding. Dairy animals suffering from downer cow syndrome and milk fever are drenched with wine. In cases of milk fever, stockowners may also cauterize the tips of the horns.

To treat mastitis, the affected area is washed with a lukewarm aqueous decoction of neem leaves and then massaged with coconut or sesame oil. In addition, a drench of one part powdered *Datura alba* root and two parts jaggery is administered twice daily until the animal is cured. Oral administration of camphor and banana is also recommended. Physical methods, too, are employed in treating mastitis. For example, milk collected from the affected quarter is poured on burning coals in a vessel placed under the udder. The fumes thus generated reportedly afford the animal some relief; likewise for cauterization above the base of the tail and below the external genitalia.

Dairy animals that fail to go into heat are fed fruits of the marking-nut tree. A deficient sex drive in adult bulls and male buffalo is countered with a month-long daily drench of equal parts of sesame or linseed oil and sugar, or of one part powdered catechu to five parts ghee. Some stockowners also feed 250g to 500g of wheat, barley or millet (*Pennisetum glaucum*) sprouts twice daily for 30 to 45 days (Gupt 1961, Patel 1967). Yet another preparation consists of 1.25kg of gram pulse in one litre of cow's milk soaked for four to six hours and then diluted with

500ml of water and reinforced with jaggery. The bulls are rested throughout the treatment period. After natural service or artificial insemination, repeat breeders are drenched with castor oil or sugar to ensure that they will conceive. Also, red silica may be rubbed on their bodies.

Dietary deficiencies

In western India, cotton-seed cake has long been fed to farm animals as a nutritional supplement. Linseed or sesame oil is given to working bulls and calving animals. Besides providing a concentrated source of energy, these oils have an antizymotic action. Weeds can also play an important role in animal nutrition. In some regions of Gujarat State, for example, farmers with large fodder needs leave extra space between crop rows; the weeds that grow up between the rows are harvested as fodder. Jowar millet is harvested for green fodder after it has been exposed to two or three rains so as to prevent hydro-cyanic acid poisoning when the sorghum is consumed. To test the safety of this fodder, the first time it is harvested, it is fed to less productive or old animals.

Other health problems

Cattle and buffalo with gout are fed camel-bone meal. *Citrus medica* or a decoction thereof in water is given orally for retention of urine; an alternative is cauterization on the perineum. An aqueous decoction of *gokhru* (*Hygrophila spinosa*) seeds and tea granules is used as a diuretic. Tea granules alone serve as an antitoxin for *Ricinus communis* poisoning. Topical applications of alum or its aqueous solution are used to treat rhinitis. A lotion prepared from *Tamarindus indica*, *Rubia cordifolia* and henna leaves in water is poured on the forehead of animals bleeding from the nose.

A topical preparation of 540ml of *karanj* (*Pongamia glabra* Linn.) oil, 180ml each of garlic and onion extracts, 80ml of lemon juice, and 10g each of turmeric and camphor is used to treat ringworm in cattle. The preparation is applied daily to the affected areas after cleaning them with a decoction of *babul* (*Acacia arabica*). To be successful, treatment generally requires 12 to 15 days (Sharma and Dwivedi 1990).

As we have seen, cauterization is a common, multi-purpose therapeutic technique. In addition to the uses cited earlier, it may be applied to the affected parts of rheumatic bullocks. It is also used for lameness and dengue fever (Patel 1967). Surgical removal of ear tips is another common therapy for several diseases, among them tympany and contagious caprine pleuro-pneumonia. For some ailments, ear-cropping may be accompanied by sprinkling powdered black pepper into the sick animal's eyes.

Buffalo threatened with heat stroke are bathed with water. To ward against the winter cold, animals are provided beddings of dried sugar-cane leaves or paddy straw. To forestall foot-and-mouth disease, people keep dried fish in animal quarters.

Supernatural beliefs and practices also play a role in Indian animal healthcare. Many rural people believe that high-yielding dairy animals and male calves or bulls of good quality are subject to the evil eye of jealous people. Evil eye is diagnosed by symptoms such as loss of appetite, lethargy, nervousness and a sudden drop in milk yield. A garland of 15 *Terminalia belerica* fruits is tied around the afflicted animal's neck. If any fruit falls off the garland, this constitutes a positive diagnosis of evil eye. The fallen fruit is then replaced.

No further detachment of fruit from the garland indicates recovery from the evil eye (Patel 1967).

For the general prevention of animal ills, many farmers of Gujarat State seek to enlist God's aid by observing *Anuja* at least twice each year. In *Anuja*, stockowners do not sell their animals' milk for one or two days. Instead, they distribute it free to relatives, friends and saints, thus earning God's blessing and protection.

Conclusions

During recent years, stockraising has taken great strides toward meeting India's increased agricultural needs. One of the major factors responsible for such progress has been improved health coverage for farm animals. Across the past decade, veterinary services provided by government, co-operative and other agencies have been greatly strengthened; and veterinary hospitals all over the country are now staffed by trained veterinarians. Nevertheless, many areas still lack adequate access to modern veterinary services.

Fortunately, the past decade has also seen a great upsurge of interest in and research on indigenous herbal drugs in India. Major biomedical laboratories and medical organizations, plus a few veterinary institutions, are now screening numerous ethnobotanicals for pharmacological effects (see again Table 1, plus Anjaria, this volume). This work has been undertaken largely with human patients in mind. The positive results of such investigations, however, strongly suggest that many ethnoveterinary botanicals may be equally useful, since many of the same items are employed for both human beings and animals. Moreover, pharmacological evaluation of plants has mostly been performed with animal models. Hence, information about potential veterinary value can be gleaned from these experiments.

The validity of many traditional Indian remedies—including many of the treatments for microbial infections, parasitic diseases, gastrointestinal problems and reproductive dysfunctions—has already been substantiated by scientific research. And it appears that most traditional Indian herbal remedies for domestic animals are safe at the prescribed dosages. Moreover, some of these remedies are even capable of treating diseases for which modern medicine has not yet found a satisfactory or lasting solution. There is great need to unravel the mysteries of the indigenous pharmacopoeia and unearth its hidden treasures through scientific study. If research in human ethnomedicine is any guide, ethnoveterinary pharmacology has much to offer in the way of potent, inexpensive, accessible and safe drugs to treat and prevent animal health problems.

Table 1. Pharmacology of indigenous medicinal plants with actual or potential veterinary utility

Plant name	Plant part, preparation, active ingredient	Medicinal value	References
Acacia auriculiformis	Plant, without root	Antiviral	Rastogi and Dhawan 1982
Acanthus illicifolius	Methanolic extract of leaves	Analgesic, anti-inflammatory	Agshikar et al. 1979
Adhatoda vasica	Leaves	Wound healing	Bhargava et al. 1988
	Alcoholic and chloroform extracts	Antifungal	Malik et al. 1991a
Aegle marmelos	Ethyl acetate extract	Antibacterial, antifungal	Rusia and Srivastava 1988
Aerna lanata	Aqueous extract	Diuretic	Udupihille and Jiffry 1986
Aglaia roxburghiana	Plant, without root	Antiviral	Rastogi and Dhawan 1982
Allium sativum	Crude extract of bulb	Antibacterial	Sharma et al. 1977
	Alcoholic extract	Antifungal	Malik et al. 1991a, Kumar and Gupta 1984
Alpinia officinarum	Flavonoid	Antifungal	Ray and Majumdar 1976
Anaphalis controta	Whole plant	Antibacterial	Sinha et al. 1977
Annona squamosa	Leaves	Antimicrobial, wound healing	Thaker and Anjaria 1986
Arbenia nobilis	Arnebin	Antifungal	Wahab et al. 1982
		Anticancer	Katti et al. 1979
Asparagus racemosus	Root	Lactogenic, galactogogue	Satyavati et al. 1976
Atylosia trinervia	Atylosol-biphenyl	Antibacterial	Tripathi et al. 1977, 1978a
Azadirachta indica	Oil	Wound healing	Bhargava et al. 1989
	Chloroform extract	Fungicidal	Mishra and Sahu 1977 Thaker and Anjaria 1986
	Leaves	Antimicrobial, wound healing	
Bergenia lingulata	Ethanolic extract of root	Analgesic, anti-inflammatory	Gehlot et al. 1976
Bergia odorata	Leaves	Antimicrobial, wound healing	Thaker and Anjaria 1986

Species	Preparation	Activity	Reference
Blumea membranacea	Essential oil	CNS depressant	Mehta et al. 1986
		Antibacterial	Zutshi et al. 1976
Bridelia retusa	Bark of stem	Antiviral	Rastogi and Dhawan 1982
Butea frondosa	Alcoholic extract of seeds	Anthelmintic (*Ascaridia galli*)	Lal et al. 1976
Calophyllum inophyllum	Xanthones	Analgesic, anti-inflammatory	Gopalakrishnan et al. 1980
Carica papaya	Alcoholic extract of seeds, fruit juice	Anthelmintic (*Ascaridia galli*)	Lal et al. 1976
Cassia auriculata	Plant, without root	Antiviral	Rastogi and Dhawan 1982
Cassia fistula	Whole plant	Antiviral	Rastogi and Dhawan 1982
Crataeva nurvala	Ether extract of bark	Urinary disorders	Deshpande et al. 1982
Curcuma amada	Rhizomes	Antifungal	Ghosh et al. 1980
Curcuma angustifolia	Essential oil	Antifungal	Banerjee and Nigam 1977
Curcuma aromatica	Essential oil	Antifungal	Rao 1976
Curcuma caesia	Essential oil	Antifungal	Banerjee and Nigam 1976
Curcuma longa	Ether and chloroform, extracts of stem	Fungistatic	Mishra and Sahu 1977
Cynodon dactylon	Essential oil	Antibacterial	Zutshi et al. 1976
Cythocline lyrate	Whole plant	Antiviral	Rastogi and Dhawan 1982
Embelia ribes	Essential oil	Antibacterial	Zutshi et al. 1976
	Embelin	Analgesic, antipyretic, anti-inflammatory	Gupta et al. 1977
Euphorbia thymifolia	Ether extract	Antifungal, antimicrobial	Khan et al. 1988

Table 1. (continued)

Plant name	Plant part, preparation, active ingredient	Medicinal value	References
Evodia lunu-ankenda	Alkaloids	Antibacterial	Rastogi and Dhawan 1982
Grewia hirsuta	Whole plant	Antiviral	Rastogi and Dhawan 1982
Hedychinum spicatum	Essential oil	Antibacterial	Sinha *et al.* 1977
Inula racemosa	Alantolactone, isoalantolactone	Antidermatophytic	Tripathi *et al.* 1978b
Laggera aurita	Essential oil	Antibacterial	Zutshi *et al.* 1976
Leptadenia reticulata	Stigmasterol	Lactogenic	Anjaria *et al.* 1975
Lycopersicum esculentum	Ether extract of leaves	Local anesthetic	Malik *et al.* 1991b, Singh *et al.* 1978
Mesua ferrea	Xanthones	Analgesic, anti-inflammatory	Gopalakrishnan *et al.* 1980
Millingtonia hortensis	Glycosides	Diuretic	Kar *et al.* 1976
Mimordia charantia	Fruit juice	Anthelmintic (*Ascaridia galli*)	Lal *et al.* 1976
Morinda citrifolia	Ethanolic extract	Antifungal	Rusia and Srivastava 1988
Mucuna pruriens	Ether and chloroform extracts of seeds	Fungistatic	Mishra and Sahu 1977
Ocimum sanctum	Leaves	Antimicrobial, wound healing	Thaker and Anjaria 1986
Olea polygama	Plant, without root	Antiviral	Rastogi and Dhawan 1982
Palma rosa	Essential oil	Antibacterial	Zutshi *et al.* 1976
Picrorhiza kurroa	Water soluble fraction of alcoholic rhizome extract	Anti-inflammatory	Pandey and Das 1989
Pongamia glabra	Oil	Fungicidal	Mishra and Sahu 1977
Prosopis juliflora	Alcoholic and chloroform extracts of leaves	Antibacterial	Malik *et al.* 1988
	Juice of leaves	Antifungal, antibacterial	Sarvaiya *et al.* 1990

Psoralea corylifolia	Bavachinin	Analgesic, anti-inflammatory	Anand et al. 1978
	Essential oil	Antibacterial	Zutshi et al. 1976
Psychotria truncata	Plant, without root	Antiviral	Rastogi and Dhawan 1982
Rumex maritimus	Emodin	Antifungal	Agarwal et al. 1976
Salvia lanata	Essential oil	Antibacterial	Sinha et al. 1977
Sapindus trifoliatus	Aqueous extract of pericarp of dried fruits	Anthelmintic (Ascaridia galli)	Lal et al. 1976
Sapium eugnifolium	Ethyl acetate extract	Antibacterial, antifungal	Rusia and Srivastava 1988
Saussurea lappa	Alcoholic extract of root	Antifungal	Ray and Majumdar 1977
Schima wallichii	Saponin	Antifungal	Chandel and Rastogi 1978
Tephrosea purpurea	Alcoholic extract of root	Antimicrobial	Agarwal et al. 1987
Tinospora cordifolia	Aqueous extract of stem	Analgesic, anti-inflammatory	Pendse et al. 1977
Toddalia asiatica	Coumarins and alkaloids	Diuretic	Rastogi and Dhawan 1982
Vanda parviflora	Whole plant	Antiviral	Rastogi and Dhawan 1982
Vernonia cinera	Alcoholic extract	Wound healing	Bhargava et al. 1989
Vitex negundo	Ethanolic extract	Antibacterial, antifungal	Rusia and Srivastava 1988
Zingiber capitatum	Whole plant	Antiviral	Rastogi and Dhawan 1982

15. Banjarese management of duck health and nutrition

PATRICIA J. VONDAL

SOUTH-EAST ASIA has been a major regional centre of duck domestication. Ducks have been raised in Malaysia and Indonesia for at least 2000 years (Clayton 1972). In parts of Indonesia, duck farming has been an important element in the agricultural economy for centuries. One such area is Indonesian Borneo's South Kalimantan Province, where Banjarese farmers have long kept Alabio ducks (*Anas platyrhynchos borneo*), famed for their high egg production (Chávez and Lasmini 1978, Kingston *et al.* 1979, Robinson *et al.* 1977). Other well-known centres of duck farming in Indonesia include Central Java, where the Tegal duck has traditionally been herded across the island following the rice harvest from Cirebon to Jakarta, and Bali, where flocks of Bali ducks foraging in harvested rice fields are a common sight.[1]

Alabio duck farming in South Kalimantan occupies a niche in an agricultural system primarily characterized by wet rice cultivation. Because of annual flooding, however, a purely subsistence economy based on rice production is not feasible. Rural households therefore pursue a mix of economic activities. In addition to growing rice, vegetables and ducks, they also produce a number of items for sale in regional markets. These items include such things as home-made rattan furniture, woven mats and roofing materials, handmade clothing and embroidery, bamboo fish traps, and fish caught in local waterways. Like duck raising, trading is a time-honoured occupation in South Kalimantan. For centuries, Banjarese traders have bought and sold these locally manufactured and gathered goods throughout Borneo, and to Java and other islands of Indonesia.

Poultry products, particularly duck eggs, have figured in this commercial trade network for well over 100 years. Traditionally, ducks were raised under a system of extensive management in which flocks were daily herded on the many rivers, flood plains and freshwater swamps that dominate the provincial landscape. In the 1970s, however, this traditional system underwent a dramatic change. It moved from an extensive, herding regime to an intensive one entailing permanent caging of the birds. This change occurred in response to several interlocking factors. First, more and more land was put into rice cultivation in order to feed a burgeoning human population; thus, land for herding flocks became scarce. Second, the burgeoning population in the urban areas of South Kalimantan made for a sharp increase in consumer demand for poultry products. This in turn led to larger flock sizes.

The shift from extensive to intensive duck farming had immediate implications for the management of flock health. After a brief overview of the dynamics of the duck industry, this chapter describes the preventive measures that farmers have developed to ensure good health and high productivity in their flocks. The data presented here derive from 14 months of fieldwork in 1981–3 among Banjarese farmers in South Kalimantan's North Hulu Sungai Regency. This region forms the centre of South Kalimantan's poultry industry, which emphasizes production of non-fertile eggs for the consumer market.

Research was conducted in two adjoining Banjarese villages noted for their highly successful specialization in non-fertile eggs. All duck-farming households

(N=75) in each village were systematically interviewed. A formal questionnaire was administered to these households once during the dry season and again during the wet season so as to capture seasonal differences in flock management practices. The questionnaire collected data on duck rearing, marketing patterns, feed mixtures, local concepts of flock disease and methods of disease prevention, and allocation of family labour in the household poultry enterprise. In addition to these two large-scale surveys, a random sample of 10 per cent of the study households was visited weekly over a six-month period for in-depth interviews and participant observation. These families were also asked to keep daily egg-production records.[2]

Commercial duck farming in South Kalimantan

In South Kalimantan, ducks traditionally were herded on waterways, where they fed on small fish, snails, and swamp and riverine vegetation. These items are especially plentiful during the rainy season. After the yearly rice harvest, the flocks were also allowed to forage in the fields for insects, fallen grain and other vegetation. The birds were lured back to their cages at night with supplementary feed, primarily chopped sago palm. Ducks were traditionally raised for both meat and eggs. Male ducklings were sold for fattening and resale to small restaurants and roadside stalls featuring roast duck in chilli sauce. Females were sold for meat only after they passed their egg-laying prime.

Until the 1970s many households pursued a combination of fertile and non-fertile egg production, hatching and duckling raising for the consumer market. Although a tendency to specialize in one or another of these activities had been occurring for approximately 100 years in some villages, in the 1970s specialization became firmly established during the rapid evolution of a highly commercialized poultry industry. Many Banjarese farmers chose to specialize in non-fertile duck eggs, which fetch high prices in the local weekly markets. For this purpose, they purchase five- to seven-day-old female chicks from hatchery operators in nearby villages.

Gradually, these farmers created a new and highly intensive system of flock management based on farmyard caging of mature birds. At first, the birds were caged only during the cultivation season, to keep the now-much-larger flocks from invading rice fields. However, people soon noticed that, with caging and the presentation of feed, their ducks laid more eggs. Flock owners further noted that first moulting occurred at a later age in caged as distinct from herded flocks. This is important because, after the first moult, egg production permanently drops. Another benefit of caging is reduced labour costs. A family member will no longer be required to stay with the flock throughout the entire day, as the former system required.

As the benefits of the new system became apparent, it spread to all the villages in the seasonally flooded zones of North Hulu Sungai Regency, giving great impetus to the area's commercial egg industry. Now, ducks are permanently caged from the beginning of their productive life, at six months of age. However, ducklings are still herded in the traditional manner—in part, to provide them with healthy exercise (see below) and in part to conserve on feed costs.

Duck diseases and prevention strategies

Banjarese duck farmers have always emphasized disease prevention because they recognize that treatment is very difficult and largely ineffective. They also note that some diseases, though rare, are highly contagious and can wipe out entire flocks virtually overnight.

Under the new, intensive system of management, prevention has become even more important, for two reasons at least. First, in today's highly commercialized poultry industry, ducks represent a substantial monetary investment. Many Banjarese farmers in North Hulu Sungai Regency now rely almost exclusively on egg sales for the economic support of their households. Their duck farms are truly commercial enterprises. Second, with permanent caging and the consequent concentration of animals, the threat of disease is much greater. In particular, if proper attention is not paid to sanitation, disease can rapidly spread in confined flocks (IEMVT 1987).

It is probably safe to say that, given their centuries-old tradition of duck raising, local farmers themselves are the best source of information on duck health and disease prevention in the regency. At present no clinically trained veterinarians are stationed there. While some livestock health services are available from the government-run regency-level animal husbandry office (Dinas Peternakan), Banjarese villagers do not frequent this agency because of its distant location and the high cost of its services. Moreover, people know that the office staff have no training in duck diseases. The poultry services that the regional office does provide are limited to the extension of medicines and information for chickens, particularly for the exotic breeds introduced by the national government with the aim of upgrading local breeds.[3] Thus, in managing their flocks' health, Banjarese farmers draw on their own experiences, beliefs, and ancient store of knowledge about the requirements of Alabio ducks.[4]

Common diseases of the Alabio duck

The principal ailments known to affect ducks in Indonesia include: bacterial diseases such as salmonellosis, fowl cholera and bacterial infections of the digestive tract; viral infections such as Newcastle disease and infectious bronchitis; pneumonias of various etiologies; and illness arising from contamination and toxins such as aflatoxicosis (Hetzel and Sutikno dan Soeripto 1981, Kingston and Dharsana 1977, Nari *et al.* 1979, Prodjoharjono 1977, Soedjai 1974, Witono *et al.* 1981).

With the exception of pneumonia among ducklings (see below), the diseases that are reported to affect Alabio ducks generally have low mortality rates. Ailments vary somewhat according to the age of the bird. In general, young animals are more susceptible to disease than adult ones. Moreover, the fact that they are herded may expose ducklings to wild waterfowl and the diseases they carry. In consequence, Banjarese farmers apply different management strategies to ducklings than to mature birds. Significantly, epidemics with mortality rates of up to 50 per cent are very infrequent (Robinson *et al.* 1977, Vondal 1984), and during the 14 months of field research, there were no outbreaks of epidemic disease in any village in the regency.

Ducklings are susceptible to chills, colds, and more serious ills such as infectious bronchitis, sinusitis and pneumonia (IEMVT 1987, Prodjoharjono 1977, Rahardi and Kastyanto 1982). The chicks are particularly vulnerable during the first four weeks of life (Robinson *et al.* 1977, USDA 1973, Vondal 1984). Banjarese indicate that ducklings with colds (*balawa*, literally 'cold') may be sick for five to 10 days but do not become seriously ill. Informants add that colds typically occur with the twice yearly change of weather—at the onset of the dry season in April or May and at the beginning of the rainy season in September or October—when hot afternoons are often followed by cold nights. Banjarese clearly recognize the role of environmental stress in precipitating disease.

Ducklings that catch pneumonia are said to have *lumpuh* 'paralysis'. The clinical signs of *lumpuh* include loss of appetite; closed, runny eyes; and a hunching up of the wings into a frozen position (the 'paralysis'). Reportedly, the most serious bouts of colds and pneumonia occur among ducklings that have swum in water that suddenly changes from warm to cold. This often happens at the onset of the rainy season, when a hot day may be followed by a night of cold, heavy rain. Ducklings that swim the following morning are especially susceptible to *lumpuh*, say informants; and mortalities are high then (Kingston *et al.* 1979, Vondal 1984). However, other ducklings merely catch a cold for a few days. Several informants note that only the weaklings die.

Colds, pneumonia and other respiratory ills were formerly common among both immature and mature ducks. But with today's system of permanent caging at six months, these ills are now relatively rare in mature birds. Constant confinement protects them from stressful changes in water temperature. However, permanent caging favours other ills. Research indicates that the major health problems in older ducks in South Kalimantan are, in order of importance, salmonellosis, botulism and various forms of bacterial endoparasitism (Robinson *et al.* 1977). The principal symptoms of these ills include diarrhoea (*bahera*), lassitude, loss of appetite, moulting of protective feathers and depressed egg production (IEMVT 1987).

Permanent caging increases the chances of mature ducks' contracting these diseases. Large numbers of birds are confined in small enclosures; feed and water are set out in common dishes; and some feed components are stored in bulk in containers within the cage. These practices make for rapid build-up of faecal material in cages and dishes; and feed kept in prolonged storage under tropical conditions is especially vulnerable to rot and mould. Under these conditions birds can easily develop salmonellosis or botulism. Also, they may ingest internal parasites directly from faeces in their feed or in the bedding of their laying boxes. (Layers often peck at or eat their bedding, which is composed of such items as fresh banana leaves and swamp plants.) These diseases are then transmitted via the close contact in cages, particularly in large common units or overcrowded habitats (Cumming 1980, IEMVT 1987).

Disease prevention strategies

Banjarese farmers are very concerned with preventing disease in order to obtain consistently high levels of egg laying. Management practices reflect their concern. The major elements in Banjarese prevention strategies for duck diseases are: exercise for ducklings, so as to promote lifelong fitness; subdivision of flocks by age, size and health status; careful attention to good nutrition at all stages in the flock life cycle; and good hygiene in feeding, watering and caging. Because diseases differ according to the age of the duck, so do prophylactic strategies. Banjarese farmers uniformly state that the quality of care given ducklings is very important because it has a direct bearing on their health and productivity as mature layers. Flock owners aver that their careful care of ducklings results in more disease-resistant adult birds.

Exercise As noted, Banjarese believe that exercise plays an important role in duckling health. Once chicks are 45 days old, they are herded in fields and swamps where they scavenge for a wide variety of food. Farmers say the exercise of herding makes the birds more fit and more resistant to seriously debilitating disease. Some farmers provide additional exercise within the cage by tying strings on the sloping walls just above the ducklings' reach; the chicks constantly stretch up and hop about in an attempt to snatch at the bobbling strings. Farmers say this pastime exercises the muscles of the hindquarters, which figure in the ease of egg laying when the birds mature.

Subdivision of flocks Ducklings are separated from mature birds, either in a different cage or in a major division within a shared cage. This is done because ducklings require different feed from mature layers (see below). As the ducklings begin to mature at two-and-a-half months old, farmers build low bamboo partitions within the cage and separate birds of similar size into each division. Separate feed and water bowls are placed in each subdivision of the cage, and this practice is maintained throughout the life of the flock.

This subdivision strategy prevents larger ducklings from bullying smaller ones at feeding time. Differential growth rates within a flock can be perpetuated if smaller ducklings must compete with larger ones for feed. Farmers say that if ducklings are not thus separated, the result is a flock with many undernourished birds that are more prone to disease and therefore more likely to become poor layers. By dividing the flock by size, most ducklings will attain more or less equal body weight at maturity.

Mature ducks are penned together in a single cage, but they are separated by low partitions so that every 15 to 20 birds have their own feed and water dishes. This ensures each animal ready access to plentiful feed and water. This number seems to be optimal for controlling crowding, too. Farmers know that birds are overcrowded when the creatures begin to turn on each other, pecking and fighting among themselves within the cage.

Finally, to prevent the spread of contagion, farmers quarantine both ducklings and adults if one or more of the birds has clearly contracted an infection. Also, sick ducklings receive special attention, primarily in the form of extra feed, to nurse them back to health.

Nutrition Feed components are selected on the basis of their contribution to flock health and productivity. As with any animal, good nutrition is a key factor in preventing disease. Banjarese thus feed their ducks a rich, home-made mix of local freshwater snail meat, steamed fish, cooked rice, rice bran (*dedak*), and nowadays a multi-vitamin protein additive with the commercial name of Concentrate (see below). This feed mixture is the same for both adult and young birds, but duckling feed contains a higher proportion of fish. Flock owners say that, without the extra ration of fish, ducklings will not grow quickly and be healthy. Ducklings that are herded during the day are supplemented with a morning and evening ration of this mixture in the cage. Nutrient analysis of this feed shows that it furnishes a high-protein diet appropriate to young ducklings (Kingston *et al.* 1979).

For all caged birds, feed is presented three times a day, always at regular hours. Flock owners say that if the feeding schedule is varied, the birds become agitated and their egg production suffers. At each feeding, the feed is freshly mixed. The fish are caught locally every day. The rice is freshly cooked. And the bran, which is purchased at the weekly market, is always carefully inspected for quality and freshness. The principal indicators of freshness are a 'clean smell' and a lack of lumpiness. By 1981, several poultry feed shops in North Hulu Sungai Regency offered 'already complete' commercial feeds for sale. But farmers do not trust the freshness of store-bought feed. They emphasize that mixing one's own feed from locally available ingredients is the only way to guarantee freshness. In any case, people consider commercial feeds too expensive by comparison with their own, hand-mixed ones.

The use of 'Concentrate' is a recent innovation. According to local sources, this additive was first adopted by an entrepreneurial farmer who discovered it for sale in 1979 in the marketplace in Banjarmasin, the capital of South Kalimantan Province. 'Concentrate' contains protein, minerals and a multi-vitamin. It is manufactured by several major poultry feed companies in Java, and comes in different formulae for birds of different ages. Banjarese farmers, however, use the adult version for all age groups.

'Concentrate' quickly became a popular substitute for fresh fish during seasonal declines in local populations. The additive has also come to be regarded as an excellent tonic for promoting rapid growth in chicks and for preventing flock disease generally. Farmers report that duckling illness and mortality have declined dramatically since the advent of 'Concentrate'. They assert that it is especially helpful in protecting duckling health at the beginning of the rainy season, when fishing is poor and water temperatures fluctuate drastically. By 1981, all the market towns frequented by the region's duck farmers regularly carried 'Concentrate'. The stores also offer a number of other vitamin and mineral preparations and medicines for chickens and ducks. However, farmers continue to use only 'Concentrate' because of its perceived efficacy in disease prevention. Significantly, their name for this commercial dietary supplement is *obat* or 'medicine'.

'Concentrate' is also fed as an appetite enhancer, along with vegetation like *Hydrilla verticillata*, known locally as *ganggang*. This is a common freshwater swamp plant whose leaves float on the water. It is added to the feed of both ducklings and adults because farmers have observed that the birds often poke their heads out of their cages to peck at *ganggang* leaves as they float by. Laboratory analysis of the chemical composition of *Hydrilla* reveals a high (20 per cent) protein content (Murtisari 1983).

During the year, the type and quantity of feed components are changed according to their seasonal availability. The successful farmer is consistently able to provide his flock a nutritious diet by gradually introducing and replacing feed components while always keeping the protein amount constant. For example, as the local freshwater fish population declines with the onset of flooding, farmers gradually substitute salt-dried freshwater or marine fish. Banjarese have long known that sudden dietary shifts cause moulting, which temporarily suspends egg production until new feathers are grown.

Hygiene Along with 'freshness', farmers say cleanliness and dryness of feed are important in disease prevention. They clearly understand the relationship between contaminated feed and flock illness. They know from experience how quickly feed components become *sudah tua* 'rapidly spoiled' (lit. 'already old'). This is their way of glossing the fact that, in tropical climates, aflatoxins can build up rapidly in mouldy feedstuffs. If ingested, these toxins lower duck productivity and disease resistance, and can lead to death (Cumming 1980, Hetzel and Sutikuo dan Soeripto 1981, Nari *et al.* 1979). Rice bran, in particular, can spoil quickly in tropical temperatures and humidities. It is therefore purchased weekly and then stored in a well-ventilated place. All other components of the basic feed mixture are either collected daily or checked daily to ensure freshness. Furthermore, feed dishes are rinsed out every day.

People are also well aware that dirty water is bad for both young and mature birds. So the water in all cages is changed three times a day. All old water is discarded, and clean water is never dumped on top of old water. When the annual flooding occurs, water sources close to home become brackish. People therefore travel to open water free of flooded vegetation to collect fresh, clean drinking-water for their birds.

Banjarese are equally cognizant of the importance of cage sanitation in preventing disease. They recognize that faecal matter can contaminate food and water and lead to illness. So they construct the floors of duck cages from criss-crossed bamboo slatting. This design allows faeces to drop out of the cage (Plate 1). For chicks, the slats are placed closer together to give the birds a firm footing and keep them from getting their feet caught between the slats. When ducklings are two-and-a-half months old, the flooring is replaced with larger slats placed farther apart, to accommodate the increased number of faeces generated by the growing birds.

Duck cages are typically raised on stilts over permanent or semipermanent rivers or swamp water (Plate 2). Fallen faeces thus do not lie mouldering beneath the cage. Instead, they are cycled through the aquatic life below, which is in turn eaten by the ducks. For birds of all ages, floors are washed and scrubbed twice a month to remove all the accumulated faeces and feed. And all cages are constructed with high ceilings and generous spaces between the wall poles near the ceiling to allow for maximum ventilation. Finally, farmers

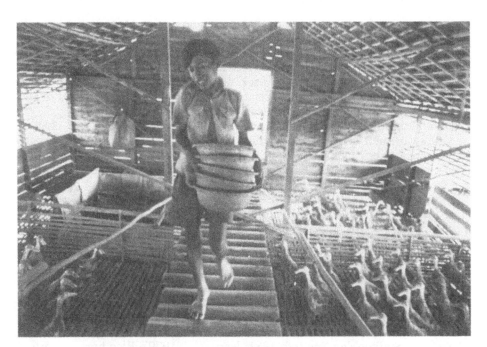

Plate 1. *Duck cages are built with water-resistant bamboo in an open-slat construc-tion so that wastes fall to the water below. To ensure good ventilation, the upper half of the side walls is also slatted. Note the interior divisions that separate ducks by size, for controlled feeding. The boy in the photo is bringing in tubs of fresh feed. (Photo by Victor Caldarola)*

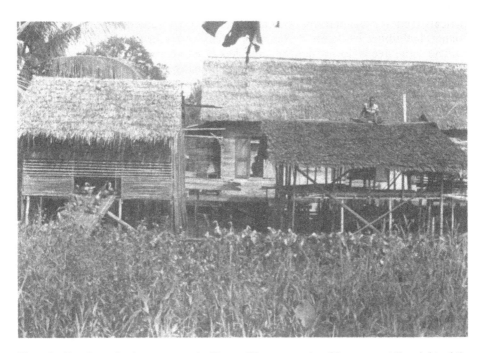

Plate 2. *Bamboo duck cages are built on stilts over water. The cage at the right of the photo is under construction. The gate to the left has been opened to allow immature ducks out for daily exercise and foraging. (Photo by Victor Caldarola)*

replace the soiled bedding in laying boxes every week or so. This practice is important because layers peck at and eat their bedding.

Conclusions

Banjarese duck farmers' methods for preventing disease have heretofore received little attention. In the absence of trained veterinary assistance for ducks in this region, farmers' own health-management measures are crucial to the continued success of their commercial poultry industry. Most Banjarese involved in commercial duck egg operations share a basic stock of ethnoveterinary knowledge about disease prevention.[5] While they are largely unaware of specific disease etiologies, they do know that poor nutrition, rotting feed, dirty water and filthy cages prejudice flock health and productivity. They are also aware of various environmental stresses that promote disease, and they take steps to prevent, avoid or ameliorate these conditions. Their careful attention to flock health and nutrition results in an impressive productivity figure of 210 to 245 eggs per bird yearly.

Many farmers continue to experiment with ways to improve their flocks' well-being in order to increase the productivity and profitability of their poultry enterprises still further. As their enthusiastic adoption of 'Concentrate' demonstrates, Banjarese are open to new livestock technologies that prove superior to old ones if they are cost-effective and fit comfortably into local production and resource systems.

Recent literature on livestock development for small farmers suggests a critical need for evaluation of a number of little-studied aspects of poultry raising, including: workable systems for intensive poultry production in tropical climates; the feeds for which an area has a comparative advantage; and the possibilities for inexpensive, locally-made housing and equipment (McDowell 1989). As McCorkle (1989) points out, ethnoveterinary research can often suggest effective animal health interventions and practices that take advantage of local knowledge and experience. In terms of affordability, ease of comprehension and application, cultural acceptability and other factors, indigenous practices can sometimes provide more appropriate solutions to animal health problems than 'modern', Western technological interventions.

The intensive duck-raising strategy developed by Banjarese farmers in South Kalimantan embraces many low-cost and highly successful methods of poultry management and disease prevention based on local resources and livestock savvy. These practices may be adaptable to other rural populations in the tropical developing world who are interested in intensifying their poultry production systems. Transfer of the indigenous knowledge and technology elaborated by the people of South Kalimantan may be especially feasible and appropriate in other areas of Asia engaged or interested in more highly commercialized village-level poultry farming.

Notes

1. For further information on the history of Indonesian duck husbandry and the breeds involved, consult Clayton (1972), Direktorat Jenderal Peternakan (1979 and 1982), Siregar (1982) and Soedjai (1974).
2. For greater detail on the field site, methodology, and social, cultural, and economic context, see Vondal (1984, 1987 and 1989). The summary presented here of the development of a highly commercialized, intensified system of household duck farming is largely drawn from the analysis in Vondal (1987).
3. Although ducks are considered hardier than chickens and less prone to disease, national poultry development strategies in Indonesia have centred on intensive chicken raising and the introduction of exotic breeds. But for villagers, the exotics are difficult and expensive to manage and care for, and they are notoriously susceptible to disease (Gunawan 1989, Ibrahim and Abdu, this volume).
4. To the extent possible, corroboration of farmers' views and statements was sought in the scientific and applied literature on duck husbandry and from the Duck Programme of West Java's Centre for Animal Research and Development, whose scientists have conducted controlled experiments with the Alabio duck and short-term fieldwork on duck farming methods in North Hulu Sungai Regency. However, it was not possible to validate all of the emic information on the basis of these sources. Many fruitful and fascinating aspects of local husbandry remain for future research.
5. Of course, not all farmers possess the same level of knowledge about diseases and disease prevention. Hence differences in flock productivity are found.

16. Sheep husbandry and healthcare among Tzotzil Maya shepherdesses[1]

RAÚL PEREZGROVAS

THE TZOTZIL MAYA Indians inhabit the highlands (c. 2000m) of Mexico's remote, southernmost state of Chiapas, on the border with Guatemala. Over the past 400 years, Tzotzil women have developed their own Chiapas breed of sheep, along with a husbandry system that allows these animals to survive and produce in their difficult, mountainous environment. The Tzotzil system of ovine husbandry and healthcare derives from a mix of ancient Mayan ethnomedicine and cosmology with herding techniques learned from the early Spanish priests and landlords. Today, sheep and sheep's wool play a central role in Tzotzil economy and society, with Indians placing a very special value on their relationship with these animals.

The Tzotzil adopted sheep from their Spanish conquerors sometime during the first half of the sixteenth century.[2] The Chiapas breed is descended from the Spanish Churra, Manchega, Lacha and Castellana breeds,[3] and it has maintained the genetic potential that keeps its Spanish ancestors near the top of the milk production list (Perezgrovas et al. 1989:22). Although its wool production of about 1.2 kg per year seems low by Western standards (Razgado 1989:34), the breed yields a longer, coarser fibre that is easy to process by hand. And although Chiapas sheep are small,[4] more than 400 years of adaptation have made them exceptionally hardy and disease-resistant. Indeed, no other breed has been so far able to survive the difficult highland environment.[5]

Its hardiness and other characteristics make the Chiapas sheep a very promising animal for genetic improvement through selective breeding. In fact, numerous government agencies have attempted to introduce improved animals plus modern husbandry techniques into the Indian-managed flocks. To date, however, these attempts have all failed. So far, they have had nothing to offer that represents any real improvement within the context of Tzotzil production systems and the Indians' own traditions and values of sheep raising, including shepherdesses' unique understandings of their animals. Sadly, anthropologists studying Tzotzil culture have paid little heed to animal husbandry, while animal scientists and veterinarians have neglected the culture. Worse still, few such technical specialists are trained to deal with the small-scale, family livestock operations typically found among indigenous groups.

This chapter examines practices and beliefs in Tzotzil husbandry and healthcare of sheep from an integrated perspective that incorporates synchronic and diachronic, anthropological and veterinary, and emic and etic points of view. The research reported here was conducted as part of a larger, on-going programme of the Sheep Research Group of the University of Chiapas and its Centre of Indigenous Studies. The unifying goal of these efforts is to collect and analyse data useful for re-thinking and re-designing conventional approaches to improving sheep production among the Tzotzil and other peoples who pursue small-scale stockraising within a unique cultural context.

After an overview of subjects, methods, the research setting, and Tzotzil husbandry systems, this chapter concentrates on the Indian shepherdesses' healthcare perceptions and practices for one of the common sheep diseases that were to be investigated during the study as a whole: fasciolosis or liverfluke disease. These ethnoveterinary concepts and management strategies are then analysed for their likely effects on the prevalence of this disease, as well as for their historical origins. The conclusion offers some insights and recommendations for ethnoveterinary research and livestock development efforts generally among stockraising peoples like the Tzotzil.

Subjects and methods

Although the Tzotzil Maya are officially citizens of the Mexican Republic, in fact they inhabit a different world. They have their own language, history and social and political structures. They reside in 14 municipalities of Chiapas state, each of which has special costumes and traditions. The study reported here was conducted among Tzotzil of the municipality of San Juan Chamula, which has the highest ovine population density in Mexico (Pérez Inclan 1981:11). The data presented in the following pages derive from a number of sources: historical research and literature reviews; participant observation; firsthand, in-field examination of animals, grazing locales and livestock quarters; and formal but open-ended interviews with 38 Chamulan shepherdesses. Fieldwork and interviews were carried out from January 1986 to July 1987 in 30 different hamlets spread throughout the municipality. Together, these hamlets represent every major agro-ecozone to be found in San Juan Chamula: dry lowlands, humid pine forest and high-altitude highlands.

Collecting the interview data was not easy. Among the Indians of this region, every outsider is to be distrusted. Moreover, Tzotzil social mores forbid women to speak to certain types of people, but especially to men who are not members of the community. The author was able to overcome these cultural constraints through the assistance of a 12-year-old bilingual girl from a Chamulan hamlet. Shepherdesses were willing to talk to this young female assistant whereas they would likely have refused to be interviewed by a male outsider. Thus, the assistant conducted the interviews while the author listened silently, evaluating the responses for sincerity and accuracy. (Most interviewees did not realize that the author could understand their answers in Tzotzil.)

The interview protocol covered a diversity of topics: family composition, home economics, sheep management, toxic plants, the weaving process and religious beliefs. (For greater detail on the survey instrument and its findings, consult Perezgrovas 1990.) In the open-ended interview format used for this study, interviewees were allowed to expand on any relevant subject that interested them. Most interviews took place seated in the open air at a site where the women could keep an eye on their grazing flocks. During the interview and with the shepherdess' permission, each animal present was routinely inspected, along with the pastures where the flock was grazed and the wooden shelters in which they were quartered. In addition, samples of plants that interviewees viewed as medicinal, harmful or nutritious for their sheep were collected for later identification and analysis.[6]

Specifically for ovine diseases, the following information was elicited: the illnesses known to the interviewee and their local names; the clinical signs and causes she recognized; seasonality of the disease's occurrence; ages of animals affected and mortality rates; any known remedies and their preparation, dosage and mode of administration. Whenever permission was granted—almost always after a great deal of persuasion by the female research assistant—samples for copro-parasitologic examination were also collected.

Profile of Chamulan households and husbandry systems

On average, 10 to 20 households make up a hamlet in San Juan Chamula. Typically, each family has a one-room adobe house with a tile roof, a small kitchen off the main house, a patio, a wooden shelter for sheep, a garden for vegetables and fruit trees, and an agricultural plot of about 0.25ha for basic foodcrops such as maize. The typical family of San Juan Chamula is headed by a 42-year-old man whose main activity is farming his own land plus doing waged agricultural labour off-farm. His wife is 38 and looks after three or four children. Although men are considered the centre of the Tzotzil patriarchal social structure (Pozas 1977:119), women are in fact responsible for maintaining the family nucleus. Unlike the men, Tzotzil women mainly speak the native Tzotzil Maya language and they maintain their traditional dress and way of life. They care for and teach the children, keep the house clean, collect plants and herbs, prepare the food, make the family's woollen clothes and of course tend the chickens and sheep.

Family flocks average 10 sheep (with a usual range of two to 24) consisting of three rams and seven ewes. Most of the animals derive from an initial pair of sheep given to the Indian couple at marriage. Chamulan families earn up to 40 per cent of their annual income directly or indirectly from sheep raising (Wasserstrom 1980:34), primarily via an active trade in wool and woollen garments woven by the women on the indigenous backstrap loom. Weaving has long been part of the Indian culture, with the elaboration of cotton garments dating back at least 2500 years. Given the economic importance of wool processing and weaving among the post-Columbian Tzotzil, live sheep are rarely sold; and Tzotzil religion prohibits the consumption of mutton. (When a sheep dies, it is simply left out for the dogs and coyotes to eat.) Moreover, sheep are believed to have souls and to experience emotions such as happiness and sadness just as humans do.

Women hold all decision-making authority over sheep, their husbandry, and the resulting products. Women assign a name to each animal in their flock; they build, move, and maintain the animals' wooden shelters; they see to the daily grazing and watering; they shear at the proper time;[7] they treat their flocks' health problems and pray to the Holy Shepherd, John the Baptist, for the animals' well-being and productivity; they make all the family's durable woollen clothing, for both daily and ceremonial use and for sale; and they teach all this to their daughters. It is very common to see a Chamulan shepherdess seated on a promontory where she watches her sheep and washes, cards, spins and weaves wool, while a little girl sits next to her, learning how to perform these same tasks (Plate 1).

The grazing day runs from about 9:30 a.m. to about 5:30 p.m. Throughout the day, each animal is staked and the stake is moved three or four times. During the rainy season (June to November), communally owned pastures are used. In order to protect the ripening maize fields that the flock passes on its way to the day's rainy-season grazing site, each animal is muzzled with a hand-made grass muzzle. With the first frost around early December, forage in the communal pastures disappears (Ley *et al.* 1986:32). During the subsequent dry season

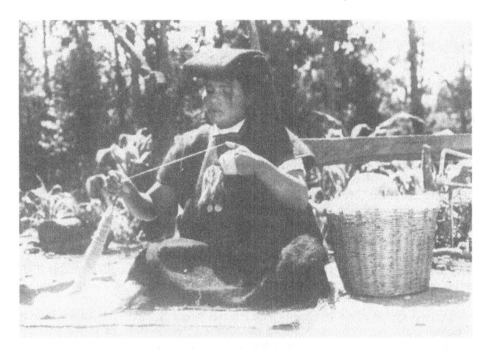

Plate 1. *A Maya shepherdess spins as she oversees her flock.*

(December through May), the animals graze the harvested maize fields. Later in the season, the flock is moved to the forest, where it can browse.

At night, the sheep are kept in wooden shelters of approximately 6.5 square metres. About half of the women interviewed said they move the structures every six weeks. The shelters are generally rotated within the vegetable garden in order to incorporate the manure into the soil. Those who use fixed shelters instead remove the manure every eight to 10 weeks and distribute it on their maize fields. Half of the sheep shelters inspected were roofed—with grass, cardboard, wood or tile, in that order.

The flock is watered once or twice a day, depending on the temperature. Instead of trailing their flocks to wells or streams, however, most shepherdesses (90 per cent of interviewees) water their sheep from a bucket, almost on an individual basis. Once a week, the animals are given locally-made mountain salt and, when available, crop surpluses such as potatoes left from the seeding batch or squashes. Special care for the animals is provided only at parturition. For a few days after lambing, the ewe is tied close to the house and fed some maize gruel.

Tzotzil shepherdesses' concepts of ovine disease: the case of fasciolosis

In what is likely a Maya–Catholic syncretism, Tzotzil Indians perceive life as a constant struggle between good and evil, with the gods of the heavens pitted against the demons of death and destruction from the underworld. They believe that both such forces are the ultimate source of, and often the solution to, sickness and death in both humans and animals. For example, to protect a new-born sheep against the evil eye, women tie around its neck a red ribbon that the Holy Shepherd has blessed in the local church. (For a detailed overview of Tzotzil ethnomedical concepts in relation to cosmology and ideology, consult Holland 1978:118–68. See also Ochiai 1985.)

However, shepherdesses are well aware of more naturalistic causes and characteristics of the principal illnesses of their sheep. For all such diseases, shepherdesses can describe the clinical signs and provide the other information requested in the interviews, such as morbidity, mortality, ages and types of animals most affected and season of major presentation. In evidence, Table 1 presents a summary of interviewees' responses for a number of the most commonly cited sheep diseases. Here, a single disease—fasciolosis—is used as a case example to illustrate the nature of Tzotzil ethnoveterinary knowledge and practice.

Fasciolosis or liverfluke disease is enzootic in the Chamula region, with its major occurrence during the dry season (Perezgrovas and Pedraza 1985). It is caused by *Fasciola hepatica*, a leaf-shaped trematode that infects various ungulates, especially sheep and cattle. The parasite depends on sufficient moisture and certain snail species for its development. Adult flukes live and reproduce in the bile ducts of their vertebrate host. Their eggs are excreted on to the pasture in the host's faeces. With warmth and moisture, small larvae called miracidia hatch from the eggs. The larvae then infect a snail host and develop through several stages into cercariae. The cercariae leave the snail and encyst themselves as metacercariae on aquatic or wet vegetation. Ungulates become infected when they feed on the infested vegetation (after Fraser 1986).

The course of fasciolosis depends on the number of parasites an animal ingests. Sheep may die after six to 10 weeks of acute or subacute liverfluke disease. Chronic infection is characterized by anaemia, submandibular oedema (commonly known in English as 'bottle jaw') and reduced lactation and failure to thrive. The oedema is not directly caused by the parasite. Rather, it results from pathological changes such as disturbed circulation, which is associated with a reaction to circulating parasite products (communication with Schillhorn van Veen). Submandibular swelling can also occur in other diseases, such as haemonchosis (common stomach worms).

Tzotzil shepherdesses, however, understand submandibular oedema as a particular sheep *disease* rather than as a non-specific disease *sign*. Ultimately, modern science may prove this concept correct, in that the oedema is probably caused by derived biochemical mediators (akin to certain prostaglandins) which appear to occur in a number of diseases including fasciolosis and haemonchosis. Further supporting this concept is the fact that the 'bottle jaw' rapidly disappears after treatment with anti-inflammatory drugs [editors' note]. Nevertheless, for Indians the swollen jaw is also the major diagnostic sign of the eponymous disease. (See Delehanty, this volume for greater detail on the ethnoscientific implications of this distinction.) For simplicity of presentation, the remainder of this section adopts this emic, discussing submandibular oedema as though it always resulted from fasciolosis.[8] That is, the following description of ovine fasciolosis is couched in terms of the Indians' concept of a disease that they usually call simply 'water necklace' or 'water bag' (*lik vo*, where *lik* means 'bag' or 'necklace' and *vo* means 'water') in the same way that an English-speaking sheep raiser may talk of 'bottle jaw' as an ailment in its own right. While *lik vo* is the most common Tzotzil name, other terms are *lik yaal* 'liquid bag' or 'saliva bag' and *lik a-lel* 'juice bag'.

Tzotzil attribute 'water bag' in sheep to two main causes. One is 'sadness' (see

Table 1. Common diseases among traditionally raised sheep in highland Chiapas, as identified by Indian shepherdesses (N=38)

Common Tzotzil name[a]	English equivalent[b]	% of sample citing	Reported mortality	Sheep most affected[c]	Causes cited	Treatment
Tsoj	Diarrhoea	80	Moderate	All	Natural	Plants
Obal	Coughing	67	Low	All, in winter	Natural	Ritual
Xuvit	Nasal worm	67	None	All	Either	None
Lik vo	Bottle jaw/submandibular oedema	63	Low	Adults	Either	Plants, rituals
Co'oc	Fever	60	Low	All	Natural	Ritual
Ic	Wind	37	Low	Adults	Supernatural	Ritual
Cacal sat	Evil eye	20	Low	All	Supernatural	Ritual

[a] Here, only the most frequently encountered name is given; see text.
[b] These are only rough equivalents, not exact translations or glosses.
[c] 'All' refers to adults plus lambs. Interviewees were not asked to draw any finer distinctions such as neonates, yearlings, or juveniles.

below). The other—and the most often mentioned—is an animal's ingestion of various plants that grow near wells, rivers, meadows and maize fields. The Tzotzil names for these plants and their botanical classifications are presented in Table 2, according to the frequency with which interviewees cited them. In particular, Tzotzil shepherdesses associate 'water bag' with sheep's eating any of a group of small herbaceous species that grow in humid places and are known generically in Tzotzil as *nixnam* or 'lake flower'.

Another plant that shepherdesses consider 'very dangerous' is *esparo* (*Rumex acetosella*), known in English as 'sheep sorrel' (King 1966:175). This small plant is found not only in humid areas but also near maize fields; thus sheep are very likely to ingest it. Shepherdesses say it can kill a sheep within a month, although three to four months is more common. Interviewees explain the plant's action as follows. In the rumen, the *esparo* leaves are not regurgitated and ruminated; instead they move to the liver, where they change colour from green to the purple-grey characteristic of liver flukes. Sheep sorrel in fact undergoes certain changes in acidic soils such as those of highland Chiapas—its leaves become smaller, redder and narrower as they age (ibid.). This peculiarity doubt-less figures in shepherdesses' associating *esparo* with flukes. In any case, after the leaves are ingested, they are believed to turn into 'animals'. As such, they are motile and thus can invade and 'rot' the liver. The result is that the ovine host stops eating, becomes emaciated, and grows water or juice under the jaw. Interviewees claim they have observed these leaves turn into living creatures when, at Carnival or some other major ritual event, a bull or a cow is slaughtered for feasting. At necropsy, they note that the sacrificial animal's liver is discoloured and brittle and that, when the liver is crushed, the little leaf-animals come out and move. (Recall that Tzotzil do not eat mutton; hence most of their knowledge of ruminant anatomy derives from cattle.)

Tzotzil women say the second most common cause of 'water bag' is 'sadness', a frequent affliction of both livestock and people. When sheep 'know' or 'feel' that something is amiss, they become sad. Their unhappiness is most often evidenced by the appearance of 'juice' under the jaw. According to intervie-wees, sadness can be triggered by situations such as the following: when the flock is tended by someone other than its shepherdess–owner; when an owner talks or even thinks about selling animals—women say the creatures can sense this; when husband and wife argue and fight about domestic matters and their

Table 2. Plants Tzotzil associate with 'water bag'

Tzotzil name	Botanical name
Nixnam	Sisyrinchium scabrum SC
Cuchara nixnam	Viola nannei
Nat nixnam	Cardamine flaccida
Cocom nixnam	Polygonum punctatum
Esparo	Rumex acetosella L.
Canis	Trifolium amabile HBK
Cocom jobel	Berula erecta (Huds.)
	Aster exilis
	Aster subulatus
Yamachauk	Arracacia bracteata
	Thalictrum guatemalense

'anger' is transmitted to some of their sheep; and when animals are under the care of a lazy, inattentive shepherdess.

To treat 'water bag'—or for that matter, any livestock disease—Tzotzil do not turn to prescription drugs. Indeed, they rarely use such costly medications even for themselves. Home remedies, prayers and rituals are more common. Among the treatments that interviewees described for 'water bag' are the following.

o The most popular therapy is drenching across several days with an aqueous decoction of 13 sprigs of *Eupatorium ligustrinum*. Known in Tzotzil as *pomchate* (*pom*: incense or honey; *cha*: bitter; *te*: tree), this shrub is commonly found throughout the highlands of Chiapas. *Pomchate* is known for its anti-inflammatory properties, and is also used in human ethnomedicine— most notably as part of a steam cure given by local healers to reduce swelling (Laughlin 1975:91). The *pomchate* drench is also used for ovine diarrhoea.

o Garlic (*Allium sativum*) is a multi-purpose botanical in Tzotzil ethnomedicine for both humans and livestock and for both natural and supernatural ills. Freshly ground garlic is generally used as a topical anti-inflammatory. For sheep with 'water bag', however, three small cloves are mixed with *pox*, home-made sugar-cane alcohol. This mixture is then administered orally once a day over several days. Shepherdesses say this preparation also relieves bloat.

o Following the same schedule, a mixture of salt and dried, toasted maize may be used instead. Maize is a semi-sacred item in Tzotzil cultural and ethno-medical systems. Its 'soul' is said to be in close contact with both the gods of the heavens and the lords of the underworld. Thus it is commonly used in healing as well as other rites (Laughlin 1975:61, 225). However, shepherdesses report that this remedy for 'water bag' is less effective than the first two.

o Another oral preparation given only once is 13 chilli peppers (*Capsicum annum*) blended and mixed with water. However, this remedy is used for liver illness generally, rather than specifically for 'water bag'.

Because 'water bag' may sometimes have a non-naturalistic cause—for example, sadness—a ritual treatment may be called for in order to detect and then correct the source of the sadness. The most commonly reported such treatment is the following.

o The shepherdess leads the sick sheep to a trail crossing, places the animal on the ground, and then crosses its legs, front to rear and left to right. While holding the sheep in this position, the woman takes off her own, preferably much-used, woollen sash and ties it around the animal's belly for a minute or two while cinching the sash tight with three strong pulls. At the same time, she calls out in very strong language 'requesting' that the sadness leave her sheep and go away down any of the trails. Afterwards, she unties the sash and throws it away, and must never pick it up again. No other people or animals should be nearby during this procedure, since the illness could enter them instead of departing down one of the trails. This ritual treatment is used for cases of sadness generally, as well as for another livestock ill known as 'wind'.

Discussion and analysis

Although ovine fasciolosis is enzootic in the Chamula region, copro-parasitologic counts in the Chiapas sheep managed by Indians are surprisingly low by comparison to sheep (Chiapas or any other breed) kept on-station under experimental conditions. The latter must be treated regularly with commercial anthelmintic and other products in order to avoid high mortality. In contrast, research on a sample of Chiapas sheep showed no infection by *F. hepatica* in lambs under six months old; and the occurrence of detectable fasciolosis in adults was consistently low during the dry season (Lucero 1990, Perezgrovas and Pedraza 1985: 22). Given the facts that, first, sheep do not appear to develop resistance to liver-fluke infection (Fraser 1986:211) and, second, that Chamulan environmental conditions clearly favour the development of *F. hepatica*, these low parasitic burdens in Indian flocks may be best explained by reference to shepherdesses' husbandry and healthcare practices.

Although Tzotzil shepherdesses are unaware of the complex life-cycle of *F. hepatica* (its eggs, snails, miracidia and cercariae), research reveals that they hold a highly practical and effective working knowledge of ovine fasciolosis. This knowledge allows them to understand, and somehow control, the disease. What do they know or do that helps them prevent or manage fasciolosis, and how did they acquire this knowledge and expertise?

Tzotzil shepherdesses correctly associate 'water bag' with animals' consumption of plants near water sources. As noted above, aquatic plants are indeed the most likely to be infested with the metacercariae of *F. hepatica*. Tzotzil knowledge in this regard might have some origin in Spanish pastoral tradition, as well as in local empirical observation. As early as the eleventh century, Spanish shepherds were advised by the *Mesta*[9] to keep their animals away from 'wet weeds and corrupted waters . . .' in order to avoid sicknesses (Manrique 1968:375). A number of Tzotzil beliefs and practices—some of which are quite unique—in fact do serve to control 'water bag' by minimizing animals' contact with aquatic and hydrophilic plants and with the humid areas where they flourish.

One such practice is muzzling each animal while driving the flock to pasture during the rainy season. This obviously prevents the hungry animals' ingestion of 'dangerous' (that is, metacercariae-infested) plants as the flock is trailed through the humid areas and maize fields where such vegetation grows. Muzzling is a uniquely Tzotzil technique. There are no precedents for it in Spanish pastoralism. If nothing else, the size of Old World flocks (up to several thousand head) would have precluded this kind of individual handling.

Beliefs about 'water bag' developing in sheep that become sad and sick because of their owner's (or more likely, a non-owner's) laziness and inattention are also uniquely Mayan. They have management implications similar to those just described above for fasciolosis control. Namely, a conscientious shepherdess will not allow her animals to stray close to places where dangerous plants are found.

Also of practical value in controlling fasciolosis is shepherdesses' method of watering their sheep from a container, instead of allowing the animals to drink directly from streams or springs. This breaks the lifecycle of *F. hepatica*, because the sheep thus cannot ingest the plants on which the metacercariae are encysted. Given the high rainfall and numerous streams and wells in the Tzotzil region, this practice cannot be explained by exigency. It seems more likely that its function is disease control. It is probably a long-standing Tzotzil husbandry technique; anthropological studies from the 1950s describe how Tzotzil women watered their animals from clay pots (Pozas 1977:168). Certainly, it finds no precedent in Spanish sheep raising. Again, Old World flocks were far too large to be afforded such individualized attention.

Another clearly beneficial practice is regularly moving or cleaning the animals' shelters. This makes it difficult for parasite eggs and larvae to reach infective stages. This practice finds a rough parallel in the Spanish custom of rotating transhumant herds on farmers' fields (Manrique 1968:375). Although this was done mainly to manure the soil, it also helped control parasitism.

In contrast to these control methods, the value of Tzotzil therapies for ovine fasciolosis is more difficult to assess. Leaving aside ritual treatments, the salt-and-maize feedings doubtless produce some beneficial nutritional effects. The action of the other ingredients in Tzotzil ethnomedicines for 'water bag' is unknown. To the extent that they have anti-inflammatory benefits, they may at least reduce the oedema [recall earlier editors' note]. Certainly, both garlic and hot peppers are common remedies for endoparasitism worldwide [editors' note]. But to the author's knowledge, none of the Tzotzil's ethnoveterinary remedies have been pharmacologically tested, although the Sheep Research Group plans to conduct some basic tests on *pomchate* in the near future. However, inter-viewees note that even this popular botanical is not always effective in the long term. They say the bag of 'juice' may reappear later on. This observation accords with the characteristics of chronic fasciolosis.

Implications for livestock development and extension

For decades, innumerable government agencies—both anthropological and agri-cultural—have sought to 'help' the Tzotzil shepherdess with all manner of 'modern' technology: new weaving instruments, synthetic fibres and chemical dyes; different breeds of sheep; improved management methods; vaccines and prescription veterinary drugs. The list is long. Yet she still weaves only with the coarse Chiapas wool on her backstrap loom, using dyes of earth and plants; raises only her small, thin and commonly despised Chiapas sheep, giving each such 'soul' meticulous personal attention; cures her animals with herbs, prayers and rituals; and thanks her gods regularly for the wealth and well-being that her flock provides.

After some years of experience (learning-mistakes included), the Sheep Research Group at the University of Chiapas concluded that a new approach to livestock development in such contexts was needed. Scientists and developers must take a different, more humble attitude that includes '. . . the willingness to understand the culture of recipient peoples, to look for the good in these cultures, to search for the reasons of traditional ways, to restrain excessive missionary zeal which leads to inability to see alternatives, and to take the time and trouble to prepare oneself, technically and emotionally, to work in a foreign society' (Foster 1962:260).

As this chapter has shown for just one among many diseases, local people often know much more about animal health and husbandry than developers might imagine. The Sheep Research Group has come to appreciate this fact, and to build upon local knowledge systems and their associated practices in selecting, designing and targeting its research and development (R&D) efforts. For example, as a result of the findings reported here, the group judged that fasciolosis was not a priority health problem among Indian-managed flocks. Shepherdesses were already taking effective (and cost-effective) steps to control the disease. The group therefore re-focused its health-related R&D on more pressing problems. Also, now that they are aware of Indians' ethnoveterinary pharmacopoeia, scientists have begun field trials to test a number of local plant-based treatments to determine if these could be effectively deployed against some of these priority problems.

In sum, the Sheep Research Group has come to recognize that any proposed interventions to improve the health and productivity of local flocks would be wise to build upon the strengths of the traditional management system still practised by Indian shepherdesses today. Indeed, this system has achieved what neither early Spanish sheep raisers nor contemporary government agencies could—the development and survival of a hardy sheep breed under difficult environmental and management conditions. All it took to do this some four centuries ago was another 'new approach' to sheep raising, which the Tzotzil invented largely on their own.

The value of a more technically and emotionally sensitive and more culturally informed approach for development efforts in animal husbandry and healthcare around the world has been highlighted in a number of recent publications on ethnoveterinary research and development (Mathias-Mundy and McCorkle 1989, McCorkle 1986, 1989, Ibrahim and Abdu, this volume). But in Mexico, until only very recently, developers adopting this stance were labelled 'crazy anthropologists', 'misfit veterinarians', or worse. Yet in the case of Tzotzil sheep raising, it seems clear that an integrated, interdisciplinary approach is a must. Conventional approaches to livestock development that ignore local knowledge, practices, beliefs and attitudes and that are suitable only for large-scale, Western-style production systems have uniformly failed. It is time we learn from local people's generations of stockraising experience, their disease terminology and idioms of animal healthcare, their home remedies, and even their understandings of animal feelings and fears. Only then can we begin to design appropriate and socio-culturally acceptable interventions to help keep a few more livestock 'souls' 'happy' and thus healthy and productive.

Notes

1. The research reported here was supported by the Centro de Estudios Indígenas, Universidad Autónoma de Chiapas, México. Research would not have been possible without the unstinting assistance of Maruch Gómez, however. Visiting Indian hamlets with her was more than just fieldwork; it was also an enjoyable learning experience. I am also grateful to her mother Paxcu and her sisters Luch and Veronica for their help. Thanks are also due Lorena Soto and Tim Killeen for their assistance in plant classification, Emilio and Noemi Oyarzabal and Ruth Lucero for technical analysis, Karen Langner and Linda Tia Saide for their comments on a draft of the manuscript, and Donna Johnston for manuscript preparation.

2. As part of a more comprehensive analysis of sheep husbandry in Tzotzil communities, the author and colleagues are at work on a reconstruction of how and which Spanish breeds first reached highland Chiapas. For a brief overview, see Villalobos and Perezgrovas (1989:5–14) and Sarmiento (1989:4–9).

3. Until the twentieth century, the peripheral location of Chiapas state and the rough terrain of the highlands kept the Tzotzil region largely isolated from the rest of Mexico. Thus the Chiapas breed evolved without any influence from the more recently introduced Merinos so common elsewhere in Mexico.

4. Live weights for ewes and rams respectively equal about 25kg and 31kg (Perezgrovas and Pedraza 1984:11).

5. Government agencies have attempted to introduce purebred Rambouillet and Columbia sheep into traditionally managed flocks, but all such animals died within a matter of weeks. A more recent experience showed that some F1 Romney Marsh X Chiapas crosses produced under controlled conditions and introduced experimentally into

Indian flocks managed to survive. However, they can do so only with constant de-worming.

6. Scientific names of plants were obtained from Laughlin 1975 and other sources; see Note 1.

7. Shearing has a clearly ritual character. It is not a pre-programmed activity; instead, women determine when the wool on a given sheep is long enough for shearing. On average, however, an animal is shorn twice a year.

8. Interestingly, based on faecal examination of a sample of Indian-managed Chiapas sheep, the action of stomach worms in producing bottle jaw can largely be ruled out.

9. The *Mesta* was the largest and most important association of shepherds in Spain. Founded in AD 1273, it provided its members with practical husbandry and healthcare advice, regulated transhumance and trading patterns for sheep, and set wool and mutton prices (Klein 1920).

17. Care of cattle versus sheep in Ireland: South-west Donegal in the early 1970s[1]

EUGENIA SHANKLIN

THE PEOPLE OF Ireland's County Donegal—both English- and Gaelic-speaking, Protestant and Catholic—live dispersed across one of the more inhospitable landscapes of western Europe, in the north-westernmost reaches of Ireland. Theirs is a cold and rocky land with mostly thin, poor, acid peat soils. The climate is almost as bad as the soil: gale-force winds, a growing season constrained more by rainfall than by temperature, and extreme variations both in rainfall and in the length of the frost-free season. These agro-climatic features make cropping difficult. Stockraising therefore forms a key part of Donegal farmers' centuries-old adaptation to their harsh climate and limited natural resources. Indeed, Donegal farmers operate two kinds of livestock production systems simultaneously: one a highly controlled and intensive regime of cattle raising, the other an extensive, range-stock system of sheep raising.

Archaeological research indicates that cattle keeping was the primary subsistence mode in Donegal even before the arrival of the Celts in the third century BC (Orme 1970). Although the Celts came with both cattle and sheep, for them, cattle were the measure of all things. This attitude persisted in Donegal at least through the early 1970s, when the fieldwork on which this chapter is based was conducted.[2] Cattle were unquestionably the prestige animals while sheep were considered a cash crop of little consequence. Accordingly, calf mortality rates in the region were the lowest in all of Ireland, while lamb mortalities were among the highest (AFT 1969 Part 2:61–2). The ways in which attitudes toward the two species differ are illustrated in the following incident.

> During the author's field research in Donegal, a man assigned to care for a relative's cattle over the winter allowed the herd to roam freely until neighbours complained; then he confined the cattle to a paddock without making any provision for adequate feed. Several of the creatures starved to death and were left unburied. A county official found the remainder of the herd in an acutely emaciated state. Some of the animals were so debilitated that they had to be destroyed. The culprit was legally charged with cruelty to animals and taken to court, where he was given a heavy fine and a suspended prison sentence. The presiding judge expressed great indignation about the whole affair, noting that he had never before tried such a shocking case. Yet it struck no one as odd that what is defined as cruel and unusual treatment of cattle is the norm for sheep.

Elsewhere, the economic and other ramifications of Donegal farmers' attitudes towards cattle and sheep have been described in detail (Shanklin 1985, 1988, 1994). Here, the focus is on Donegal farmers' husbandry and healthcare practices for each species, and the emic logic behind them. This logic might be simply a curiosity were it not for the fact that, to be effective, researchers, developers or extension staff seeking to devise and institute new husbandry and veterinary techniques must first understand the reasons behind stockraising methods that have persisted over long periods of time. The present chapter is offered as a case study of this principle, which holds for livestock development worldwide.

Below, nutrition, feeding and housing practices—so important for animal health—are first compared for the two species. Then farmers' understanding, experiences with, and management of bovine versus ovine disease are described. Although the emphasis throughout is on farmers' own perspectives and rationales, these are also examined etically. Finally, the implications of farmers' differential attitudes and practices toward cattle and sheep are explored in terms of development emphases on short-term market profit versus producer concern with the longer-term sustainability of their stockraising enterprise.

Research setting, methods and subjects

Arable land and crop choices are very limited in Donegal. According to an extensive government agricultural survey of west Donegal (AFT 1969),[3] oats and a forage barley are the only grains that can be grown; potatoes and vegetables are cultivated for home consumption. Neither farmers nor government extension staff consider cropping economically viable. Instead, stockraising constitutes the major source of farm income. At the time of fieldwork, most households owned a dozen or so chickens and an occasional goose; and under a government-sponsored programme, a few farmers were experimenting with the reintroduction of swine raising, which had been abandoned since the turn of the twentieth century. But cattle and sheep are the mainstay of Donegal's farming systems. In the 1970s, the previous small Shorthorn breed of cattle had been replaced by Aberdeen Angus or by Angus x Shorthorn or Hereford x Shorthorn crosses, thanks to the highly efficient artificial insemination services in the region. A few farmers were also beginning to consider Charolais, then a newly introduced beef breed; and two dairy farmers in the research sample kept Holsteins. Sheep are of the hardy and highly territorial Scottish Blackface breed. The Blackface had replaced an earlier breed (which no one could name) that required better care.

Cattle are raised mainly to supply the household with milk. Only a few households in the region practised commercial dairying, supplying milk to surrounding villages. Ultimately, though, all cattle are sold as beef to buyers from Northern Ireland or to local butchers; no one slaughters cattle on the farm. Sheep are raised primarily for sale to northern buyers as meat animals or, in one on-going government experiment, as feeder lambs. Sheep are slaughtered for home consumption only for special occasions, such as holidays like Easter Sunday or major family celebrations like weddings.

The number of cattle and sheep kept by a household depends directly on the kind and extent of land available to it. Rough, unfenced mountain pastures that were formerly communal lands are used almost exclusively for sheep. The more fenced land, good hill grazing, and lush, rich lowland pastures that a household owns, the more cattle it maintains. At the time of field research, most families in the region had three to seven head of cattle, two to three of which were cows; the average flock of sheep was fewer than 30 breeding ewes (AFT 1969 Part 4:7).

Field methods included participant observation, directed interviews, documentary research and formal surveys and questionnaires. One of the most useful forms of participant observation proved to be attending sheep-dippings with a local dipping inspector. Another was reviewing the local chemist's stock of veterinary pharmaceuticals. For survey and questionnaire administration, a non-random stratified sample of 30 farmers was selected to represent the variety (as versus the average) of livestock production systems in what is an ecologically and ethnically diverse region. For example, although the vast majority of farms (3 200 out of 4 500) in Donegal are classed as smallholdings (one to 12 hectares), the 30 farms sampled also included medium-sized (12 to 30 hectares) and large ones (over 30 hectares). Stock holdings varied, too: some of the sample farmers raised only cattle, some only sheep and some both; one family in the sample had neither cattle nor sheep but was experimenting with raising swine. Moreover, the sample included both ordinary and 'model' farmers, with the latter identified as such by local agricultural agents.

Three out of five households in the sample spoke Gaelic as a first language. Field research revealed some differences between English- and Gaelic-speakers' vocabulary and knowledge of livestock health problems. For one thing, Gaelic speakers were often unaware of veterinary controversies or of emerging health-care problems discussed in English-language circles and bulletins. This situation reflects a more general lack of communication between Gaelic speakers and the government (one that could be easily remedied by bilingual extension materials, however). For another thing, Gaelic appeared to have fewer disease names than English; and Gaelic terms that did exist tended to be broader and more descriptive.[4] Field interviews were conducted in both languages; but since all but one sample household understood spoken English, when communication threatened to break down, English was used. Below, livestock diseases are referenced mainly by the local English names used in Donegal; these are given in apostrophes upon first occurrence. Gaelic terms are indicated where relevant and/or if they were in common use.

Sample members were systematically queried about their knowledge and practices of animal husbandry and healthcare. Questioning began with the livestock diseases described in an Irish veterinary manual. However, it quickly became apparent that many of the animal health problems common in other parts of Ireland did not exist in south-west Donegal. Conversely, it was necessary to add a category of livestock disease not mentioned in any manuals or surveys: supernaturally-linked ills. Many sample members waxed eloquent on this subject—albeit usually when recounting their 'neighbours' experiences rather than their own.

Grazing, feeding and housing

With proper nutrition and shelter, livestock can withstand all but a few of the parasites and diseases in Donegal's harsh environment. In the absence of adequate nutrition and shelter, the animals are more prone to sickness, accidents and predation. Donegal farmers' different management of these factors for cattle versus sheep constitutes one of the clearest reflections of people's distinct cultural attitudes towards the two species.

Throughout the year, cattle are generally kept near the house and byre (barn), where they receive supplemental feeds of commercially available cattle meals or concentrates and whatever hay is available. Cattle are also the first beneficiaries of the rich 'aftergrass', that is, the grass that remains or springs up after haying. The hay itself—which is in short supply and of low quality—is usually given only to cattle. This is particularly true during the winter, when the cattle are housed in the byre.

Adequate bovine nutrition in Donegal largely hinges on the factors involved in the production of hay for the winter months. These factors include the quality of the hay meadows and their forage, the weather conditions when the hay is made, and the technology used. According to official studies, the local hay is poor or substandard (AFT 1969 Part 2:57). Donegal farmers take issue with this assessment, however. As one man put it, 'We've heard about poor quality hay since these people [official resource surveyors] started coming here . . . But what they don't seem to understand is that the problem here . . . is between poor-quality hay and none at all, as often as not, given our weather.' In the past, the hay crop was sometimes completely destroyed by the region's frequent storms or early frosts. Today, tractors and other modern farm machinery plus pasture-improvement techniques (liming, re-seeding, manuring or fertilizing) ensure that no matter how bad the year, at least some hay will be saved.

In sharp contrast to cattle, sheep are generally left to fend for themselves on open pastures; and few Donegal farmers give hay or supplemental feeds to sheep. Thus, ovine nutrition is almost entirely dependent on the year's climatic conditions. Generally sheep must survive on whatever forage nature provides. Not surprisingly, malnutrition is the primary cause of lamb losses. As one farmer noted when he grew impatient with the interview queries about sheep diseases: 'Whatever the disease that causes the sheep to die, the real cause is starvation'. In Donegal, ovine losses ranged as high as 40 per cent in a bad year, and 30 per cent in a good one.

The other key variable in Donegal livestock nutrition is the type of land available for grazing. For obvious reasons, this is more important for sheep than for cattle. All sample members who kept sheep were asked to estimate their flock losses for a year, were they to begin with 100 lambs. Predictably, respondents with access only to the rough, unfenced mountain pastures that had formerly been communal lands produced the highest loss estimates (25 per cent to 40 per cent). Farmers estimating 20 per cent or fewer losses all possessed partially or completely fenced land and some good hill grazing. Respondents who gave estimates of 10 per cent losses or fewer all owned lush, rich lowland pastures and all fed their sheep supplementary concentrates during especially harsh winters and before lambing. Clearly, farmers are not unaware of the problems sheep face; but most people are simply indifferent.

Management of disease

For both cattle and sheep in Donegal, the most important health problems are parasitism, deficiency diseases and a variety of infectious diseases. Sample members also cite supernaturally-linked ills, but official studies do not mention these. Because cattle are watched carefully, most stockowners quickly detect any signs of poor health in this species. Just the opposite is true of sheep, since they are left largely unattended in open pastures throughout the year. Thus, sheep often are not seen to be suffering until an ailment is far advanced or until they are found dead in the pastures of unknown causes.

Endoparasitism
Farmers say liverfluke disease or simply 'flukes' (*Fasciola hepatica*) is the most prevalent bovine parasite. The AFT survey concurs with their assessment. It found that flukes constituted the 'most important parasitic disease of cattle in the area' and that 'nearly all cattle are affected sub-clinically on farms where clinical cases are occasionally observed' (AFT 1969 Part 2:65).[5] If they cannot

identify recognizable signs of any other disease, Donegal farmers automatically drench any cattle that seem 'low' with a flukicide. All cattle owners surveyed also employed a regular regime of fluke prophylaxis. Most dosed twice a year, in spring and autumn, although the government agricultural service recommends three times a year—in October, December and April or May (ARTAI 1965:4). While a few interviewees said they dose for flukes throughout the year or according to faecal analyses, government reports generally accuse farmers of underdosing and/or of dosing too infrequently (for example, AFT 1969 Part 2:65), with the result that the infection persists.

Farmers readily admit they do not follow the government's recommendations; but they argue that this is for good reason. They have observed that the officially recommended dosage seems to put cattle off their feed temporarily. They also explain that overdosing can be as harmful as the parasites themselves, leading to seriously debilitating effects and even death. Many respondents averred that the dosage prescribed on the drug label for a lactating cow would be too much for Donegal cattle, which are smaller than most other breeds in the British Isles. Thus farmers prefer to err on the side of caution in drenching. They calculate that three-quarters of the normal amount of flukicide is usually enough for the local cattle. Based on field observations, however, cattle in south-west Donegal are perhaps only about 10 per cent smaller than their mates elsewhere in Britain.

For Donegal sheep, liverfluke is again the most common and universally treated parasitic ill. As with cattle, any unthrifty sheep are dosed with a flukicide on general principle. Most farmers also follow an annual prophylactic regimen for flukes in sheep. But these regimes are highly idiosyncratic by comparison with cattle: 17 per cent of sheep owners in the sample say they dose 'constantly', 3 per cent do so four times a year, 20 per cent twice or thrice, 10 per cent once or twice, and 3 per cent according to faecal analysis. Officials recommend dosing in October and then monthly until lambing; but no sample member reported this regimen.

Most interviewees were aware that certain pastures can aggravate fluke problems in both species (AFT 1969 Part 4:35). This is especially true for pastures with peat soils, which are more moist than most; thus they offer favourable conditions for fluke reproduction (see also Perezgrovas, this volume). Usually sheep are grazed on the peat pastures while cattle enjoy the low-lying and better-drained meadows. Sheep are therefore more often exposed to fluke infestations. The AFT reports that ovine fasciolosis is usually chronic, that 'mortality is never high' but that the disease is 'aggravated by the marginal nutritional status at which many flocks are maintained' (Part 2:65). Several interviewees echoed this observation, noting that flukes can never really be eliminated and that stockraisers' precautions merely control it.

A few farmers knew of other endoparasites of cattle such as roundworms—perhaps because the labels on the flukicide bottles note that the medication also destroys roundworms. Within the sample, 37 per cent said they treat their cattle regularly for roundworms, usually along with fluke dosing. However, most respondents did not know that roundworms can and often do cause significant economic losses. Neither did most farmers recognize lungworm infections, known locally as 'hoose' (whether this is Gaelic or English is unclear), even though this parasite is quite common in the region. Most of the sample believed wrongly that hoose could be combated with the same drugs used for flukes and roundworms; but in fact in south-west Donegal in the 1970s, the only lungworm treatment available was an injectable formulation.

Apart from liverflukes, the only other endoparasite that sample members considered of any consequence for sheep was 'gid', caused by larval tapeworms (*Taenia multiceps multiceps*). High and moderate prevalence of gid were respectively reported by 6 per cent and 20 per cent of sheep owners in the sample. Among the latter, only a third were aware that dogs carry this parasite. Technically, the process is as follows: sheep ingest the embryos of tapeworm eggs voided in dog faeces; when the embryos become larvae, some may encyst themselves in the sheep's brain and spinal cord, producing 'giddiness', head staggers, stumbling, circling and other central nervous system signs. Gid is the only ovine disease that all farmers agree should be referred to a veterinarian. The cure consists of boring a hole in the sheep's skull and extracting the cysts. All the interviewees knew about this procedure; after watching the veterinarian perform it, a few tried it themselves. But an animal's chances of surviving this operation are about 50/50. Knowing this, farmers seldom bother with it unless the animal is a special pet.

Ectoparasitism

The major ectoparasite of Donegal cattle is generally known in local English as 'cattle grubs' or 'warble flies' (*Hypoderma* spp). In spring and summer, the flies lay their eggs in the hair covering the lower parts of the animal's body. The eggs hatch and the larvae bore into the skin, eventually settling on the animal's back, where they pierce breathing holes. At maturity, the insects force their way out via these holes, thus irreparably marring the hide. Warbles cause thousands of pounds of damage to cattle hides each year (Ogg 1977). Heavy fly infestation also greatly reduces milk (as well as meat) production, although this was not widely appreciated in south-west Donegal.

At the time of field research an animal with warbles fetched as much as £15 less than an uninfected one. This figure is 10 to 15 times greater than the treatment fee that was charged during a government campaign to eradicate warble infestations in the area in the late 1960s. The treatment consists merely of pouring a small amount of Derris wash over the backs of the animals. The campaign required all cattle to be treated for warbles at the time of tuberculin testing. After the campaign had been under way for two years, however, the National Farmer's Association (NFA) demanded that the government provide treatment *gratis*. Because the NFA and the government could not agree on a fee, mandatory treatment was ultimately suspended. Subsequently, cattle showing signs of warble infestation were denied entry into Donegal's principal cattle market in Northern Ireland. Consequently, Donegal farmers had to sell their infested but otherwise healthy animals locally for a much lower price.

Despite such financial losses, many Donegal farmers eschewed both government supervised and home treatments for warbles. Within the research sample, only 13 per cent of the farmers (including all those who customarily sell at the local Donegal market) voluntarily treated their cattle. The majority mistakenly believed that the campaign to eradicate warbles had made continued treatment unnecessary. Although this was of course the goal of the campaign, it was not achieved. Monolingual Gaelic speakers were generally unaware of the problem or the controversy around it given the general lack of communication between them and the government services. But farmers who spoke English and who understood the controversy roundly condemned both parties to the dispute. In any case, the majority of people either preferred to 'take their chances' with warbles, or were confused about or ignorant of the economic importance of the problem. This must have cost them dearly, since field research indicated that one in 20 of the cattle sold at the local mart in Donegal and three to four of every 10 sold at the then-just-opened Dunkineely market were infested.

Deficiency diseases
Both cattle and sheep are subject to several deficiency diseases in Donegal. But because cattle are cared for so assiduously, farmers detect and correct such problems promptly in cattle. Almost all sample members knew the signs of the major deficiency diseases affecting both cattle and sheep: copper and cobalt deficiency or, in local parlance, 'swayback' and 'pine', respectively. However, few people had ever had any cases of either disease in their cattle. These problems likely are largely avoided by the local practice of providing cattle (but not sheep) with mineral blocks and concentrates. In the few cases in which a veterinarian diagnosed one of these deficiencies in cattle, the owners dosed or gave concentrates to their animals regularly thereafter, and the problem did not recur.

For sheep, 27 per cent and 30 per cent of respondents respectively drenched for swayback and pine. But almost all practised the ancient Donegal custom of moving the sheep to different pastures. Other interviewees who reported occasional cases of these deficiencies said they usually did not take any special measures. This may in fact be an appropriate management decision, in that some of the flukicides used in Donegal are labelled as containing traces of copper and cobalt.

A once-common deficiency in cattle and apparently the only one for which there is a specific Gaelic term is *crupan* or, in the local English, 'bog lameness'. The technical name is aphosphorosis. Sometimes, too, people describe this condition by reference to its major symptom, a depraved appetite. Many local women recalled how cattle would often devour clothing hung out to dry. Seventeenth-century writers reported *crupan* as a serious problem, as did most of the older farmers surveyed. The traditional cure was to move affected cattle to higher, or at least different, pastures. (Sheep are routinely transferred, in any event.) But for many years now, *crupan* has been rare because of the widespread use of chemical fertilizers, which have a high phosphorous content; these are spread over the low-lying pastures on which cattle are kept. All of the sample (although curiously *not* the local veterinarian) knew that fertilizers can correct this deficiency, although not many knew why.

Another condition farmers recognize is 'grass tetany' (hypomagnesemia). Scientists suspect that this condition results from insufficient magnesium due to an imbalanced intake of other minerals; they note that it is most common in adult cows and ewes, especially those in heavy lactation and on lush grass pastures. Cattle that develop this disease die quickly. In such cases, farmers call in a veterinarian to diagnose the cause. But only 13 per cent of the sample had ever found this condition in their herds, and only 10 per cent had ever had a veterinarian treat their animals for it. Grass tetany can also occur in ewes, especially those on rich pasturage. But no one had ever observed this condition in sheep, probably because sheep are seldom grazed on rich pastures.

A final deficiency problem recognized for sheep is 'twin lamb disease' (hypocalcemia or toxaemia). Defined by a ewe's inability to sustain two lambs, the disease is typically triggered by inadequate or sharply fluctuating feed regimens in late pregnancy, as when storms or other weather conditions interrupt feeding or limit forage resources abruptly. Although sheep are exposed regularly to such conditions, the disease is nevertheless rare in south-west Donegal because twinning is rare. Only 13 per cent of the sample bothered to give extra feed or supplements to a ewe with twins.

Other diseases

Bacterial, viral, and protozoan diseases of cattle seem less a problem in south-west Donegal than in other parts of Ireland. This may be due in part to local farmers' meticulous attention to bovine health, which is favoured both by cultural attitudes towards cattle and by the region's small-scale production systems. Tuberculosis, for example, was easily eradicated in Donegal in 1963, whereas in the south it continued to present serious health hazards until 1966. Dysentery and trichomonosis, a venereal disease, are virtually unknown; and mastitis, the plague of dairiers, is rare.

Farmers (especially those with little fenced land) also take great pains to avoid cattle injuries. Among other tactics, they keep the animals awake at night in the byre to avoid accidents that might result from crowding. Such practices also help forestall 'blackleg' or blackquarter, a clostridial disease of cattle in which bruising is sometimes a predisposing factor [editors' note]. Blackleg was reported as having occurred in the cattle herds of 30 per cent of respondents, and it was treated by the veterinarian.

Twenty per cent of the sample reported cases of 'scours' (protozoal or, less commonly, bacterial diarrhoea), particularly in calves. Cures range from veterinary treatments to, more typically, home remedies. A common example of the latter is simply drenching with boiled water. (No one mentioned taking the calf off milk, a step recommended by veterinarians.) Of course, fluid replacement is an important part of any diarrhoeal therapy, in that it helps combat dehydration. There was no mention of scours occurring in sheep or lambs, again probably because sheep are left unattended most of the time so there is less opportunity to observe their health problems.

For Donegal farmers, however, the most widely known and dreaded 'other' disease of cattle is 'redwater' (babesiosis or piroplasmosis), also known as *murrain* (a Middle-English term meaning 'plague'). Redwater is an especially virulent, tickborne protozoan disease that afflicts only cattle; the ovine equivalent does not occur in Ireland [editors' note]. Government surveys report that the local cattle have some natural immunity to redwater, whereas 'Cattle introduced into the area or transferred over a considerable distance within the area show acute symptoms of redwater' (AFT 1969 Part 2:68). As usual, however, farmers disagree with government findings. They maintain that animals 'bought-in' from only a short distance away are susceptible to *murrain*. Indeed, in every case of redwater reported by sample members, the afflicted stock had come from within a radius of 15 miles. In point of fact, the distribution of *Babesia*-carrying ticks can be highly idiosyncratic, such that both infested and non-infested farms can be found even within very delimited areas [editors' note]. Interestingly, farmers did not attribute redwater to ticks or to genetic susceptibility. Rather, they viewed it as one of the many dangers of cattle transfers, and an especially inexplicable one since wasting and death are very rapid.

For sheep, the most common 'other' disease is 'braxy' (malignant oedema). An especially virulent clostridial disease that kills sheep almost overnight, braxy is sometimes linked with predisposing injuries such as wounds from fighting among rams or lacerations of the vulva from parturition. Virtually all Donegal farmers vaccinate against this disease as there is no known cure. Respondents recalled how their fathers and grandfathers lost more sheep to braxy than any other cause before today's highly effective vaccine was developed. 'Pulpy kidney' (Type D enterotoxaemia) is another clostridial disease that, like braxy, is characterized by rapid onset and frequent fatalities in sheep. Within the sample, 27 per cent vaccinated against it regularly; 7 per cent reported occasional cases. According to agricultural agents, lamb dysentery (Types B and C enterotoxaemia) is rare in Donegal. However, 17 per cent of the sample vaccinated ewes prior to lambing, so that antitoxins will be passed to new-borns in their dams' colostrum.

At the time of field research, 'sheep-footrot' (virulent, malignant or contagious footrot) was relatively new to Donegal. Whatever its source, its spread was helped by the growing pressures on land resources that have led to overgrazing, which can promote the muddy and mucky conditions that contribute to foot-rot. In the early 1970s footrot did not yet seem to be a very serious problem, and it was still unknown in the county's Gaelic-speaking areas. Although people evinced little concern about prophylaxis, they discussed possible therapies at great length. One common remedy they mentioned was a footbath of Bluestone (copper sulphate). Within the sample, 17 per cent had used this on their sheep; another 13 per cent had occasionally had a sheep with footrot.

'Orf' (contagious ecthyma) is a zoonotic viral disease that attacks only sheep, primarily lambs and juveniles. The chief signs are redness, swelling, and the formation of bloody sores and scabs in the buccal area (see also Brisebarre, this volume). While orf itself is rarely fatal, excessive sores can cause sheep to stop eating. Orf can also prevent lambs from suckling if their dams have lesions on the udder. Thus it can cause serious debilitation and even death by starvation. Only 10 per cent of the sample treated orf when they saw it; 7 per cent had seen the odd case in their own flocks. The traditional remedy was to rub turf soot on the sores, a 'cure' that apparently did no harm. Although a vaccine was available, few of the sample were aware of it, and none had ever used it. Typically, though, the disease disappears on its own in a week or two. Apparently humans can acquire a partial immunity to orf by handling sheep. The doctor in Donegal noted that he had never seen a serious case among local people. In contrast, the only two workers at a government experiment station who had no prior experience with sheep became very ill with this disease; one even had to be hospitalized. The few farmers who do contract orf consult a doctor instead of a religious healer (see later sections). According to the local doctor, there is no real cure for the condition in humans, but penicillin will clear up the secondary infection.

A minor ovine disease but one with a long history in Donegal is contagious conjunctivitis (Gaelic *dullnamollog* or 'moon blind'). Farmers diagnose it by the formation of a white film over one or both eyes. Some people are skilled at snipping out a small piece of the film and then pulling away the rest with a needle and thread. This is a very delicate but effective operation. Other home remedies include putting ground glass, household bleach, acid or still other materials into the sheep's eyes. Used prophylactically, such measures might conceivably have some beneficial effect by causing an inflammation just before the disease hits, thereby accelerating healing [editors' note]. In any case, if one sheep is discovered to have *dullnamollog*, the whole flock is promptly treated. People did not know the cause of this disease, although several speculated that wet weather can bring it on. In fact, it can have various etiologies, usually bacterial in young lambs and chlamydial in adults [editors' note]. Farmers made no mention of an equivalent disease for cattle.

Another minor but ancient ill of sheep in Donegal is photosensitization, which results from the consumption of plants with substances that cause hypersensitivity to ultra violet (UV) rays. The Gaelic name for this is *galornacat* 'disease of the cat' because the condition can cause a sheep's ears to wither and drop off, leaving stubs that resemble cats' ears. Folk remedies abound, but the most common is to rub buttermilk on the ears. In fact, sheep usually recover on their own; losses are due to secondary infections. The best 'cure' at present is penicillin, although neither the local veterinarian nor the chemist understands why; nor did they know of the connection between penicillin and the secondary infections. Ethnoetiologies of *galornacat* vary. Unaware of its connection with UV, many Donegal farmers relate it to the wind or to high mountain grazing. More knowledgeable individuals attribute it to sheep's consumption of the tiny sun-dew plant, which grows on wet, marshy lands. Recent experiments at the Agricultural Institute's Sheep Research Station in County Galway indicate that the sun-dew plant is unpalatable even to semi-starved lambs. However, there is evidence linking photosensitization with mycotoxins produced by fungi that sometimes thrive in association with the highly palatable bog asphodel, which grows on the wet, acid moorlands where sheep are often grazed. Thus this ethno-etiology may not be far wrong.

Finally, two tick-borne diseases are common among Donegal sheep. 'Pains' (tick pyaemia) is an endemic staphylococcal disease of lambs characterized by pyemic abscesses in the joints and elsewhere. Farmers dip their lambs against this ill about a month after birth. Nevertheless, shortly thereafter many lambs may contract 'pains' and die. Mortality rates can be high. 'Louping ill' (ovine encephalomyelitis) is a tick-borne viral disease of the central nervous system that affects sheep of all ages. A vaccine for it was once available in Donegal, but during the 1960s the vaccine was taken off the market due to production difficulties and irregularities. Dipping is now recommended instead. The dips are largely efficacious and hence today few sheep are lost to louping ill. Nevertheless, most of the sample expressed indignation at the withdrawal of the vaccine.

In general, Donegal farmers consider vaccines infallible and dips fallible, not without reason. Dips often fail for a variety of possible reasons. First, the margin for error is much greater in dipping as versus vaccination; vaccines generally come in ready-made doses, but dips must be 'mixed up'. Second, farmers often purposely prepare a more dilute solution than is prescribed because, as with flukicides for cattle, most believe that strong dips can harm the sheep. Third, Donegal farmers have their own dipping 'styles'; many dip their sheep for only 30 or 45 seconds, rather than the full minute recommended by government agricultural agents. In consequence, the compound does not fully penetrate the wool. Neither do Donegal farmers always comply with the laws that fix the frequency and dates of annual dippings. Fourth, the dipping compounds themselves may be at fault. Several respondents waxed eloquent about the 'substandard' products used in the county dipping pit. Many also complained that the government has outlawed the best dips. Some men have even travelled to Northern Ireland to obtain compounds with ingredients (for example, DDT) they deemed more powerful but that are illegal in the Republic. Fifth and finally, dips have only a transient effect as compared to vaccines.

Supernaturally-linked diseases

Other unexplained dangers that befall livestock are sometimes ascribed to the evil eye, as when cattle run amok (sometimes due to panic at the sound that warble flies make in summer) or fall into ditches for no apparent reason, or as when sheep are found dead in the fields and farmers cannot identify the cause. Before professional veterinary services were widely available, it is likely that such events were much more frequently explained by reference to supernatural phenomena. Indeed, priests were sometimes called in on an emergency basis to dispel the evil eye in cattle. This ill was not believed to strike sheep, however. Vestiges of these and other beliefs still linger (although priests no longer make house calls). Even sceptics take precautions like identifying others' cattle as their own if, at a market or fair, a person believed to have the evil eye inquires after their animals. On several occasions, interviewees reported—always as a joke— that in order to ward against redwater in cattle transfers, 'some' Catholics took the precaution of sprinkling holy water on cows they purchased from Protestants, thus ritually neutralizing the dangers associated with livestock transfers (see also Brisebarre, this volume). As with evil eye, however, no one reported such practices in any contexts involving sheep.

There are, after all, inexplicable accidents and to-local-eyes strange afflictions even now. An example is ringworm, a zoonotic disease of cattle. In the 1970s, most people in Donegal believed (correctly, according to the local doctor) that there was no effective medical treatment for humans who contract ringworm. So they consulted folk healers whose remedies consisted of reciting odd prayers, reading certain pages of the Bible in a prescribed order, and the like.

Analysis and conclusions

To summarize, in terms of nutrition and feeding, cattle are fed and stabled over the winter and sheep are not. For most farmers in south-west Donegal, it is that simple. One would have to be 'daft' to do otherwise. AFT findings bear out this production choice: '[The] level of winter nutrition is more than adequate for the minimum nutritional requirements of dry cattle including dry cows and is almost sufficient for moderate fattening of dry stock. If the sheep on these farms were fed from the same reserves, then the nutritional requirements of the total live-stock would not be adequately satisfied' (AFT 1969 Part 2:61). Thus, both farmer attitudes and experiment-station studies of nutrition and feeding suggest that the people of south-west Donegal learned long ago that feeding sheep imperils cattle production, the farm's economic mainstay. This is a risk too great to take. For Donegal farmers, this principle seems so obvious as to require no comment. But to an untutored outsider, its expression can seem as bizarre as court cases over the inhumane treatment of cattle, but not sheep.

Similarly, with regard to livestock disease, cattle receive immediate treatment for most ills, and even professional veterinary care. (The one exception to this statement—warble infestation—seems to be related to farmer confusion about the incidence and importance of a disease that somehow came to be misper-ceived as a political matter.) In contrast, attention to ovine health is much more limited and haphazard, and sheep are almost never accorded professional veter-inary care. For example, for the major parasitic ill of both species (liverfluke disease), if there was regular (but reduced) dosing for cattle, there was irregular (and reduced) dosing for sheep. Overall, not even half the survey sample dosed their sheep regularly or adequately for flukes or other endoparasites. In the case of deficiency diseases, in the rare instance that these were diagnosed in cattle, the animals were promptly provided with mineral blocks and feed supplements; and in difficult cases, a veterinarian would be called in. But fewer than a third of the sample treated sheep for deficiency diseases; only a very few ever provided them with minerals or supplementary feeds; and the idea of calling in a vet for such problems was unheard of.

Indeed, farmers of south-west Donegal seem mostly indifferent to deficiency and infectious diseases in their sheep, unless they can be easily and inexpensively treated. Virtually the only instance in which the word 'all' could be applied to farmers' management of ovine health is that of braxy, where all interviewees said they vaccinated against it. (As it turned out, however, at least one of them lied.) Despite their complaints about dips, with the exception of braxy Donegal farmers were rarely willing to invest in vaccines for sheep. For example, one vaccine marketed at the time of field research immunized sheep against seven diseases, including all the clostridial group plus other ills that sample members had never heard of. This vaccine was not commonly used, however, because of its expense.

Certainly, economic considerations play a role in farmers' different attitudes towards and management of cattle versus sheep. One head of cattle is worth some 10 sheep (Attwood and Heavey 1964:250). And while a visit from the veterinarian costs only about 1/50th of the value of a full-grown cow, for an adult sheep this figure is approximately one-fifth. At first glance, then, simple economic explanations for Donegal farmers' different approach to bovine and ovine healthcare might appear to suffice. History tells a different tale, however, as the following incidents reveal.

> During the 1930s, the government prohibited the sale of livestock outside the country. Since Donegal's primary livestock market was Northern Ireland, cattle fell in value until they were almost worthless. Calves fetched a mere 10 shillings, and a good cow went for just a few pounds. During this time, however, local veterinarians say they received no fewer calls for services for cattle than they did during the period of research reported here (although they noted that they were not paid as often). No one neglected sick or hungry cattle, despite the fact that for nearly a decade, cattle had very little monetary value. Of course, they continued to produce milk and occasionally to serve as draught animals. But in contrast to cattle, sick, starving sheep were ignored, even though sheep did not lose their value because of a lively trade in contraband wool.

Donegal farmers of today reconfirmed this stance when asked under what circumstances they would call in a veterinarian. Respondents indicated that, for cattle, they would seek veterinary services in any and all cases in which they could not themselves immediately identify and treat the problem. But they said they almost never had recourse to veterinarians for sick sheep. Respondents tendered a variety of explanations for this: they weren't sure what disease the sheep might have; they tried curing the animals with home remedies; or, most frequently, they observed that whatever the precipitating cause of a sheep's ailment, the real cause was starvation—and what could a veterinarian do about that?

The distinction between cattle and sheep is maintained in other ways, too. In farmers' differential response to zoonoses, there are hints of an almost sacred versus secular division between the two species. People consult religious healers if they contract ringworm from cattle; but they turn to medical doctors if they catch orf from sheep. Lending further credence to such a division are verbal and ritualized protective acts taken to ward against supernaturally-linked ills in cattle; but there are no such practices or beliefs concerning sheep.

Such economic and ideological distinctions between livestock species are neither illogical nor unusual, as research in other parts of the globe attests (Perezgrovas, this volume, Primov 1992, McCorkle 1994). Their importance lies in their immediate implications for the extension of new husbandry and healthcare techniques to stockowners who draw them. These distinctions often dictate what or how much people will be willing to invest in improving their management of one or another livestock species. In the case of south-west Donegal, techniques to enhance bovine production are much more likely to be accepted (so long as they are not politically entangled) than are interventions to improve ovine husbandry and healthcare. The latter are apt to be ignored, particularly if they require extra work or expense, such as increased dipping or costly vaccinations. While most stockraisers are well aware that better feeding and veterinary attention would increase lamb survival rates and overall ovine production and productivity, they choose not to take such measures.

Livestock developers have often characterized such production decisions as 'irrational'. Conversely, stockraisers often find many of the proposed interventions of developers just as irrational—or in the words of Donegal farmers, 'daft'. When it comes to livestock development in such contexts, two kinds of logic may be at odds: the farmers' logic, based on centuries or even millennia of stockraising experience; and the developers', wherein 'Local systems are judged inefficient because they do not respond to the goal of market production. There is no serious consideration of the possibility that there may be other, more appropriate models for evaluating production systems' (Primov 1992:54). In south-west Donegal, the model is a simple but shrewd one: maximize production from cattle and minimize losses from sheep. Put another way, one species is raised with the goal of ensuring long-term consumption and cash needs rather than short-term money profits, while the other species is deployed so as to take maximum advantage of annual agro-ecological opportunities with minimal risk to the stockraising enterprise as a whole. In some years, extra money will be made on the sheep; in others, they may fetch little or nothing.[6] But in any event, nothing much has been invested in them so nothing much will be lost. Meanwhile, there will always be cattle, to provide the household with milk and some longer-term economic security.

As researchers have found in cognate systems of mixed livestock production in other parts of the world, 'It is very difficult, to say the least, to improve upon this strategy' (ibid.). Farmers of south-west Donegal echo this observation in contrasting their ovine management system with that demonstrated at government experiment stations: 'The government puts everything in and takes nothing out; we put damn all [very little or nothing] in and take everything out'.

This is a fairly accurate assessment. Hundreds of years ago, Donegal stockraisers empirically sorted out most of the key production factors in their environment. While each new generation is free to make adjustments, the fundamental principles of south-west Donegal's livestock production strategy became culturally routinized, reinforced by legal precedent and ideological belief. The region's system of mixed livestock production is one that was designed to last. And it *has* lasted—for at least 2000 years. A production strategy that permits 'everything to be taken out' (albeit something of an over-statement) will be retained until a new strategy can be demonstrated to be better. As of the early 1970s, for the people of south-west Donegal, none had been demonstarted.

Notes

1. The field research on which this chapter is based was conducted during 14 months between 1970 and 1971, funded by a grant from the National Institutes of Mental Health. The author would like to thank the editors of this volume for their comments on earlier drafts of this chapter and for the prodigious amount of work involved in their critical technical review.
2. Rural life has changed significantly since then, especially after Ireland joined the European Economic Community. The ethnographic present tense used throughout the text should be understood as referring to Donegal's situation preceding this event.
3. This survey used a random sample of 249 farms drawn in the Glenties Rural District of West Donegal, an area of approximately 411 square miles or 263 000 acres.
4. For example, in Gaelic a broad range of symptoms/illnesses that involve wasting are described by a single term which translates as 'pining'. It is also interesting to speculate whether—as in the case of footrot—the lack of a Gaelic term for a specific disease may signal that the disease was introduced in more recent times (see also Schillhorn van Veen, this volume).
5. Indeed, records of liver condemnations at slaughter between the years of 1968 and 1971 indicated that approximately 90 per cent of all adult cattle in Ireland were infested with flukes (Nuallian, 1973).
6. One point that farmers made over and over during field research was that they think in terms of seven-year cycles, believing that good and bad years will average out across any one cycle. There was no general agreement as to when these seven-year cycles began or ended. Most respondents seemed to date their individual cycles from the time they began farming.

18. Ethnoveterinary R&D in production systems

CHIP STEM

SUSTAINABLE ECONOMIC PROGRESS in the Third World cannot be achieved merely through technology transfer from the so-called developed countries. Indeed, the transfer of 'miracle' but alien technology has created development white elephants around the world. Worse still, attempts at direct technology transfer have often severely disrupted traditional systems of production, leaving people with even less than they had before they were 'developed' (Grigg 1985, Halderman 1985, Horowitz 1980, Howes 1980, Packard-Winkler 1989, Scott and Gormley 1980, Skinner 1989, Swift and Maliki 1984).

In arid and semi-arid Africa, stockraisers face severe production constraints related, among other things, to population pressures that have forced more and more people on to less and less land; much of the better traditional grazing areas have been settled by farmers, significantly reducing available pasturage (Campbell 1984, Dupire 1972, Swift and Maliki 1984, White 1986, 1987). Moreover, with the decreased rainfall of recent decades, many parts of Africa have experienced declines in livestock productivity (Bernus 1975, Day 1989, Lamb 1986, Malo and Nicholson 1990, Sollod 1990, USDA 1981). At the same time, there is growing evidence that government policies aimed at permanently settling pastoralists and encouraging them to adopt Western-style ranching techniques are exacerbating problems in both pastoral production and the environment (Halderman 1985, Hogg 1986, Little 1985a, Penning de Vries 1983, Stryker 1984). In fact, where pastoralists have begun to adopt modern ranching methods, environmental degradation is often at its worst (Campbell 1984, Hogg 1983, Little 1985b, White 1987).

This realization has stimulated a renewed interest in and respect for the efficiency, advantages and inherent sustainability of traditional livestock production systems (Bernus 1981, Bernus *et al.* 1983, Horowitz 1981, 1983, McCorkle 1989a, 1989b, Rhoades 1986, Salzman 1983). Such systems typically feature risk-averse strategies that give producers a reasonable assurance of long-term success, even though production in any given year may be less than its short-term productive potential (Stryker 1984). Recent research suggests that what many dryland livestock producers need is not major innovations but rather targeted, incremental changes that reduce or eliminate some of the more important risks and constraints to animal health and production, without drastically modifying the overall system (Horowitz 1983, Sollod *et al.* 1984).

In order for these incremental changes to be identified and introduced in a sustainable fashion, however, the entire system of livestock production must be understood to the fullest possible extent, including its social, cultural and ideological matrix (see, for example, the chapters by Ibrahim, Ibrahim and Abdu, Lawrence, and Perezgrovas in this volume). Ethnoveterinary research and development (R&D) has a critical role to play in this regard. Here, ethnoveterinary R&D

(sometimes also termed veterinary anthropology) is defined so as to embrace not only disease factors but also epidemiological, socio-cultural and biophysical aspects of animal health and production. Such a production-systems perspective is imperative if appropriate incremental changes are to be successfully effected. Only thus can researchers and developers pinpoint and address the real constraints, as perceived by producers and as validated by rigorous scientific investigation within the production system itself. Otherwise, R&D invites the transfer of inappropriate technology—technology that turns out to be technically, economically and culturally unsustainable over the long term.

This chapter has two goals. First, drawing upon ethnoveterinary R&D by Tufts University's Program of International Veterinary Medicine, it outlines key considerations in designing and conducting ethnoveterinary studies. Second, some of the practical benefits of applying the results from such studies to the design of appropriate and sustainable livestock interventions are discussed. Throughout, the principles, findings and benefits of ethnoveterinary R&D are illustrated with firsthand experiences from Tufts University fieldwork in Burkina Faso, Kenya, Morocco, and Niger between 1981 and 1995.

The design and conduct of ethnoveterinary R&D[1]

As many of the chapters in this volume attest, ethnoveterinary R&D typically entails surmounting major cultural and linguistic barriers. This means that particular attention must be paid to making study design and implementation socio-culturally sensitive if findings are to be truly useful in shaping development interventions (Sollod *et al.* 1984). Research goals and procedures must be well thought-out and clearly articulated from the start.

First, of course, research instruments must be carefully selected or devised to embody the study goals. Otherwise, they will not capture the data needed. In preparing surveys and other instruments, scientists should always build upon information already available about the society, culture and animal health and production strategies of the target population. The extent to which these topics have been previously documented helps define the scope of the study. Reliance on the work of others can save considerable time and expense. One example of how such pre-preparation and literature review can be useful is the following.

o Among the Samburu of Kenya, veterinary researchers found that referring to the work of historians, demographers, developers and especially anthropologists on gender-related divisions of labour in the household allowed them better direction and focus of their survey instruments and sampling. Among Samburu, women are largely responsible for collecting and preparing the plants used in traditional veterinary treatments. When men were questioned on this subject, however, they did not refer the researchers to the women in their household who perform these tasks. Instead, the men offered answers of their own. When the research team later interviewed household women, it was discovered that the men's answers had often been inaccurate or inappropriate (see also Heffernan *et al.* this volume).

In the above example, if researchers had failed first to consult the anthropological and other literature, they might well have overlooked or misrepresented women's role in animal healthcare. Consequently, the full extent of Samburu ethnoveterinary knowledge might have been underestimated.[2] But by first consulting previous research, a project can ensure that all relevant actors are included in the research design from the outset, thus ensuring more accurate and complete data collection.

Whether reviewing the literature or gathering preliminary secondary data, however, past fieldwork and assumptions should always be verified with live-stock producers. The following case is instructive.

○ In both Morocco and Niger, a lack of definitive diagnostic data on *Clostridium perfringens*-induced enterotoxaemia had led the government and some scientists to assume that this disease is not a major constraint to pastoral production. (The lability of the toxin involved makes it difficult to diagnose under field conditions.) Consequently, the livestock services did not offer a vaccine against it. Still, *C. perfringens* enterotoxaemia produces classical signs; and when it is observed with the appropriate epidemiological indicators, experienced animal health specialists can confidently diagnose it in the field. However, ethnoveterinary research demonstrated that grass-induced enterotoxaemia is indeed an important disease of sheep in certain regions. In part, this finding resulted from the fact that, in both countries, pastoralists themselves accurately recognize this disease and can describe it in detail. Such information from herders led the R&D team to recommend increased government attention to this problem (Fine *et al.* 1990, Stem 1986c). As a result, the government of Niger funded a national veterinarian to learn how to produce the appropriate vaccine.

The next step in ethnoveterinary R&D—actual data collection—often uses surveys. Survey instruments may consist of questionnaires, open-ended interviews or a combination of the two. Tufts researchers (for example, Heffernan *et al.*, this volume) and others (for example, Casley and Kumar 1988) have found that a combination of methods works best (see also Grandin and Young, this volume). Specific questions should be routinely asked of all respondents: which diseases of each species do producers consider the most important; which treatments work best and which routinely fail; what special measures do livestock producers take during droughts. Many questions, however, are best asked in an open-ended format, because this approach often elicits information or raises topics that might otherwise be overlooked. Yet it is these topics that can often be immediately useful in implementing interventions as in the following example.

○ Open-ended interviews with agro-pastoral Peul (Fulani) in Burkina Faso and Niger revealed that they use a reportedly effective, traditional vaccination against contagious bovine pleuro-pneumonia (CBPP) (Wolfgang 1983). This finding served as an extremely useful point of departure later on, in explaining and mounting a herder-based animal-health extension programme that included (see below). It is doubtful that a closed questionnaire would have unearthed this information.

Of course, when conducting any kind of interviews or surveys, language and cultural barriers can cause interviewees to interpret researchers' questions in many different ways. To cross-check answers, interviewers should always re-phrase their questions about a given topic at several points in the interview. This strategy allows for discussion of seemingly discrepant answers with respondents, thus preventing misunderstandings of the questions asked or the answers given. A good example is the following.

○ While investigating the causes of drought-related animal mortality in Niger, researchers identified a wide variety of diseases that contributed to high mortality rates among small ruminants. But when herders were asked about what had killed their animals, they almost invariably answered that it was 'hunger' or 'lack of feed'. Re-phrasing and re-posing this question revealed that respondents really meant that lack of pasture and feed had made their animals more susceptible to diseases that are frequently fatal. When the question was clarified, herders reported that malnutrition *per se* accounted for only 17 per cent of drought-related mortality in sheep and 7 per cent in goats. For goats, interviewees described 12 causes of death other than hunger. And for both species, they indicated that enterotoxaemia was the most important cause   (Cord *et al.* 1986).

Re-phrasing and re-posing questions is especially important if a translator is involved in interviews. It is vital that the translator understand the intent of each question correctly. Also, her/his demeanour and approach are important. Translators from the same ethnic group as interviewees are more likely to be sensitive to and respectful of respondents' customs and attitudes. Translators should be sure to share this cultural knowledge with the research team, too; and they should coach the team in proper etiquette in approaching interviewees. This will help avoid unintentional *faux pas* that may trigger refusals to participate in the study or lead to wrong answers. Above all, translators should be instructed (and reminded frequently) that their role is not to interpret, but to translate. Insofar as possible, they should repeat questions and answers exactly as stated, so as to prevent misunderstandings on the part of both researchers and respondents.

○ In Niger, the Tufts University team discovered that one translator sometimes re-interpreted people's answers, or did not ask the questions in detail, or gave his own answers to the questions posed. The result was that certain data had to be rejected.

   Ideally, translators should also be the same sex as interviewees.[3]

   In the Moslem nations of Morocco and Niger, researchers found that women frequently refuse to be interviewed by men. And men do not always take a female translator seriously; sometimes they even give her purposely false or misleading responses.

Almost invariably, stockraising and thus ethnoveterinary R&D involves both women and men. In fact, fieldwork teams have demonstrated that, globally, the role of women in animal rearing, healthcare and marketing is far greater than previously supposed (Heffernan *et al.*, this volume, McCorkle *et al.* 1989, see also Horowitz and Jowkar 1992 and Jowkar and Horowitz 1991). The relative roles of males and females in stockraising have obvious practical implications for conducting research, designing interventions, and staffing and implementing extension and training programmes in livestock development. Some instructive examples follow.

○ Among Twareg herders residing within a 150km radius of Tahoua in central Niger, women do the milking. However, 250km to the north, Twareg males assume this task (Bernus *et al.* 1983). In both areas, young boys are often responsible for milking goats, while men milk the camels. Thus, an extenison programme to promote recognition, treatment, and prevention of mastitis, for example, would be confusing and largely ineffective if directed to Twareg men in the Tahoua region or, conversely, to women among the northern Twareg.

o As noted earlier, interviewing Samburu men about ethnoveterinary botanicals yielded imprecise data because it is actually the women who collect these plants. On the other hand, Samburu women cannot give detailed information about administering these indigenous drugs because that is usually the job of men (Heffernan *et al.*, this volume).

In addition to gender roles, differences in socio-economic status must also be taken into account in designing and conducting ethnoveterinary R&D. Most livestock development projects try to include beneficiaries from middle- and low- as well as high-income groups of stockraisers (see Grandin and Young, this volume). Yet it is all too easy to focus on the wealthier producers. They are usually better educated; they often speak the official language of the country; they are more accustomed to, and more sophisticated at, dealing with outsiders; and their community stature and local political standing dictate that they be the first to be contacted. However, for many of the same reasons, these wealthier individuals' production systems are likely to differ greatly from the poorer people's in their community. Thus, interventions designed on the basis of information collected solely from higher-income producers may well be inappropriate for the broader population. If a project is to benefit middle- and lower-income people too, then study goals and design must be such that statistically reliable data are gathered from *all* economic classes of producers.

o In Niger, when wealthier herders were asked about the need to treat their animals for internal parasites, they responded that it was necessary to treat all their stock with anthelmintics. Likely they answered as they did partly because of their comparatively frequent contact with government livestock agents, who tend to emphasize regular anthelmintic treatment. Poorer herders who had less contact indicated that treatment for gastrointestinal parasitism was *not* necesssary. As it turned out, they were more likely to be correct for this region of the Sahel (see below).

Another reason why it is important for ethnoveterinary R&D to examine a cross-section of the economic strata engaged in livestock production is to determine how widespread a given healthcare or management practice is. This information is invaluable for identifying special or minority practices that may merit extension to a broader range of stockraisers. For example:

o During the 1982/3 drought, Twareg herders in Niger varied markedly in the strategies they adopted to keep their animals alive. One might suppose that wealthier Twareg—who began with larger-than-average herds—would also end the drought with more animals than poorer herders. However, the most successful herd-survival strategy was one in which Twareg entered the drought with a minimum core of reproductive stock and sold off or lent out their remaining animals. This strategy worked for all economic classes of Twareg who had viable herd sizes of > 5 TLU tropical livestock units per family at the beginning of the drought (Cord *et al.* 1986). If researchers had ignored economic differences among herders, these findings would not have come to light.

Lessons such as the foregoing can be fed into extension programmes and used for the benefit of livestock producers as a whole. Of course, socio-economic status can also be a key variable in stockraisers' use of extension services. For instance:

○ Throughout Kenya, Morocco and Niger, research shows that wealthier herders tend to use livestock extension services and to accept changes introduced from outside more frequently than do middle- or low-income stockraisers. The reasons for this may include poorer producers' lack of transport and hence access to extension workers, their imperfect understanding of the extension services available, the price of drugs and the general tendency of extension to concentrate on larger farmers.

Such findings suggest that any extension programme aimed at improving the livelihood of *all* classes of livestock producers should make a special effort to reach the poorer ones.

The uses of ethnoveterinary R&D

Ethnoveterinary studies constitute an extremely effective way to initiate research and development in any livestock production system. Ethnoveterinary work should begin as early as possible in a project because it is one of the best entrées into a stockraising society. People are almost invariably enthusiastic about discussing their production savvy, their animals and especially their herds' health. Rarely is a producer unwilling to take as much time as the investigator desires to explore such topics. Such producer-researcher dialogue communicates a sincere interest on the part of latter in the health and well-being of the former's herds and in the constraints that producers themselves consider most critical (Sollod *et al.* 1984). Ethnoveterinary research can thus play a key role in building the mutual trust and respect that ultimately lead to successful and sustainable development.

Among other factors, the frequent, positive contact that an ethnoveterinary study engenders between producers and R&D personnel can make field trials[4] and livestock interventions much more readily acceptable to stockraisers. In large part, this is because the practices and strategies tested will respond directly to problems that producers themselves have identified as important. If they don't, people will be understandably reluctant to lend their animals to the trials.

○ The Niger Integrated Livestock Production Project (NILPP) sought to work with Twareg and Peul who had a history of steadfastly refusing to participate in field trials (Stem 1986a). But after a sustained ethnoveterinary study in which project personnel demonstrated their commitment to understanding and tackling animal health problems that herders themselves considered important, both ethnic groups changed their minds. They even allowed their animals to be ear-tagged for purposes of long-term identification and tracking during field trials.

Or course, balanced field trials mean that not all animals in the herd or flock can receive the intervention being tested. This may pose problems for producer participation. If stockraisers think a trial could harm their animals, they will naturally be reluctant to participate. On the other hand, if people believe the intervention will be useful and advantageous, they may want all their animals included in the trial. A good solution is the following.

○ Research on vitamin-A deficiency among Twareg and WoDaaɓe herds in Niger (see below) found that directly involving herders in the assessment of trial results led people to agree to leave a group of untreated or placebo-treated controls. Herders appreciated the explanation that, by doing so, they could judge for themselves whether a given intervention was of value.

This more participatory approach has an added benefit in that such judgements are of critical importance if people are expected to spend money to adopt the interventions. Beyond facilitating field trials, the trust that preliminary ethno-veterinary R&D inspires also allowed the NILPP to use more sophisticated, double-blind experimental designs. These more scientific methods made for greater reliability and replicability of results and for more confident and broadly applicable final recommendations than might otherwise have been possible.

Ethnoveterinary studies can also help streamline field-level epidemiological investigations, thus conserving limited project resources. If performed by an interdisciplinary team with appropriate field experience, a detailed ethnoveterinary study will usually provide a fairly comprehensive list of a region's most important livestock diseases and nutritional problems, or at least of their clinical signs and post-mortem findings (Grandin and Young, this volume, Sollod *et al.* 1984, Stem 1985). This list can then be confirmed by more in-depth field study and epidemiological investigation. Moreover, ethnoveterinary research may uncover important diseases that might otherwise escape detection. In addition to the case of enterotoxaemia noted earlier, consider the following.

○ Among cattle and sheep in the Sahel, vitamin-A deficiency may be easily missed due to the fact that it is evidenced primarily only during the dry season or in drought years. If researchers happen to make their observations only during periods of high rainfall, they may overlook this problem unless they also make sure to consult herders about other seasons or years. Likewise for diseases that appear only during the rainy season if—as is commonly the case—researchers gather data only during the dry months when travel to the field is easier.

Ethnoveterinary studies can also make important technical inputs to livestock development initiatives, via the discovery of traditional techniques of disease treatment or prevention that may approximate, equal or surpass those of their Western counterparts in a given situation. Nearly all of the chapters in this volume illustrate this point. Further examples from Tufts University experiences include the following.

○ Twareg and Peul have long used simple but effective vaccines to protect their herds against some epidemic diseases such as CBPP (see also the chapters Köhler-Rollefson, and Schillhorn van Veen).

○ Twareg report that several indigenous plants are effective in combating endoparasites of small ruminants (particularly haemonchosis) and camels. These plants include *Cucumis* spp., *Boscia senegalensi*, and the fruits of two plants known as *imaglenanoru* and *inalinadil* in Tamashek.

○ Herders in Niger frequently repair distal leg fractures by splinting with flat pieces of wood wrapped in cloth (Plate 1). This technique is often very successful. Moreover, it obviates the need for expensive and cumbersome plaster or fibreglass splints.

Indigenous techniques and pharmaceuticals such as the foregoing should be

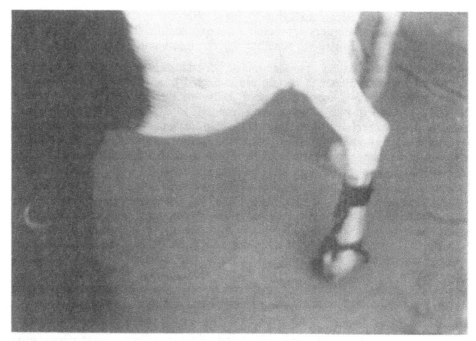

Plate 1. *A traditional Twareg splint applied to a metatarsal fracture in a sheep (photo by C. Stem)*

properly evaluated and compared to their Western veterinary equivalents, to determine if they can serve as cost-effective options that can be taken up by more and/or more different groups of producers (see also McCorkle and Bazalar, this volume). Of course, for any intervention to be successful over the long term, technical soundness alone is insufficient. The intervention must also be socio-economically worthwhile. In designing workable interventions, one common socio-economic consideration is the seasonal availability of pastoral labour.

o Dry-season forage bottlenecks are a well-known constraint on animal production in central Niger. Hence, developers might urge that producers make and store hay at the end of the rainy season. But at this time of year, labour is in very short supply. Families typically split up in order for some of their members to trail part of the herd to lusher rainy-season pastures farther north. Meanwhile, there are many new births in the herd, and the young animals demand extra care. In addition, this is the time of year when people are busy preparing for and then enjoying the most important annual festivals and holidays. Thus, unless ways can be found to free up additional labour or to reduce the labour demands of other activities, herders will probably reject recommendations that they make hay during this season.

Likewise for disposal patterns for crop by-products and residues. These must be examined carefully before any change is proposed, because such products are frequently used in other sectors of household production, where they may have great social and economic importance.

o Among Intawellen (the Twareg artisan class), women use millet chaff and bran to stuff leather pillows. The pillows are given as gifts, sold in the market or used at home. Before recommending that Intawellen feed a portion of these by-products to their livestock as a nutritional supplement, developers must first ascertain that this practice would not unduly compete with other uses. Otherwise, the household economy could be harmed rather than helped.

In every country where Tufts has conducted ethnoveterinary research, live-stock producers have demonstrated a keen understanding of the socio-economics of many of the nutritional and veterinary inputs in their production systems. A further example is the use of anthelmintics in extensive stock operations in semi-arid and arid zones.

○ Throughout West Africa, for several decades researchers and government livestock services have recommended mass anthelmintic treatment for gastro-intestinal parasites. There is ample evidence that such endoparasites are highly prevalent and numerous in the sub-humid and humid zones; most of the same parasites also occur in the semi-arid and arid zones of West Africa. Yet among Nigerien stockraisers of the Sahel, for instance, ethnoveterinary research revealed a great reluctance to adopt regular whole-herd anthelmintic programmes. Interviewees stated that it is not worth the trouble and expense to treat animals that are not clinically ill. Herders further pointed out that, with their communally-grazed pastures, it is virtually impossible to assure that all animals in a given area have been treated, and treated effectively. Thus, they reckon that an individual producer's routine use of these costly drugs would be futile.

Sahelian herders' social and economic calculation is borne out by research. In a double-blind study in a semi-intensive agropastoral production system in the semi-arid portion of Niger (Lindenmayer *et al.* 1988), animals were compared on performance indicators of morbidity, mortality, weight gain and reproductive performance. These indicators were measured biweekly, beginning with the late dry season and extending through the rainy season and both the early and late dry seasons, for a total of 11 months. In addition, the market values of individual animals in both the treatment and placebo groups were compared. Analysis revealed no statistically significant differ-ences between the two groups. Moreover, when the cost of an anthelmintic programme was calculated, the treatment group was less productive than the control animals. Furthermore, regular de-worming of the treatment group had no effect on market value.[5]

The foregoing study resulted in a pragmatic and cost-effective recommenda-tion to the Nigerien livestock service: that—except among sedentary livestock producers or where stock are regularly exposed to liver flukes—anthelmintics should be recommended only if animals show clinical signs of intestinal para-sitism. This is but one example of how veterinary interventions that may seem logical from the viewpoint of one ecozone—or one gender, socio-economic group or culture—can be impractical, uneconomical and unacceptable under other conditions. To take another example:

○ Disposable needles and syringes are a standard part of Western veterinary technology. But in nomadic contexts, such equipment is expensive and impractical. For one thing, re-supply is very likely impossible. In any case, it is culturally unacceptable to throw away something that is useful and of considerable relative cost. But under pastoral conditions in the Sahel, it is difficult to keep non-disposable needles and syringes clean. Thus, instead of improving the health situation, such inappropriate equipment can pose a health risk.

In-depth ethnoveterinary research can often suggest preferable alternatives. One example comes from ethnoveterinary R&D on vitamin-A deficiency in cattle in Niger (Stem 1986b). This case also aptly illustrates how veterinary interventions must be carefully designed within a holistic, production-system framework that spans socio-economic, ecological, and still other factors such as the availability of livestock services and inputs plus public health policy.

o Dry-season vitamin-A deficiency represents a principal and long-standing constraint to animal production throughout the Sahel (for example, Sollod *et al.* 1984). The condition is evidenced by night-blindness, which typically occurs about five to six months into the 8.5-month-long dry season. At this time, green forage containing the vitamin-A precursor, B-carotene, is scarce. Cattle and sheep are most severely affected.[6] Niger herders report that, in most years, at least 10 per cent of their cattle and sheep become night-blind. For individual herds, this figure can range as high as 65 per cent; and severely afflicted animals frequently die (Remillard *et al.* 1990, Stem 1986b). Stockraisers often water their animals in the cool of the night, but it is difficult to herd night-blind animals to the well. Instead, affected animals often must be watered separately. As their condition progresses, the creatures also become day-blind and too frightened to move more than a few feet. Thus they are unable to graze and to keep up with the rest of the herd.

To prevent and treat this deficiency, many herders try to force their animals to consume green shrubs, including the toxic *Calotropis procera*. When enough such browse is available, this is an effective treatment. However, *C. procera* can be quite toxic; and much of the time, other shrubs are scarce or unpalatable. Hence, herders must often seek other solutions. Another traditional treatment for night-blindness in both humans and animals is to place a piece of fresh goat's liver in the eyes. This is an 'insightful' treatment since liver is the main body depot for vitamin A. Moreover, due to browsing, goats have higher hepatic levels of vitamin A than other animals. Herders say this liver treatment is at least temporarily effective, especially if an animal has only recently become night-blind. Another temporary cure is to pour injectable vitamin A into the palpebral conjuctiva. But herders correctly note that, with both these therapies, the condition often recurs—presumably because adequate levels of vitamin A are not sustained within the bloodstream.

If animals can reach the livestock service, they can receive direct injections of the vitamin. However, livestock posts are few and far between in the pastoral zone of Niger, and transportation is extremely limited. Another alternative is oral vitamin-A boluses. But they are not always available. Moreover, bolus administration entails handling each animal individually—a very time-consuming task in a production system constrained by labour shortages. In addition, bolus administrators risk being gored. Finally, the boluses are very expensive for pastoralists.

Herders' detailing of all these considerations during initial, ethnoveterinary studies led scientists to conduct field trials on a newly developed water-soluble vitamin-A powder, comparing this alternative to the injectable and bolus forms. Since the powder can be mixed into the drinking-water, whole herds can be treated much more easily and safely than with either injections or boluses. Also, the powder is cheaper. Herders' participation in these trials was outstanding, and they were enthusiastic about the product's success and convenience in both treating and preventing vitamin-A-induced night-blindness. A further benefit of this effort was that it encouraged herders to participate in later and more complex trials, thus advancing the research agenda as a whole.

Veterinary auxiliaries

The foregoing example suggests one of the major ways in which participatory ethnoveterinary R&D can contribute to improving animal health and production on the micro-economic level. That is, it often suggests a least-cost approach to disease treatment and control. Of course, in order to introduce such technology packages or control programmes on a large scale, extension services are required. Yet in production systems where people and animals are scattered over vast areas and where transportation and infrastructure are limited, health-care extension is a difficult and costly job. An effective alternative to conventional extension, however, is a network of veterinary auxiliaries (Sollod and Stem 1991).

Veterinary auxiliaries are livestock producers who are trained and equipped as primary animal-healthcare and husbandry specialists (Plate 2). As herders themselves and as co-ethnics of their clients, they share the same social, cultural and linguistic background; and they are easily accessible by fellow producers because they generally live and work in the same vicinity. Furthermore, auxiliary programmes are consistent with the principle of self-help among rural people. Also, they are more likely to reach poorer stockraisers, in addition to rich or middle-income groups. Third World governments and development experts alike agree that this auxiliary approach to livestock development promises both effectiveness and sustainability (Haan and Nissen 1985, Sollod *et al.* 1984). After initial training and drug and equipment provisioning, the only recurrent costs of a veterinary auxiliary programme are for occasional field-level supervision and continuing education.

Ethnoveterinary studies have a useful role to play here, too. For one thing, the social, cultural, and economic investigations that form part of ethnoveterinary R&D can suggest who among livestock producers might prove the best candidates for becoming veterinary auxiliaries (Grandin and Young, this volume, Halpin 1981, Schwabe, this volume, Schwabe and Kuojok 1981, Sollod and Stem 1991). For another, once the study has catalogued herders' existing skills and knowledge, the curriculum for auxiliaries can be more appropriately and efficiently designed in terms of content and level of sophistication. Reinforcement of useful items in the traditional corpus of empirical health and production knowledge reduces the volume of information that must be transferred to both trainees and clients.

This approach makes the job of extension easier and more successful. Ethnoveterinary savvy—such as that attested by traditional vaccinations, splinting techniques, or ethno-diagnostic and therapeutic skills (as for vitamin-A deficiency)—can be referenced to help explain modern veterinary alternatives

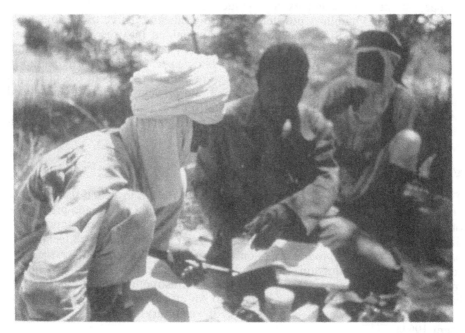

Plate 2. *Farmers and herders can be trained as veterinary auxiliaries to provide primary animal healthcare and management advice. (Photo by C. Stem)*

to stockraisers and, where desirable, to help incorporate such alternatives into the production system (Bernus 1969, Wolfgang 1983). As discussed throughout this chapter (and indeed, this whole volume), building upon herders' existing expertise markedly increases the chances that the incremental changes to be introduced will be acceptable and sustainable.

At the same time, veterinary auxiliaries are able to provide up-to-date information on the animal disease situation in areas that the government livestock service cannot otherwise reach (Schwabe, this volume, Stem 1985). One such case is provided by the Niger Range and Livestock Programme (NRLP) in central Niger.

○ The NRLP instituted a system of 'vetscouts' to provide continuous animal healthcare to a region of the country that until then had had contact with formal veterinary services only during the brief period of the annual vaccination campaign. In addition to regular healthcare, the vetscouts provided epidemiological monitoring among the remote, nomadic peoples of the region. Using simple pictographic reporting forms, 65 Twareg and WoDaaɓe vetscouts spread over an area of approximately $50000 km^2$ kept monthly records of diseases they encountered and treated among nomads' herds. When the auxiliaries reported to the government livestock service or pharmacy to purchase fresh drugs and supplies, their treatment records were collected and forwarded to a centrally located facility. There, only one trained employee was needed to enter the data into a simple computer programme that tracks disease occurrence and treatments administered.

This vetscout approach provided an invaluable but highly cost-effective and thus sustainable animal disease-surveillance system and stock inventory tool. Three years after the training programme was completed, over 75 per cent of the veterinary auxiliaries were still operative. (For more detail, consult Sollod and Stem 1991 and Stem 1985 or 1986c.)

Conclusions

Ethnoveterinary investigations have repeatedly demonstrated that a major concern among most pastoral producers is greater access to livestock health services. This chapter has suggested some of the ways in which ethnoveterinary R&D can facilitate, accelerate, refine or strengthen the scientific design, participatory implementation and policy outcomes of field trials, plus systems of veterinary extension and epidemiological intelligence.

With the growing economic crises that many Third World nations face (for example, Haan and Nissen 1985), maintaining even the present level of services is difficult. In such countries, it is unrealistic to expect public-sector funding for livestock development to increase significantly, even though current government spending is already less than proportional to the contribution that the livestock sector makes to African economies (ibid.).

Innovative techniques and programmes that enhance services to livestock producers without adding to government fiscal burdens are sorely needed. Drawing upon ethnoveterinary knowledge and practice, both research and extension can sift out, reinforce and promulgate viable strategies that targeted producer groups may find more acceptable. Wherever appropriate, rather than importing alien technology, developers should build upon tools and techniques that have been developed and 'tested' locally by stockraisers themselves (see, for example, Ibrahim and Abdu or Vondal, this volume). Innovations developed on-site are always more likely to work because they are generally both culturally and economically more appropriate. Furthermore, using findings from ethnoveterinary R&D as a basis for veterinary auxiliary programmes, herders' empirical health and husbandry skills can be tapped to provide efficient, cost-effective services to stockraisers in pastoral production systems. These strategies can extend the frontier of animal healthcare in the developing world well beyond its present limitations.

Notes

1. Throughout this section, general principles of good research design and fieldwork are illustrated with specific reference to ethnoveterinary medicine. Thus, this section is illustrative only. It does not pretend to constitute a thorough-going introduction to field methodologies and approaches. For the latter, readers should consult the vast literature on this subject in anthropology, sociology, veterinary epidemiology and international development. To name just a few useful works, Werner and Schoepfle's (1987) two-volume set furnishes an excellent overview of many of the topics discussed in the text. Devereux and Hoddinott (1993) provide case studies of different techniques under developing-country conditions, with some studies devoted specifically to livestock research. Nichols (1991) supplies a basic 'how-to' of survey methods for fieldworkers. For insights into the selection of ethnoveterinary field assistants, see Grandin and Young, this volume [editors' notes].
2. In general, Tufts University teams have found that male heads of households may respond incorrectly or incompletely to questions regarding the livestock-related activities of women. Thus it is imperative to interview both genders.

3. If for some reason this is not possible, however, experience indicates that it is usually easier for women investigators to reach both female and male respondents.
4. Naturally, good field trials should always actively involve livestock producers and their animals in their real-world production context, because trials performed at government ranches or on experiment stations are likely to be of questionable practicality. However, potentially dangerous interventions should always first be tested off-farm, lest human or livestock well-being and project credibility suffer.
5. In evidence of such recommendations and/or the distribution of such parasites, see: Akerejola *et al.* (1979), Bembello (1970), Bohnel (1971), Fabiyi (1970), Graber (1966, 1967, 1972), Gretillat (1976), Hart (1964), Mishra *et al.* (1979), Morel (1959), Schillhorn van Veen (1980), Schillhorn van Veen *et al.* (1976), Sprent (1946), Tager-Kagan (1984), Vassiliades (1981, 1984) and Vassiliades and Toure (1975). In arid and semi-arid Africa, it appears that recommendations for regular anthelmintic treatments have been based more on the presence of parasite eggs in faeces, rather than on the parasites' effect on animal production. Moreover, most of the scientific studies that have been performed have not realistically represented livestock production in the field.

One of the better-designed production studies to date in the Sahel (Vassiliades 1984) conducted extensive investigations of the effects of anthelmintic treatments on sheep production and mortality rates in Senegal. However, considerable experimental bias may have been introduced because sheep from different villages were used in the treatment as versus the control (placebo) groups. In addition, all sheep in the treatment village were treated—something that is impossible to obtain under real-life production-system conditions on communally-grazed land. Finally, all such studies should be conducted across a number of years so as to account for the Sahel's considerable intra- and inter-annual variation in rainfall and hence in parasitic disease [editors' note].
6. As browsers, camels and goats usually show signs of vitamin A deficiency only during periods of protracted or especially severe drought. This is because browse furnishes more B-carotene than grasses and is typically available year round.

19. Collection and use of ethnoveterinary data in community-based animal health programmes[1]

BARBARA E. GRANDIN AND JOHN YOUNG

THIS CHAPTER DESCRIBES and analyses the elaboration and use of an ethnoveterinary data-collection instrument in Maasailand, along with the instrument's subsequent application in the Kenya Livestock Programme (KLP) of the Intermediate Technology Development Group (ITDG). In collaboration with various community-based non-governmental organizations (NGOs), the KLP assists in the design and establishment of self-sustaining community-based programmes of animal health training and extension (CBAHPs). ITDG itself is an international non-governmental development agency whose mission is to enable poor people to develop and use productive technologies and practices that give them greater control over their own lives and contribute to the long-term development of their communities.

Since 1986, the KLP has been involved in five major CBAHP efforts.[2] Two are located in cropping areas: one among WaMeru farmers in Meru District (Young 1987) and one among WaKamba farmers in Machakos District (Njeru 1991). The other three have been conducted in Baringo (Young 1988), Samburu (Iles 1991) and Isiolo Districts (Grandin n.d.) among, respectively, Pokot, Samburu, and Turkana and Borana pastoralists. Each of these projects is in a different stage of development; but in each, the KLP has assisted with needs assessment (emphasizing the needs of the poorest households) and with project design and technical input into the development and use of veterinary training materials and methods that build upon local veterinary knowledge and practice.

In reflecting on its work with various projects, the KLP has outlined a minimum data set required to conduct a needs assessment and then to design and monitor the progress of CBAHPs (Grandin *et al.* 1991). The aim of collecting this data set is to understand:

o Intra-community wealth differences, so as to define the range of variation in animal management patterns by households of different economic standing, and to ensure that programme benefits reach poorer farmers.
o Principles of local social structure, in order to provide equal opportunity in recruitment of CBAHP trainees and the delivery of services.
o The major crop and livestock production practices in an area, and the role and importance of various livestock species to households of different economic standing, as well as to different sexes within the household.
o The main constraints to livestock production.
o The level and range of local vocabulary and knowledge with regard to livestock diseases, their symptom and syndrome recognition, etiologies, and the traditional and modern treatments known and used.
o The effects on community livestock production of national policies regarding, for example, veterinary services, drug regulations, and price controls on livestock inputs.

The depth of KLP data collection has varied from very rapid appraisals (Young 1988) to more intensive surveys (Njeru 1991, Young 1987) according to the wishes of the NGO partners, the time and resources available, and the particular project's needs. Thus, to collect its minimum data set, the KLP uses an array of techniques that are purposely flexible enough to be adapted to each project's requirements, yet standardized enough to provide the basic data required for programme design and implementation and to permit comparisons across projects.

Ethnoveterinary data-collection techniques span both informal and formal, general and specific methods. Informal and/or general techniques include literature reviews, participant observation, and free-flowing discussions with farmers, project personnel, government veterinary staff and NGO workers.

The primary formal method of data collection is wealth ranking (Grandin 1988). To do this, key informants rank community households according to their relative economic status as this is locally or emically defined. The ranking task captures the general differences between richer and poorer households. It is also used to elicit specific differences across wealth ranks with regard to aspects of animal management and health, such as size and composition of livestock holdings, perceived production problems and needs, and access to veterinary services. Depending on project resources, this information can be supplemented and double-checked by a modicum of household-level survey data.

Another key technique is progeny histories. In essence, these are animal genealogies that record the fate of all offspring born to a selection of animals in a herd/flock. When compiled, these histories provide basic information on patterns of animal offtake, fertility and mortality (cause, age, seasonality). Such histories are best begun with the dam of an animal currently in the herd/flock in order to provide more longitudinal data. This approach avoids the biases inherent in more conventional interview protocols, which often span only one year (Grandin 1984a, Young 1987).[3] Together with wealth ranking, progeny histories indicate which local livestock production problems might be amenable to appropriate technological interventions for which types of households, thus ensuring that some benefits will flow to poorer members of the community.

The focus of the present chapter, however, is the ethnoveterinary interview guide (hereafter EIG), which is applied in a flexible manner to collect mainly the information outlined in the fifth item bulleted above. Ethnoveterinary data collection has been a component of the KLP since its inception in 1986. The programme works from recognition of several basic facts about livestock production and healthcare systems. To wit: most stockraisers have at least some understanding of their animals' diseases, as well as ways of classifying, recognizing and treating them; however, the type, depth and breadth of veterinary knowledge can vary significantly across and within cultures as a function of numerous historical and contemporary factors;[4] and CBAHP training will be more successful and retained better if—rather than relying automatically or exclusively on Western-scientific etiological and diagnostic principles and terminology—training also builds on producers' existing animal healthcare concepts and vocabulary.[5]

The EIG was explicitly created in order to elicit its local understanding. This instrument was initially developed and implemented in Kenya's Maasailand by the first author, based on careful pre-testing, refinement, and verification with clinical case studies by a veterinarian (Grandin 1984b). The EIG also served as the basis for ILRAD's ethnoveterinary investigations in coastal Kenya (Delehanty, this volume).

Briefly put, the EIG provides substantial amounts of information useful for mounting animal healthcare initiatives. It identifies key actors, categories, concepts and recognized disease factors in ethnoveterinary systems. It generates a precise lexicon of local disease names and related terminology. For each disease chosen for detailed investigation, the EIG provides information on what animals are affected; how people diagnose the ailment; local understandings of its etiology, contagiousness and seasonality; and whether traditional or modern treatments for it are well-known and available. Applied to a diversity of individuals, the EIG gives a good idea of what veterinary information is in general circulation (as compared with what is restricted to specialists) and of how consistent this information is throughout the community of producers. Moreover, the EIG can be modified to capture all such insights at whatever level of resolution is desired.

Of course, a certain degree of ethnoveterinary intelligence could be collected merely by talking with stockraisers informally. But an organized interview guide administered by a skilled and sensitive fieldworker forestalls biases, omissions and misunderstandings; and it provides data that can be systematically compared both within and across sites. Based on the authors' firsthand experience in the development and use of the EIG, this chapter outlines: the interview guide and its components, along with the rationale behind them; typical responses plus potential biases in the instrument's administration; the interviewer skills and sensitivities required for gathering ethnoveterinary information; ways to record, organize and analyse the data collected; and the uses of EIG findings for designing and implementing CBAHP projects as well as other types of livestock development efforts.

The ethnoveterinary interview guide

The EIG consists of two parts. The first section is designed to collect basic background information on animal healthcare and husbandry in the region and to identify the livestock diseases that are locally named and recognized. This information is needed before the second part of the EIG can be applied: a list of 10 open-ended questions or question sets tailored for use in individual interviews about specific diseases.

As with any formal data-collection instrument, the EIG evolved and changed as it was applied in different contexts. One beauty of the instrument is that it can be pursued at whatever depth is required for the specific project. Farmers and pastoralists alike are usually quite happy to talk about their animals' health. Rarely are there any gaps in the conversation; instead, people usually provide more information than any investigator can absorb. Rather than detail all the variations on the EIG as it has been applied in each site, here the general methodology is outlined, illustrating from a model EIG (Figure 1). Throughout, however, some of the ways in which the instrument has been or could be modified are noted, to illustrate how the basic format can be altered so as to respond to different project structures, needs and resources.

Part I: Background information
Livestock information The goal of this first step is to gain a basic understanding of actual production practices in the community by asking general questions of a wide spectrum of key informants. In addition to men and women farmers and herders, key informants might include project staff, field agents of the government veterinary or livestock service, traditional healers, local livestock traders and butchers. Particular attention is paid to the division of labour and decision-making within households with regard to livestock management and healthcare. This information is necessary for choosing knowledgeable and representative

Part 1: Background information

Livestock information

- Who in the household is responsible for, manages, or treats sick animals?
- What are the local seasons of the year and their relevance for livestock disease?
- What species of livestock are kept, and what breed, age, or other categories are considered relevant for animal health?

Disease names

- Elicit the names of all livestock diseases in the area, by species, seasons, and other locally relevant variables
- Cross-check all terms for duplications, overlaps, confusions and omissions.
- Decide which diseases warrant further investigation in Part II.

Part II: The question list

1. What species, breeds, ages and sexes of animals are affected by this disease?
2. Is there seasonality or other timing to the appearance of the disease?
3. Does it usually affect one animal or a group of animals at the same time? Does it spread from animal to animal (i.e., is it contagious or infectious)?
4. What causes the disease: natural/physical causes, supernatural/non-physical causes or both? Describe.
5. Are there ways to prevent/avoid this disease? If so, what are they?
6. Describe the main symptoms, if possible in their order of progression and timing. What is the first symptom seen, and when? What is the second symptom seen, and when? Also, what is the symptom, if any, that makes you decide it is this specific disease?
7. Are traditional treatments available? Basically what are they? Where/how are they obtained? What happens when they are used (please be as specific as possible)?
8. Are modern treatments available? What are they? Where/how are they obtained? What happens when they are used (please be as specific as possible)?
9. What usually happens if the animal is not treated?
10. When did you last have (or for cropping areas with few livestock per household, hear of) an animal with this disease? What did you do and what happened to the animal?

Figure 1. *The ethnoveterinary interview guide*

informants for the second part of the EIG. Informants for Part II should represent a mix of stockraisers by age, gender, location and any other factor (for example, religion, ethnicity) shown to be important in livestock management.

In selecting the mix of informants, it is important to distinguish cultural ideals from actual behaviour. For example, Maasai informants said men have primary responsibility for animal healthcare and make most veterinary treatment decisions. Field research largely confirmed this statement, but it also revealed that Maasai women have healthcare duties too, particularly for young stock. WaMeru farmers made statements similar about males to Maasai's responsibilities. But subsequent KLP monitoring of WaMeru use of veterinary services showed that, because many men were away from home for long periods, women actually decided if or when to seek veterinary assistance. The lesson here is that, in each culture, background interviews (and thereafter, the EIG question list) should be conducted with women as well as men, emphasizing the livestock problems for which each gender is responsible. In the Maasai case, for example, the emphasis in interviews with women should be on young stock and lactating animals. In cases like WaMeru's, equal or even greater numbers of women as versus men should be interviewed because women's knowledge (especially of symptom recognition) and beliefs about animal disease and healthcare will be critical for sound project design and implementation.

A basic understanding of local seasons constitutes another part of the background information necessary for CBAHP design and implementation, since outbreaks of certain diseases often follow seasonal conditions. In addition, it is important to determine local categories of animals as defined by age, reproductive status, physiology, coat colour or any other characteristics that people consider to be strongly related to disease susceptibility, severity, incidence and seasonality. Such categorizations of livestock are important for understanding responses to the second part of the EIG.

For example, Maasai draw three such distinctions. The most important is the type of grazing group, which can be glossed as 'herded just around the homestead', 'herded with other young stock' and 'herded with the adult stock'. Grazing groups are closely correlated with animal age, and Maasai have different words for the same disease when it affects animals of different ages. To illustrate, *enkeeya oltao* refers to pneumonia in calves aged one to three months; but the word for pneumonias in older calves and adult cattle is *ilkipiei*. Maasai's other two important distinctions are physiological status (especially weaned versus unweaned) and 'fatness'. Along with Borana, Maasai observe that several diseases preferentially attack fat animals. Such categorizations are best collected specifically in the context of disease incidence, as many languages (particularly pastoralists') have very elaborate classifications of livestock types.[6] But only those distinctions that people believe have implications for animal health are of interest for CBAHP design and implementation. All such background information can simply be recorded 'freestyle' in notebooks.

Disease names In this second step, informants are asked to name all the livestock diseases they can think of, using their native-language terms. Often this procedure works better with small groups rather than with individuals, as one person's stories and ideas may spark the mind of another. Several separate groups should always be consulted. To obtain as complete a list of disease names as possible, more knowledgeable individuals representing different ages and genders should be included. Whether it is possible to interview men and women together in the same group depends on the culture, however. For example, Samburu women will not usually contribute to a discussion if men are present, whereas Turkana women will.

As each disease name is elicited, it can be recorded in notebooks or, better, on index cards. The authors have found the latter technique more useful in fieldwork, for a variety of practical reasons. The backs of the cards can be used to jot down comments about each disease as it is named. In subsequent interviews with new individuals or groups, the cards from previous interviews can be glanced through as each name is mentioned in order to check for overlaps, duplications or discrepancies in terminology. This way, the new informants can be asked to provide on-the-spot clarification. Moreover, unlike notebook pages, cards can be readily sorted and re-sorted as new information emerges. Finally, the index cards make it easy to pull together the diversity of disease names later, for cross-checking and analysis (see later sections).

Along with differences in knowledge and experience between informants, differences in language, dialect or other linguistic features (for example, degree of colloquialism) may give rise to diversity in disease names. The Samburu project, which included both Samburu and Turkana speakers, is illustrative. There was considerable overlap and interchange among disease terms in these two ethnic groups, particularly in areas where Samburu and Turkana were in close contact. It was essential to sort out all these terms in order to apply the second part of the EIG. Fortunately, in many cases, disease names seemed to have a straightforward translation between the two languages. In other cases, Turkana tended to use Samburu names for diseases and vectors found in more humid areas, such as East Coast Fever (ECF) and ticks. Conversely, Samburu— who had only recently begun to learn camel raising from their Turkana neighbours—often used Turkana terms for camel diseases.

Another problem in sorting out local disease names is that a given word may refer to more than one ill. Often, such words are the names for body parts. For example, in KiKamba, *metho* 'eye' denotes both conjunctivitis and eyes inflamed by a spitting cobra. However, WaKamba clearly recognize these as separate and unrelated conditions, and they add adjectives to distinguish them when needed. Among Maasai, the word *oltikana* appears to refer collectively to ECF, heart water and redwater. Significantly, all three of these diseases are tickborne, and they manifest similar clinical signs at onset. Although Maasai maintain that these are basically the same disease, they can add adjectives to *oltikana* to make finer distinctions. Conversely, stockraisers may sometimes class the scientifically 'same' disease as two different ailments. For example, on the basis of clinical signs that vary with animal age, WaMeru farmers distinguish *ikai* from *itaa*; but both are manifestations of ECF.

In the elicitation process, care must also be taken to avoid several potential biases in responses. One is seasonality (see also Stem, this volume). That is, producers are most apt to mention the diseases that are prevalent at the time of interviewing. Therefore, for each species, informants must also be specifically queried about diseases that occur in other seasons and/or year round. Because of time pressures, the Samburu project omitted this part of the elicitation process. Instead, it used a single-visit household survey, which was conducted in the dry season. However, it was soon discovered that virtually all the diseases named in the survey were dry-season ailments. In consequence, a separate effort had to be mounted later in order to elicit the names of wet-season diseases and to assess their importance relative to dry-season ills.

Another potential source of bias is producers' tendency to give only the names of the most 'serious' (that is, fatal) diseases. It is therefore imperative to ask specifically about chronic and non-fatal diseases that can lead to production losses. The translation and phrasing of questions is especially important in this regard (ibid.). To illustrate, in the Samburu survey mentioned above, two pairs of assistants administered the household questionnaire which asked, among other things, when the household last had a sick animal. Despite pre-translation and review of the questionnaire, the two pairs of interviewers used different phrases for 'sickness'. As a result, one pair was told only of animals with serious illness while the other was told of mild and chronic ailments as well. By influencing the diseases reported, the interview phraseology also influenced the reported time of the last disease occurrence.

Groups should also be asked whether there are diseases that strike only periodically. Otherwise one might miss major epizootics that occasionally sweep through an area, or conditions that appear only under unusual climatic circumstances. Depending on the nature of the project, these may or may not be pursued in detail, but it is useful to know about them. In the Maasai study, for example, one disease was eliminated from further investigation when it turned out that it was known to have occurred only once, after devastating floods following upon a 1962 drought. While such a disease might be scientifically interesting, it clearly is not a top CBAHP priority. Still, even a rare disease may sometimes merit study as an index of the depth and range of stockraiser knowledge. For example, the same study revealed that although no outbreaks of rinderpest had occurred in the area since about the early 1950s, older Maasai were quite knowledgeable about this disease (*olodua* 'pancreas'); and every single informant noted that the few animals that recovered were immune for life. They also knew that the government had a vaccine for *olodua*, although they could give no specifics about it.

To address the foregoing or other potential biases, informants can be asked to rank diseases according to various parameters, for example, morbidity, mortality, depressed productivity or ease of treatment. Such rankings can yield important insights, which are sometimes significantly different from the perceptions of government veterinary staff or even traditional animal healthcare specialists. Illustrating for cattle diseases in Meru, Table 1 shows how farmers, traditional healers and government staff can vary in their assessment of disease importance and hence healthcare priorities. In this Meru example, all agree that worms and pneumonia are important; but only farmers consider mange and *nyongo* 'liver' (probably referring to a gall-bladder condition linked to chronic anaplasmosis) as problems. Both veterinarians and farmers consider foot-and-mouth disease (FMD) a somewhat serious problem, but for different reasons. The former worry about the threat that FMD poses to national exports of animal products. But the latter are more concerned about the extra work and trouble of having to quarter and feed a lame animal at home instead of grazing it with its fellows. In prioritizing animal health problems, besides productivity and mortality, stockraisers usually also take into account management factors that government personnel may not.

In any case, in designing a CBAHP, the perspectives of *both* producers and the government veterinary service need to be considered. Part I of the EIG will elicit these. Part I also reveals gaps in local knowledge, as signalled by the absence of names for diseases known to occur in the project area. For example, groups like the Digo of coastal Kenya, who have only recently taken up cattle husbandry,

Table 1. Most common diseases of cattle as reported by different groups in Meru[a]

Common local names	English names	Farmer groups	Traditional healers	Veterinarians and health assistants
Njoka	Helminthosis (worms)	+++	+++	+++
Nthiana	Anaplasmosis	+++	+	+++
Mauri	Pneumonia	++	++	++
Meetho	Conjunctivitis	++	+	+
Ikai, itaa	Theileriosis (ECF)	+	++	+ (1984)
Mutombo	Trypanosomosis	++	−	+
Kurema njau	Dystochia	+	++	−
Ugere	Mange	++	−	−
Nyongo	'Liver' (see text)	++	−	−
Ikunguri	FMD	+	−	+ (1984)
Kunguru	Gid	+	−	−

[a] Code: +++ very common, ++ common, + uncommon, − not reported. The dates in parentheses represent the last outbreak of the disease recorded by the government veterinary service.

cannot name or accurately describe trypanosomosis in cattle. Obviously, such findings have immediate implications for planning CBAHP activities. If stock-raisers do not realize that an animal is sick, they will not seek treatment.[7]

At the conclusion of data collection in Part I, the complete roster of disease names that has been elicited can be winnowed down to focus on the problems that seem most common and that are of greatest concern to stockraisers. In the Maasai study, for example, this part of the EIG produced a list of 23 disease names. But for CBAHP purposes, only 15 of these seemed to warrant collecting more in-depth information in Part II of the EIG.

Part II: The question list
Furnished with the final roster of disease names, the stage is set for administration of the EIG question list. The questions are typically posed individually to three or more key informants, although small-group interviews have also been successful. The final number will depend upon project resources as well as the heterogeneity of informant responses. If three very different individuals give very similar answers, then there is less need for further interviews. If, however, they produce significant discrepancies, more informants should be queried. Usually it is best to cover only two or three diseases at a time so as to avoid informant fatigue and hasty answers. Also, it is not necessary (or even desirable) to ask the same few informants about all the diseases.

Informants should be chosen to represent the local diversity in stockraiser age, gender, wealth and residence within the community to be served by the CBAHP. In addition to ordinary producers, it is useful to include traditional livestock healers, if any practise in the area. Their responses will permit comparison of the nature and extent of generalists' versus specialists' knowledge. Moreover, the co-operation of traditional healers may be critical for later identifying efficacious local treatments (see concluding section). Of course, understanding ordinary producers' veterinary knowledge is of primary importance because they are the ones who will be using the CBAHP and who therefore must perceive it as useful. For example, do producers recognize a given disease but, perhaps unlike healers, they do not know how to prevent, control or cure it? Or are they unable to diagnose the disease in the first place? These are the sorts of questions that Part II of the EIG helps answer. In the process, it also captures intra-community variation in the level of local veterinary savvy.

While EIG question-list data can be recorded on fixed questionnaire-style forms, these either limit the amount that can be written in answer to any one question, or they result in forms that are mainly empty space. Therefore, the KLP recommends recording this information 'freestyle' in notebooks.

The questions The first question is *What species, breeds, ages and sexes of animals are affected by the disease?* As noted earlier, these or still other distinctions may be important for understanding stockraisers' veterinary concepts, observations and actions. In both Meru and Machakos, for instance, it is necessary to distinguish between local cattle and crossbred cattle because they are managed differently and have different disease susceptibilities.

Question 2, *Is there seasonality or other timing to the appearance of the disease?*, builds on the temporal information gathered in Part I. Answers to this question often reveal correlations (though not necessarily causal links) that producers observe between certain seasons or events and the disease under discussion. For example, farmers in Meru know that intestinal parasites are a greater problem during the rainy season. Maasai recognize that outbreaks of malignant catarrh follow upon the wildebeests' annual migration to their Maasai-land calving grounds (see Schillhorn van Veen, this volume).

Question 3, *Does the disease usually affect one animal or a group of animals at the same time? Does it spread from animal to animal (i.e., is it contagious or infectious)?* These questions are best posed in broad terms, such as 'Is it usually just one animal that gets this disease at a time or do many animals get it together? Can the disease spread from one animal to another? If so, how?' Unless the investigator's local-language skills and his/her technical knowledge about the disease are excellent, such terms like 'contagious' or 'infectious' may be difficult to translate and interpret accurately. This set of questions often leads naturally into a description of ethno-etiology, particularly in the case of vector-borne diseases. For example, Maasai associate *intorrobo* (which means both 'tsetse flies' and 'trypanosomosis') with grazing their cattle in certain areas during the seasons in which the flies occur. So they answer that sometimes only one animal will be affected, but that if there are many flies, then a number of animals may fall sick. While Maasai know that trypanosomosis is not contagious, they realize that the exposure of many animals to the vector can lead to an outbreak.

Question 4, *What causes the disease?*, inquires specifically about ethno-etiologies. Sometimes informants cite both physical (for examples, drinking water from a certain place) and non-physical causes (gods and witchcraft). However, if informants know that the interviewer is a veterinarian and/or a foreigner, they are often reluctant to mention supernatural causes because they are aware that many outsiders consider such beliefs primitive or superstitious. This difficulty can be overcome with culturally sensitive interviewers and interviewing techniques (see later sections). Often, too, producers say they don't know the answer to this fourth question. Instead, they may again cite the situational factors that they have observed to correlate with the disease. Or they may give vague answers. Among Borana, for example, a frequent answer to question 4 was 'It comes from the sky'. Yet with greater probing, informants are sometimes willing to give more concrete answers. For instance, with further questioning, it was found that Borana blamed a recent epizootic of *marchakas* (most likely Nairobi Sheep Disease) on ticks, which they say inject poison into the animals they bite. Informants further explained that new ticks carrying *marchakas* were brought into the area by another ethnic group who was migrating across long distances to escape drought and war.

Fifth, *Are there ways to prevent or avoid this disease?* In the KLP's experience, informants most commonly report preventive measures for contagious, infectious and vector-borne diseases. Measures often include isolating animals, avoiding certain pastures at certain times, instituting hygienic practices and trailing herds to a particular area or waterpoint (see Schillhorn van Veen this volume). For example, Pokot say that a good way to avoid ECF is to graze stock in a hot area; this makes perfect sense in that the tick vector does not survive in the hotter lowlands. Sometimes preventive measures are mentioned along with curative ones (see below), especially when traditional vaccinations or herbal remedies are involved. For example, in response to this question, one Maasai described how he boiled the meat of an animal affected by *empuruo* 'black-quarter' with parts of special trees (in Maasai, the *emi sigiydy* and *esere* trees) and then administered the decoction intranasally to immunize other animals in his herd.

Describe the main symptoms in their order of progression and timing if possible: what is the first symptom seen, and when; what is the second, and when; etc. What symptom (if any) makes you decide it is this specific disease? This sixth set of questions explores people's knowledge of disease progression and their diagnostic skills. Here, the attention and meticulousness of the interviewer are critical to ensure orderly recording of what is said and to probe for more details. The final query is especially important because several diseases may initially display identical clinical signs. This is the case with ECF, heart water and red-water, for instance. Maasai say they know for sure that an animal has ECF if its glands begin to swell; but before that they are not positive and so they use the general term *oltikana*. In describing the symptoms of fatal illnesses, informants also often mention post-mortem observations by way of verifying their pre-mortem diagnoses and thereby determining what parts of an expired animal are safe to eat. When Maasai slaughter a dying animal, they usually conduct a practical necropsy, paying particular attention to the condition of the muscle tissue and various organs. For example, they definitively diagnose rinderpest by post-mortem observation of a swollen liver and pancreas. In the Pokot project (Young 1988), the last question in this set was re-formulated as 'Are there any similar diseases and if so how do you tell them apart?' This phrasing speeded identification of the key ethno-diagnostic signs. Among other responses, this query elicited names for two skin diseases, *simpirion* and *moko-yon* (probably sarcoptic mange and streptothricosis, respectively). Two informants described these diseases as similar but noted that, unlike *mokoyon*, *simpirion* is contagious, covers the whole animal, causes bleeding cracks in the skin, and can be fatal. This is a good example of how the basic ethnoveterinary question list can be and has been expanded to fit various interests and time frames for data collection.

The seventh set of questions—*Are traditional treatments available? Basically what are they? Where/how are they obtained? What happens when they are used?*—covers the core knowledge of traditional veterinary medicine and its efficacy. Treatment details are not recorded at this stage; only the main ingredient(s) and/or actions involved are noted. Informants may give the names of plants, trees, or plant and tree parts, usually along with the mode of administration (for example, 'by mouth', 'in the nose', 'washing'). Sometimes nonbotanical ingredients are cited, such as Maasai's use of laundry detergent as a wash to control fleas and lice in young sheep and goats. Treatments may also consist of management actions, such as Maasai's trekking animals to salty water, or of physical actions, such as Maasai and WaMeru branding of the swollen neck glands of ECF. But sometimes informants know of no effective treatment. During the *marchakas* epidemic mentioned above, for instance, Borana said that no matter what, the sick animals would all die. One potential source of bias in responses to question set 7 should be noted: informants may be reluctant to discuss traditional treatments if they fear this will preclude their access to Western drugs. Also, the general nature of the question on treatment outcomes often yields only superficial answers such as 'Some recover, some don't'. The difficulty of generalizing about outcomes across cases is the reason for including question 10 below.

The eighth set of questions parallels the seventh, but with regard now to local knowledge of modern treatments, including types of treatments or medicines, dosages and modes of application. In the Maasai study, this set of questions revealed that although Maasai rely heavily on a wide range of Western drugs, they are not always knowledgeable about these medicines' uses and, particularly, their dosages. Sometimes producers know the generic names of the commercial drugs they use; but other times they can describe them only in physical terms. Like some First World stockraisers [editors' note], Maasai and Samburu commonly discuss drugs in terms of their colour, size, shape and texture (Iles, pers. comm.). Such informant descriptions may make it difficult for the interviewer to determine what drug is being cited. For example, it may be impossible to distinguish an anthelmintic and a tetracycline that are both yellow and slightly viscous. Finally, where some limited government veterinary service is available, stockraisers occasionally answer that they know the service has some drug but they don't know what it is.

Question-set 8 often revealed that Kenyan producers rely on poorly informed traders and shopkeepers for information about commercial drugs and their posology. At other times, responses indicated that stockraisers assume 'more is better' in terms of dosage. Unfortunately, this assumption leads at best to a waste of money, and at worst to serious side-effects or even death. Conversely, responses may signal under-dosing. For example, for mild cases of disease or with drugs that are very expensive or that people deem particularly potent, stockraisers often divide the recommended dose for a single animal among two or more (see also Shanklin, this volume). Among Samburu, for instance, Wormicid Plus™, which is very viscous, is thought to be far more efficacious than the more watery Wormicid™ (Iles, pers. comm.). In consequence, Samburu stockraisers tend to use less of the former, although the recommended dose for the two drugs is the same. Again, such practices can waste the stockowner's money. Under-dosing also raises the possibility of chemoresistance.

Sometimes, too, stockraisers administer a 'cocktail' of various medicines. While people are often strong believers in the efficacy of Western drugs, they do not always understand drug specificity; so a sick animal may be given a mixture of several medicines in the hope that one or another, or the combination, will work. Maasai and Pokot, for example, commonly combine trypanocides and antibiotics. Stockraisers may also be unaware of the proper mode of administration of Western drugs, or they may purposely choose a different mode. For example, to treat trypanosomosis in cattle, Pokot often insert a Novidium tablet into an incision in the patient's skin. However, most groups in Kenya have a strong preference for injections over oral medications, whether for livestock or humans.

Question 9 is *What usually happens if the animal is not treated?* General questions like this are often difficult for informants to answer, as many factors can influence the outcome of a disease. Thus, common and reasonable responses are 'Some animals die' or 'Some get better'. Nevertheless, the range of answers gives some sense of how often diseases are seen to be fatal, chronic or self-curing. To illustrate, for *cheptikon* (ECF), five different Pokot informants responded as follows: some animals recover after a week and some die; it [the disease] lasts for two weeks then the animal dies; it lasts two to five days then the animal dies; the animal survives only four days; fat animals will die very quickly (within 24 hours) whereas thin ones may last some time (a week or more) and may recover. Despite this variety of answers, it is clear that most Pokot see *cheptikon* as generally fatal.

Question set 10—*When did you last have an animal with this disease; what did you do and what happened to it?*—is a critical complement to the first nine in that it enquires about a specific occurrence of a given disease, rather than just general local knowledge, beliefs and actions taken. These queries produce mini-case studies of actual rather than ideal or generalized situations. (However, in farming areas where livestock numbers and hence disease occurrences are low, these questions are changed to refer to the last time the farmer has *heard* of an animal with the disease.) These mini-case studies provide a good indication of the extent to which people actually put their veterinary knowledge into practice and of the external factors that influence their actions in diagnosing and handling livestock diseases. Both general and specific approaches are necessary for a complete understanding of an individual's decision-making and action. Question set 10 uncovers deviations from the normal or expected as reported in questions 1 through 9 in terms of actions taken, outcomes and sometimes reasons. (Consider, for instance, the difference in responses that the following pair of questions would elicit: 'What do you usually do on market days?' versus 'What did you do on the last market day and why?') Responses to the second half of question set 10 have included statements like the following: 'I wanted to use an antibiotic, but couldn't find any'; 'The head of the household was away, so we couldn't do anything until he returned'; 'The animal was very old so we decided to slaughter it rather than wasting time and money trying to cure it.'

In sum, knowing stockraisers' perceptions of disease occurrence and prevalence, CBAHPs can gauge people's familiarity with the economically important animal health problems. Such information is also helpful in assessing the relative impact of different diseases on livestock production. Other things being equal (for example, dramatic clinical signs, the economic or socio-cultural value of the species affected), ethnoveterinary knowledge is usually greater for common health problems than for rare ones.

Selecting EIG interviewers
As with any interview technique (open-ended or otherwise), EIG data are only as good as the interviewer who gathers them. There is a vast literature on interview skills and innumerable works on the attributes of good field inter-

viewers—including such characteristics as honesty, motivation, meticulousness, and positive attitudes towards women and other groups. However, it must be emphasized that research on local technical knowledge makes unique demands, whether the interviewer is an enumerator, translator, research assistant or project staff member. In addition to the usual attributes of good interviewers, he or she must have some specialized knowledge and skills.

Although interviewers themselves need not be veterinary experts, they must have a reasonable grasp of the subject matter, of local animal health issues, and of the associated technical terms in the local language (see Delehanty, this volume). They should also be eager to expand their veterinary knowledge and lexicon and to record meticulously local definitions and vocabulary. Otherwise, they will not understand the purpose behind the EIG and they will be unable to conduct accurate and comprehensible interviews, to phrase their questions properly, and to probe for clear and complete answers. Nor will they be able to communicate the information from producers to the investigator or project officer, who ultimately 'translates' the interview data into more technical and analytic terms. To take a simple example, an urbanite interviewer who does not know the local-language terms for 'liver' or 'pancreas' will certainly have trouble conducting an ethnoveterinary interview. Moreover, such uninformed interviewers will misunderstand, filter out, or jumble much of what producers say. This is especially true for ethnoveterinary (or more generally, ethno-medical) data. Many other kinds of agricultural R&D deal with more factual or readily observable areas of enquiry—such as species/varieties/area of crops grown, numbers of livestock kept, or product and input prices. These topics usually can be discussed using only the ordinary vocabulary that any native speaker has already mastered or can easily 'pick up'. But this is not the case for ethnoveterinary information. Every stockraising society typically has a specialized and often highly complex set of terms and concepts for talking about ethno-medical matters.

Cultural sensitivity is another 'must' for any work in local knowledge systems. If the interviewer does not have a deep respect for local beliefs, this will inevitably be communicated in the interview process, with the result that responses will probably be more terse. In ethnoveterinary R&D, this is particularly true for questions about ethno-etiologies and traditional treatments. As noted earlier, informants may fear that, if they answer honestly, they will appear backward or superstitious or they will be denied access to desirable Western drugs. For the same reason, the presence of 'outsiders' or foreigners during the interview should be carefully assessed. It is imperative that the interviewer spend time explaining what data are wanted and why, stressing the value of the knowledge and skills of stockraisers themselves. At no time should an informant be interrupted with comparisons to Western views or practices.

A final word of caution is in order here. The mere fact that interviewers, enumerators or extension agents are from the local area does not mean they automatically have the requisite local knowledge, language skills and cultural sensitivities for studying local knowledge systems. For example, the KLP discovered that NGO extension agents in Samburu—who were natives of the district—knew far less than producers about livestock matters; moreover, a number of the agents displayed contempt for traditional knowledge (also see Roepke, this volume).

The field assistant for the Maasai study exemplifies an appropriate choice for ethnoveterinary interviewers. This young Maasai man had completed secondary school and had a keen personal interest in veterinary issues. Although he had no formal training in animal husbandry or veterinary science, he had grown up in a pastoral area where schoolchildren herd on weekends and holidays. And he was eager to learn more about pastoral production, as he felt less knowledgeable in this area than other Maasai who had *not* gone to school. Also, he displayed a deep respect for the wisdom of elders. In his fieldwork, he carefully recorded native vocabulary, particularly for unusual or complex symptoms. His interviews produced significant detail and he always pointed out and tried to resolve discrepancies like those described earlier for *oltikana*.

In fact, in most of the ethnoveterinary efforts described in this chapter, the EIG was administered by less-well-educated enumerators and/or field assistants. But, they were given rudimentary training by a project officer who also usually supervised them in pre-tests of the EIG in each site. Experience has shown that overall, the depth of producer responses varies significantly with the quality of the interviewer. Enumerators with poor training or little enthusiasm are sometimes content to write down the first thing an informant says, without prompting for more information or clarification of discrepancies; sometimes, too, they write down their own interpretations of what is said. The issue of skill in administering the EIG is clearly a critical one. CBAHP decisions must be based on producer knowledge, *not* on interviewer notions. ITDG is still reviewing its experiences worldwide to determine what are good mixes of interviewers (and trainers) of different backgrounds and educational levels, given varying project goals, schedules and resources.

Organizing and analysing the data

No matter who collects the EIG data or how they are recorded, they ultimately need to be collated and organized so the important information can be extracted. This can be done in a number of ways, depending on the use to which the information will be put and the level of detail that will be required. For example, one CBAHP might be primarily interested in trying to match Western and local disease names in order to train local drug traders and shopkeepers in drug specificity and posology. Another programme—like the KLP's Samburu project—may plan to deliver veterinary training directly to groups of stockraisers. In that case, in order to make training more efficient, it is important to know not only disease names, but also local concepts and vocabulary pertaining to clinical signs. Whatever the immediate programme goal, concrete decisions must be made about how detailed the data need to be, and then a data organization method can be selected accordingly.

The simplest method is to collate all the responses for each disease so they can be compared and analysed for commonalities and inconsistencies, the general depth and spread of stockraisers' veterinary knowledge, and topics on which local knowledge is especially strong or weak. Responses can then be synthesized into a general profile of knowledge about each disease. This can be done mentally, in writing or with a computer.

A mental synthesis is easy when the number of diseases named and the amount of information about each is small—as is often the case with peoples who rely mainly on cropping. For example, most WaMeru informants mentioned a disease they called *njoka* 'snakes', that is stomach and gut worms (helminthosis). People clearly had a general understanding that *njoka* was caused by 'snakes' in the intestinal system. However, only a few informants could describe the clinical signs in detail (weight loss, rough coat, swelling under the jaw, pale eyes and sometimes diarrhoea); most informants cited only a dramatic loss of weight. Some knew that the disease was more common in the rainy season, while others thought it occurred throughout the year; and some knew it affected young animals more than older ones. But few were able to recognize helminth infestation until it was far advanced and animals were in very poor condition.

In contrast, Pokot pastoralists described a much larger range of diseases in far greater detail. For the Pokot project, therefore, the KLP made a written compilation of all the responses to each question for each disease so that the full range of responses was permanently recorded and could be instantly compared. The results of this more thorough-going approach are illustrated for one disease (*lokurucha* or trypanosomosis) in Table 2.

Computerized coding and analysis of question-list responses is also possible. In fact, preliminary codes were developed for this purpose for the Samburu data. While one of the EIG's functions is to generate an accurate core vocabulary of critical disease nomenclature and other livestock vocabulary, the KLP soon realized that to code and enter all the data would absorb an enormous amount of time and resources. In the context of the KLP's relatively small, NGO-oriented projects, the additional information that computerization might provide was ultimately deemed not worth the while. However, this approach has been used successfully in other contexts. (For example, see Delehanty, this volume). It provides very fine-grained information and analysis, which are perhaps most appropriate for specialized scientific research efforts.

Using ethnoveterinary data in CBAHPs

The EIG data are useful at many stages of CBAHP design, implementation and evaluation. At the most basic level, it is impossible even to talk to stockraisers about their animal health problems without knowing local disease names and related terms, and how producers use them (ibid.). Beyond that, there are two decision areas where ethnoveterinary information is of major assistance: whom to train as CBAHP workers—specialist intermediaries versus stockraisers generally, and men, women or both; and what to include or exclude[8] in training and how to present the information.

Trainee selection
In Meru—the KLP's first CBAHP—the EIG revealed a relatively low level of ethnoveterinary knowledge among local farmers. Informants could recognize and name only some 10 diseases; informant descriptions of clinical signs varied greatly; and people knew of few effective treatments, whether traditional or modern. In addition, the wealth ranking, the EIG, and other studies revealed that WaMeru usually consult local specialists (*wagaa*) about livestock health problems. Only the wealthiest stockowners had access to government veterinary services. Thus, it appeared most appropriate to give intensive training to selected male and female farmers as CBAHP workers and to focus training on recognizing and treating the most common and simple livestock diseases. This system proved both effective and popular in Meru, and there has been considerable community demand for more workers to be trained.

These successes in Meru led the KLP to apply the same model to its second project, in Pokot. But Pokot CBAHP trainees soon ceased working. In retrospect, a comparative analysis of EIG and other data for the two sites would have shown

Table 2. Pokot informants' responses to the EIG question list for *lokurucha* or 'trypanosomosis'[a]

Animals affected
a) Cattle, all ages, males and females.
b) All species, but only adults.
c) Cattle, all ages, males and females.
d) Cattle and goats, all ages, males and females.
e) Cattle, any age, males and females.

Cause
a) Brought by insects.
b) Spread by flies; common where stock grazed in areas with a lot of bush and wild animals; the flies bite the animals while they are grazing in such areas.
c) Flies.
d) Ticks.
e) Biting insects; some people say it can be caused by ticks.

Signs
a) Loss of appetite and weight; slowly by slowly it kills the animal.
b) Animal smells bad; loss of milk production; loss of body condition until it dies.
c) Loss of appetite and milk; does not drink water; animal smells bad; stays in the shade and then dies.
d) Loss of weight; stops eating and drinking; body smells bad.
e) Animal stands in the shade; does not graze or drink; coat stands up and becomes rough.

Outcome
a) Can last between one day and one month, then dies.
b) Can last up to two seasons.
c) Weak animals can die after three days; healthy animals last up to four weeks.
d) Dies after a long time—one or two months.
e) Animal can live for one year and then die.

When common
a) Can occur at any time.
b) At the end of the wet season.
c) Mainly in the wet season.
d) During the rainy season.
e) *Kitokot* 'rainy season'.

Where common
a) Amaya, Orus, Kalachamoyos, Chepirokoran, Chepofurin.
b) No answer.
c) Lochoriangocowie, Kerio Valley.
d) In highland areas.
e) Kero Valley and Churo.

Treatment
a) Novidium, Berenil; recovers quickly. No traditional treatment.
b) Berenil, Novidium, Ethidum. Traditional treatment with a plant called *litwonoi* or baboon faeces.
c) Bleeding to remove the bad blood; this works if done in the early stages of the disease. Also soak the fruit of the *sognohowio* plant or the bark of the *sokwon* tree and give the infusion intranasally.
d) Soak the beaten bud of the *sokwon* tree in a small amount of water for three to five minutes, then drench by mouth.
e) Give the sick animal boiled roots of the *chepopet* tree. Slaughter a healthy sheep, boil the meat, and give the soup to the sick animal; but this does not work for most cases.

Contagious?
a) No.
b) No.
c) No.
d) No.
e) No.

Prevention
a) No prevention, only treatment; dipping [sic].
b) Avoid grazing in areas where flies are found.
c) None.
d) Dipping.
e) Do not allow animals to graze where insects will bite them.

Similar diseases
a) None.
b) *Cheptigon* 'ECF'.
c) *Cheptigon* 'ECF'.
d) *Pkison*.
e) *Toroi* 'anaplasmosis'.

What distinguishes them?
a) No answer.
b) In *cheptigon*, blood is found inside the ear.
c) *Cheptigon* is rare in places where *lokurucha* is common.
d) In *lokurucha*, loss of weight, animal stops eating and drinking; if an animal with *pkison* is injected with Novidium it dies immediately.
e) With *toroi*, the faeces become very dry and hard; the animal may not pass any faeces for three days.

---

[a] Letters identify each of the five informants' responses.

that, instead of a few selected herders, Pokot pastoralists as a whole should have been trained. In response to the EIG, most Pokot could name and describe nearly 20 different diseases; informants demonstrated a very high and consistent level of veterinary knowledge; and they often knew both traditional and modern treatments. Furthermore, there is a strong tradition of each Pokot household controlling the knowledge and skill needed to tend to its animals' health. Although local healer-specialists exist, Pokot responses indicated that herders consult them only when all else fails.

A retrospective of all KLP efforts to date reveals that they fall into two basic types according to the clientele to be served: cultivators and pastoralists. As a comparison of minimum data sets across KLP projects reveals, the needs of these two groups vary along several important dimensions, all of which must be considered in CBAHP design.

Briefly, among cultivators, human population density is high; settlements are fixed, which makes access to households and their animals relatively easy for CBAHP workers; and both livestock numbers and levels of ethnoveterinary knowledge are low. Indeed, the average farmer often does not recognize that an animal is sick until a disease is far advanced, when much productivity has already been lost and treatment is more difficult or uneconomic. In such settings, training for individual CBAHP workers will often need to be coupled with some farmer extension, so that farmers will fully use the workers' services.

In contrast, among pastoralists, human population density is low; households and herds move frequently and often far, making delivery of healthcare services extremely difficult; although animal population density is low, livestock numbers per household are high; and local veterinary knowledge is quite sophisticated. Further, in Kenya's pastoral cultures generally, herder success and to some extent pride and prestige are linked to stockraisers' ability to treat successfully the healthcare problems of their own herds. On the whole, therefore, pastoralists prefer to receive veterinary training themselves rather than rely on some (often distant) intermediary for most services. This is particularly true for routine procedures like drenching or treatment of surface wounds.

EIG background information on gender responsibilities for livestock healthcare will also help determine how best to organize and target training. In Meru and especially Machakos, Part I of the EIG revealed that male out-migration has increased women's stockraising duties overall. Therefore, in these two sites, the KLP decided to train a number of female farmers in the same classes with men. Among Samburu, however, the EIG indicated that women's pastoral responsibilities are fairly specialized. They centre on young stock and chronic diseases, because young and debilitated animals are placed in women's care to graze near the homestead, where women spend much of their day (Iles, pers. comm.). Given this gender-based difference within the Samburu production system, the KLP is experimenting with separate courses for Samburu men and women.

The decision to train selected animal healthcare workers only or stockraisers as a whole flows logically from the existing levels of local veterinary knowledge and from cultural patterns of reliance on local healers. And whether for men or women, success in CBAHP training requires an appreciation both of traditional and contemporary gender roles in stockraising.

Training approach and content
The EIG constitutes the first step towards the local-language elaboration of relevant and accurate CBAHP curricula and of training and extension materials that both draw upon and bolster stockraisers' existing veterinary knowledge and skills, whether traditional or modern. Training should always start from and be based on what people already know and think in terms of disease importance, nomenclature, symptom recognition, susceptibility, and appropriate drugs and dosages. The EIG systematically elicits all this information. With it, CBAHPs can save time and money and increase their effectiveness because trainers will know what and how much they can assume in choosing training topics and preparing materials. Moreover, building on and from local knowledge using the local language speeds learning and increases lesson retention.

To illustrate, the EIG indicated that Maasai are generally quite sophisticated about symptom and disease recognition; under field conditions, they could identify virtually any disease that a trained veterinarian could without laboratory equipment (Ndarathi, pers. comm.).[9] Thus it was clear that veterinary training or extension among Maasai could be based on their traditional vocabulary, concepts and knowledge of livestock disease. On the other hand, many WaMeru farmers do not recognize certain common diseases until they are far advanced. Recalling the example of *njoka*, trainers can capitalize on WaMeru's current but limited understanding of helminthosis by explaining that the worms are present throughout the year but that they proliferate in the rainy season. With this additional information, farmers can then choose to avail themselves of

CBAHP prophylactic measures at the beginning of the rainy season, thus greatly reducing their productivity losses from *njoka*.

The general level of agreement and detail across EIG informants in disease differentiation can further refine the approach and content of training about disease recognition. For example, unlike WaMeru and *njoka*, few Pokot need to know little more about diagnosing *psosoi* (pneumonia) in goats since they can already identify it accurately. What they cannot do easily, however, is differentiate bacterial pneumonia from contagious caprine pleuro-pneumonia. The former is often precipitated by sudden changes in the weather and is easily treatable and usually self-limiting; in contrast, the latter is a much more serious and contagious disease with unpredictable treatment response. Training could therefore focus on this distinction, encouraging herders to observe treatment response carefully so as to determine what further actions to take, if any.

In particular, EIG descriptions of clinical signs and susceptibilities by type of animal can be used to assess the match between local and Western etiological definitions of disease (see also Delehanty, this volume). Insights from analysis of the question-list data can be judiciously applied in selecting the vocabulary to be used and the information to be imparted in training stockraisers in new prophylaxes or therapies. For instance, in the case of WaMeru *ikai* and *itaa* (both manifestations of ECF), trainers can point out that they are the same disease and that regular dipping against ticks will prevent both. But just the opposite would be the case for *empuruo* among the Maasai. Maasai recognize two types of *empuruo*: plain *empuruo* (blackquarter) and *empuruo entana* (anthrax). The fact that both diseases are characterized by sudden death may explain their partial co-classification emically. While Maasai can clearly distinguish the two when called upon to do so, trainers must always take care to stress which type of *empuruo* they and Maasai trainees are discussing at any given point. Otherwise, confusion will arise when trainers explain that immunization is the only effective response to the threat of *empuruo* generally, but that the two different kinds of *empuruo* require different vaccines. The Maasai disease-name *oltikana* presents yet another situation. If the goal is to explain *oltikana* transmission and prophylaxis to producers, trainers need not worry that the local term embraces what Western veterinary science recognizes as three distinct tick-borne diseases. Instead, trainers can simply speak of *oltikana* in terms of the tick-control measures that apply to all observed cases of this indigenous disease category.

It is also critical to know what and how much producers understand about drugs and dosage rates. Again, much of this information can be obtained from the EIG. For example, EIG data revealed that both Maasai and Samburu know the names of many Western veterinary drugs and sometimes also the drugs' primary properties. An example is Maasai and Samburu recognition that terramycin is used for fever. However, the EIG also showed that these pastoralists rarely understood the alien drugs' dosage rates. Therefore, a focus on correct drug use, timing and dosages was recommended for extension efforts with Maasai (Grandin 1984b); and KLP training among Samburu was designed so as to stress proper posology, with the result that Samburu are now following recommended dosages much more closely (Iles, pers. comm., based on post-training monitoring).

Perhaps the single most important factor in the success of any CBAHP, however, is ensuring that—at least insofar as national drug and other restrictions permit—it addresses the livestock diseases that stockraisers themselves see as important. For CBAHP services to be valued by the community, they must have a visible, positive effect on common veterinary problems. The EIG quickly reveals the majority of the most common diseases, and it signals which of these are of greatest concern to stockraisers. On the whole, people know more about such diseases, so the number and depth of EIG responses about a given ailment will generally indicate its importance.[10]

Of course, the EIG will also reveal lacunae in producer knowledge and recognition of diseases. Findings such as those for *njoka* among WaMeru or trypanosomosis among Digo help CBAHP designers see where some direct stockraiser extension may need to accompany training of selected animal health workers, to ensure that their services will be used. If stockraisers cannot recognize the prodromes and syndromes of disease, they cannot decide whether or when to call upon the CBAHP worker. To a certain extent, CBAHP workers themselves can undertake this kind of information dissemination, explaining to farmers the early signs of diseases they are equipped to treat.

Other uses of EIG data

The KLP is developing still more and new ways of using EIG information. For some time the programme has been committed to incorporating local or traditional as well as modern healthcare methods into CBAHP training. The goal is to bridge the historical divide between different medical systems and to ensure that Western commercial treatments—which are often more expensive and difficult to obtain—are not needlessly recommended if there are equally efficacious local ones.

The KLP is currently exploring various ways to achieve this goal (for example, McCorkle 1994). As a first step, in Machakos and Turkana districts, the programme has begun to investigate the efficacy of traditional treatments for the more common and simple diseases, such as those engendered by worms, ticks, and biting and burrowing mites (mange). In addition to drawing upon information collected in past and present workshops and interviews, this investigation asks stockraisers and traditional healers to rank the diseases elicited in the EIG background information according to the efficacy of traditional treatments for them (see, for example, Wanyama in progress–a and b). A card-sorting technique similar to that employed in wealth ranking is used for this task. In a pre-test of this technique in Machakos, 29 diseases were ranked by two farmers of varying ethnoveterinary skills and by one traditional healer. The less knowledgeable of the two farmers (a man) knew of traditional treatments for only 12 of the diseases; the other farmer (a woman) knew of local remedies for 25; for the healer, this figure was 26. Expectedly, the healer generally ranked the efficacy of traditional treatments higher than did farmers. Overall, however, there was fairly strong agreement that quite efficacious local remedies exist for five of the diseases but not for another 11; there was uncertainty about the other 13. With additional testing and refinement, this ranking technique should enable the KLP to identify a select number of traditional treatments that are consistently reported as effective, so they can be studied in depth and, if proven, included with confidence in CBAHP training.

The KLP is also exploring the use of EIG data and approaches to epidemiological monitoring (also see Schwabe, this volume, and Stem, this volume). Kenya's shared borders with Sudan and Somalia, where civil wars have disrupted animal disease control programmes, have exposed the country to increased risk of epidemics (see Grandin, n.d. for a case study in Isiolo

District). Greater understanding of ethnoveterinary knowledge systems among stockraisers in the border areas would enable the government veterinary department to improve its monitoring for health threats by collecting information from herders in their indigenous disease terminology. The Drought Contingency Planning Unit in Turkana District, for instance, already has a network of monitors who collect a variety of data to provide early warning of drought, food shortages and other problems. Among other variables (meteorological data, food supplies, market prices for livestock), the network also collects reports of animal disease. Using ethnoveterinary terminology for this task would probably increase the accuracy of data collection.

Finally, part of ITDG's mandate is to encourage other organizations working with poor producers to adopt policies that are more favourable to such producers. In terms of animal health, this means increased access to useful veterinary medicines and information, whether traditional or modern. Thus, the KLP is actively disseminating its evidence on the sophistication and shortcomings of ethnoveterinary knowledge systems and on the effectiveness, practicality and sustainability of CBAHPs in order to stimulate both governments and NGOs elsewhere around the world to try similar approaches.

Notes

1. The authors would like to acknowledge the field assistance of the staff of the KLP and its partners, in particular: Lawrence Thiaru in Meru; John Kimanthi and Stephen Kimondiu in Machakos; Veronica Eyang and Julius Lesana in Samburu; and Dismas Ekeno, Edward Losike and Gregory Ekiru in Turkana. Special thanks also go to Elijah ole Timpaine for his help in developing the type of ethnoveterinary research described here, and to ILCA for its organizational support.
2. In addition, the KLP has been involved in a host of minor activities, including seminars, workshops, consultancies, project reviews and the provision of training materials to other organizations.
3. More recently in the evolution of ITDG's livestock work, a number of other highly participatory rapid appraisal techniques have also been adopted. These include rankings of livestock management problems and success, seasonal calendars to identify periods of increased disease risk and, in Nepal, mapping and diagramming of grazing grounds and of areas where different diseases are more common.
4. The latter might include, for example, the length of an individual's or a society's involvement in stockraising, the species and/or number of animals kept, changes in the species or breeds raised, or variations in husbandry systems—which can range in intensity from quasi-feral to highly managed.
5. This approach is to some extent self-evident. But its adoption was further encouraged by earlier ITDG work in India's Gujarat State, where traditional livestock healers were trained in simple modern medicines to add to their already considerable knowledge of, and pharmacopoeia for, animal diseases.
6. Among the Samburu, for example, Sperling (1987:359) recorded 20 different categories for cattle alone. Likewise for Evans-Pritchard's studies of the agro-pastoral Nuer. See also Köhlen-Rollerson, this volume.
7. It should be noted that the EIG identifies only diseases that manifest clinical signs. Producers do not have names for subclinical conditions because these are essentially 'invisible' to them—as well as to the often poorly trained, equipped and backstopped veterinary field agents and laboratory technicians of many developing countries.
8. Of course, in deciding what to include or exclude in training, CBAHPs must take account of government regulations concerning access to veterinary drugs and the treatment of other peoples' animals (recall the minimum data set). In Kenya, for example, many of the drugs (for example, systemic antibiotics, trypanocides) for

potentially fatal illnesses are 'scheduled', that is, their sale is restricted. Thus ordinary stockraisers cannot legally obtain or possess such drugs without a prescription. Also, while producers have the legal right to treat their own animals or the animals of others, as non-professionals practising without a licence, they are not supposed to charge a fee for their services. Because of these regulations, the KLP focused initially on diseases requiring rather simple, non-scheduled Western drugs such as anthelmintics and wound powders. However, in each KLP project, efforts have been made to establish good relations between government and community so that CBAHP workers can fairly readily access veterinary staff with the right to dispense scheduled drugs.

9. This is not to imply that there is a one-to-one correspondence between Maasai and Western disease categories, however.

10. Again, interviewers must take care to avoid potential biases in EIG responses towards dramatic but rare ills, fatal versus chronic ones, and wet- versus dry-season diseases depending on the time of EIG application.

20. Methods and results from a study of local knowledge of cattle diseases in coastal Kenya

JAMES DELEHANTY

THIS CHAPTER PRESENTS selected results from a 1989 study of the technical and contextual knowledge of bovine diseases among cattle-owning farmers of Kaloleni Division, Kilifi District, Kenya.[1] The practical impetus for the study was a decision by the Kenyan Ministry of Livestock Development to test a new infection-and-treatment method of controlling the tick-borne disease, theileriosis. In English, this disease is commonly called East Coast Fever or ECF. This chapter derives from a much longer official report that describes Kaloleni conceptions of 106 cattle diseases in support of this test effort (Delehanty 1990).[2] For purposes of illustrating the study methodology and the value of ethnoveterinary research generally, however, here results are presented only for the disease selected for this study, theileriosis. The study as a whole was designed to answer three broad questions.

○ Can information on livestock diseases elicited from farmers be gathered quickly and systematically, and subjected to analytic methods sufficiently rigorous to provide scientific support, rather than mere anecdote, to veterinary epidemiologists and others concerned with regional animal health?
○ In the absence of more precise but expensive laboratory diagnostic surveys or other measures, can such information—aggregated by geographic area, culture, production system, socio-economic characteristics of stockowners, or other pertinent variables—be useful in determining variable disease risk?
○ How can data on local disease concepts and ethnoveterinary practice be most effectively structured and presented so that they will be useful for extension of sustainable veterinary interventions?

Ethnoveterinary fieldwork centred on a set of much more specific research questions, designed to operationalize the broader issues.

○ How well do Kaloleni cattle keepers recognize the clinical signs of a range of livestock maladies?
○ How do they encode clinical signs as 'diseases'—either in local or Western-derived terms?
○ What patterns of disease occurrence do cattle raisers identify?
○ What are their ethno-etiologies?
○ What traditional preventive and curative treatments do stockowners know, and which of these do they use?
○ What Western treatments do they know of, and which do they use?

The study area

The Mijikenda peoples form the predominant ethnic group in Kaloleni Division. Linguistically, Kaloleni is a transitional area. Over several centuries, KiSwahili has made great inroads, in some areas even supplanting the indigenous KiMijikenda. As Figure 1 indicates, Kaloleni Division and its 10 subdivisions or

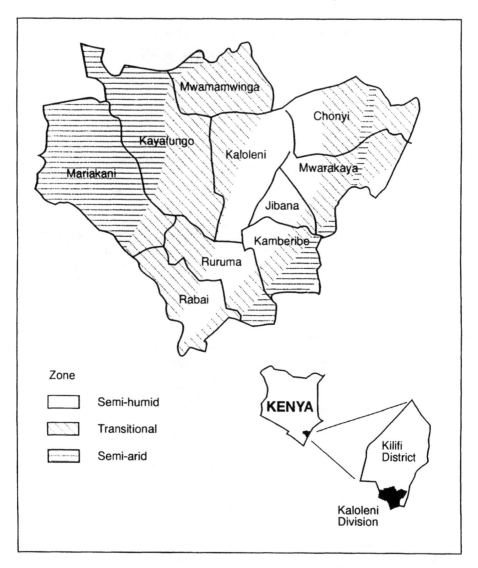

Figure 1. Map of Kaloleni Division.

'locations' span three major agro-ecozones (Jaetzold and Schmidt 1982). Annual precipitation and population density are highest along a central coastal ridge, where semi-humid conditions permit wide-scale coconut production with inter-cropped maize and cassava. Both rainfall and population density decline down-slope into a transitional zone dominated by cashew, maize and cassava. This zone gives way in turn to sparsely populated semi-arid lowlands characterized by extensive grazing and limited millet cultivation (ILCA 1989).

Cattle production is poorly developed in Kaloleni as a whole. Only one subgroup of Mijikenda have an uninterrupted history of cattle production. These are the Giriama people, who occupy mainly the semi-arid zone. While both the semi-humid and transitional zones offer an environmental complex amenable to mixed farming, a number of factors have intervened historically to focus production in these two higher rainfall areas on crops rather than on cattle.

One factor is an historico-cultural stricture against cattle, derived from pre-colonial times when pastoralist patrons required their client farmers to pledge not to raise cattle (Mathu 1988). Throughout the higher rainfall areas of Kaloleni, cattle avoidance affects farm management to one degree or another; and until recently, most Mijikenda subgroups followed this custom. Additional cultural, economic, agro-ecological and infrastructural factors that have worked to constrain cattle production in Kaloleni include: a strong local preference for small ruminants, especially goats, as a source of meat and milk for home consumption and as a medium of ritual exchange; marketing problems facing coastal farmers interested in commercial milk production; the economic importance of tree crops, which militates against animal traction and manure demand, and also limits grazing areas—especially in the densely settled, heavily cultivated coconut zone; delays in land adjudication and registration, which have impeded investment in the infrastructure necessary to develop intensive, fodder-based stockraising systems; the endemicity of trypanosomosis, theileriosis and other bovine diseases; and inadequate veterinary services (Buruchara 1988, KMALD 1986, Mochoge 1987).

Of the estimated 7000 to 10000 farms in Kaloleni Division, only 1563 or 15 per cent to 22 per cent kept cattle in 1989 (ILCA 1989). Many of these are Giriama farms. A large share of the rest adopted cattle only recently—notably in the 1980s, when the National Dairy Development Programme (NDDP) introduced an initiative to raise genetically improved cattle in zero or semi-zero grazing systems. Thus, in much of Kaloleni one would not expect to find a highly developed base of indigenous knowledge about bovine health problems.

The research reported here paid particular attention to the fledgling cattle enterprises of Kaloleni's higher rainfall areas, although dryland Giriama systems were also studied. This focus contrasts sharply with most earlier ethnoveterinary studies in Kenya, which have concentrated on pastoralists rather than farmers (for example, Grandin 1985, ITDG 1989, Ohta 1984). It thus provides an opportunity to test the proposition that ethnoveterinary research can make useful contributions to veterinary extension systems and disease control campaigns even where a large segment of the target population is not necessarily experienced or adept at diagnosis and treatment of the diseases or species of interest.

Methods[3]

Interviews were conducted with a total of 158 cattle keepers in Kaloleni. All interviews were completed within a two-month period by an experienced Giriama enumerator trained in techniques of both formal and informal sampling. An experienced stockraiser himself, the enumerator was astute, educated, highly interested in the study and fluent in each of the several Kimijikenda dialects as well as in KiSwahili and English. The enumerator carried out all data collection, initially with the author present and then later alone.

Sampling was non-random because institutional obligations dictated an emphasis on the relatively small number of Kaloleni farmers who have adopted high-production, high-cost exotic (here, *Bos taurus*) or partly exotic cattle. Hereafter, such breeds are collectively termed 'grade stock'. The study design called for interviewing all of the approximately 130 such farmers in Kaloleni; in fact, 111 interviews were completed (sub-sample A). Of these, 48 kept grade cattle only, and 63 had both grade and local stock.

In addition, 47 farmers who raised only zebu (*Bos indicus*)—hereafter termed 'local cattle'—were interviewed. Selection of this sub-sample B was informal because the available background data did not permit rigorous sampling procedures. At least three interviews were conducted with keepers of exclusively local cattle in each of Chonyi, Mwarakaya, Kaloleni, Jibana, Kamberibe, Ruruma and Rabai locations. Since these seven locations together comprise the semi-humid and transitional zones, they received broad coverage in sub-sample A. In addition, at least six interviews were conducted with keepers of exclusively local cattle in each of Mwamamwinga, Kayafungo and Mariakani locations. These locations comprise the Giriama drylands, which were under-represented in sub-sample A. The 47 interviews completed for sub-sample B exceeded (by nine) the minimum acceptable sub-sample size set during study design.

The foregoing sampling procedures provided a wide range of farmer circumstances and subcultures, with ample representation by agro-ecozone and herd composition. However, the disproportional representation of keepers of grade stock required care in analysis, because it precluded direct arithmetic generalizations to the Kaloleni cattle-keeping population at large.

At each farmstead, the principal cattle owner (almost always male) was interviewed. Occasionally the owner's spouse, a son or a hired herder was interviewed instead—typically when such persons were identified as most knowledgeable in local husbandry and healthcare practices. Interviews were conducted in the language preferred by the informant, either KiMijikenda or KiSwahili. Each interview proceeded in three steps. First, the informant provided baseline data, including his name, breeds of cattle kept, number of head, years of cattle-raising experience, membership in the NDDP, tick-control strategies employed and other background information.

Second, the informant named as many cattle diseases or health problems as possible. Informants were asked to include not only ailments they had personally encountered, but also any they remembered hearing about or encountering in any context whatsoever. This reliance on recall data was strategic. Had informants been provided a list and asked to confirm or deny knowledge of a host of maladies, each farmer probably would have cited a much larger number of health problems than was actually obtained. But the recall approach was selected in order to capture a better sense of the way disease concepts are constructed locally. Furthermore, this method focused interviews on the veterinary problems of paramount concern to stockraisers.

Third, the farmer was interviewed in depth about all or several of the cattle ills he had named. Depending upon his patience, this usually elicited detailed information on two or three maladies. This step had two parts. First, the farmer was asked about his abstract knowledge of each ill, including: its etiology; the breed, age, and sex of cattle affected; seasonality of the problem's occurrence and other conditions; the progression of clinical signs; effects on production; preventive strategies; and both traditional and modern veterinary treatments and their perceived efficacy. He was then asked to detail his most recent experience with the disease: when it had occurred; the breed, age and sex of cattle affected; what was done; and what the outcome had been. This approach distinguished informants' theoretical knowledge and ideal behaviour from their actual practice.

For data entry and analysis, a computerized data-base system was designed in which every mention of a disease name by a farmer was coded as one case.

Encoded along with each case were: the baseline data on the informant; the total number of diseases he volunteered and their names; the name of the case disease; and the precise information offered on the case disease. According to this method, an informant volunteering several disease names was associated with several cases. During statistical tabulations this required repeated entry of baseline data and the insertion of markers in order to distinguish the study population (of 158 farmers) from the much larger disease case-load.

Initially, farmers' own disease names were accepted, coded and entered in the data base as given; thus, each variation on an apparently similar or identical disease theme was coded as a discrete case. This method was followed even where variability clearly was a product of minor linguistic differences. In fact, since one objective of the research was to compile an interlinguistic lexicon of disease terms, it made sense to admit linguistic variability into the analytical matrix. Only later, during analysis and after consultation with an experienced veterinarian, were certain disease terms grouped and treated as a class (see following sections). At the study's end, the data base contained 515 cases. In other words, the 158 farmers volunteered a total of 515 identifiable disease terms, naturally with considerable duplication. Discrete disease names (before grouping) totalled 144.

Summary of data collected and preliminary steps in analysis

Baseline characteristics of the study population
Forty-two per cent of the study population preferred to be interviewed in KiSwahili, and 58 per cent in one of six KiMijikenda dialects. There was, however, a good deal of linguistic crossover. For example, some informants occasionally used KiSwahili terms in KiMijikenda interviews, while others interjected English words, especially English disease names.

As noted above, the greater number of grade cattle in the semi-humid and transitional zones dictated more interviews there. Forty-two per cent of informants lived in the semi-humid zone, 42 per cent in the transitional zone, and just 16 per cent in the drylands. Herd size ranged from one to 96 head. In general, stockraisers in the drylands kept large herds of mostly local cattle, while those in the higher rainfall zones had smaller herds (typically three to 10 head) that usually included some grade stock. Forty-four per cent of informants had five or fewer years of experience with cattle raising, while 28 per cent had more than 10 years. Keepers of zebu cattle and farmers in historically Giriama locations were the most apt to have long-standing cattle experience.

Informants' tick-control measures fell into three main categories: dipping, spraying and hand-washing with acaricides. One or another of these methods was used regularly by 78 per cent of the sample. The other 22 per cent occasionally removed ticks manually or practised no tick control at all. Notably, of this 22 per cent, 77 per cent kept exclusively zebu cattle and the remainder had mixed herds.

Since the early 1980s the NDDP has offered incentives and training to farmers willing to adopt grade cattle. Membership in the NDDP normally implies investment in the fodder crops and the fencing required to keep grade cattle in a reduced or zero grazing system. Few non-members practise such husbandry systems. Thus, NDDP membership is a reasonable index of intensive cattle management. Of the 19 per cent of the sample who were NDDP members, nearly all owned grade stock and resided in the semi-humid and transitional zones.

Analysis of disease terms reported
Overall, informants volunteered an average of 3.3 disease names each, with virtually no difference in this figure across keepers of grade-only, zebu-only, or mixed herds. However, as Table 1 indicates, the number of diseases cited per informant increased in tandem with years of experience in cattle husbandry. Of the total of 144 discrete disease names elicited, 68 were recognizably KiMiji-kenda or related vernacular phrasings, and 47 were recognizably KiSwahili. Thirteen were given in a KiMijikenda-KiSwahili patois and 16 in English.

Table 1. Number of disease names volunteered, by years of experience with cattle raising

Number of informants	Years of experience	Average no. of disease names
14	1–2	2.6
55	3–5	3.0
44	6–10	3.3
45	11–40	3.8

Table 2 displays three clusters of disease terms drawn from the complete list of 106 disease groupings analysed in Delehanty (1990). Each such cluster typically encompasses several local phrasings that may be interpreted cautiously as usually corresponding with either a precise (for example, theilerio-sis) or a more general (for example, helminthosis, diarrhoea) Western disease

Table 2. Selected theileriosis-related disease names volunteered by informants

Disease name	No. of informants reporting (x/158)	Language	English gloss
Theileriosis cluster			
ngai	58	KiMijikenda	calf theileriosis
homa	22	KiSwahili	fever
East Coast Fever	18	English	
ukongo wa kuha	8	KiMijikenda	tick disease
ugonjwa wa kupe or			
homa wa kupe	7	KiSwahili	tick disease
Helminthosis cluster			
minyoo	72	KiSwahili	intestinal worms
minyolo	12	KiMijikenda	intestinal worms
worms	4	English	
Diarrhoea cluster			
Kuharisha	16	KiSwahili	diarrhoea
kumwaga	12	KiSwahili	to pour
kufyoka	6	KiMijikenda	diarrhoea
kuhara damu	4	KiSwahili	bloody diarrhoea
diarrhoea	1	English	

characterization. Within a cluster, higher-order groupings of disease names both within and across languages can be constructed analytically. At the highest level of analysis, these taxonomic constructs can be taken as corresponding to broad, ethnoscientific categories of diseases according to the semantic features they encode, as expressed in informants' detailed descriptions of the original disease names they cited.

As a first step in delineating such categories, two or more disease names were grouped together when the differences between them appeared to arise from an informant's arbitrary choice between synonymous or nearly synonymous terms in the same language. For example, KiSwahili *ugonjwa wa kupe* 'tick disease' and KiSwahili *homa wa kupe* 'tick fever' were grouped under the former, more frequent term. Dialectal variants of terms in KiMijikenda were similarly grouped. Such variations tend to be extremely minor matters of pronunciation that are likely to be universally understood among KiMijikenda speakers. This process collapsed the original 144 disease names into 106 terminological classes.

The next step in category construction was to combine these lower-order groupings of disease names at one higher level, across languages. For example, KiSwahili *ugonjwa wa kupe* and KiMijikenda *ukongo wa kuha* both translate as 'tick disease', and informants' detailed descriptions of the two phrases were congruent. The English translation provides a convenient gloss under which to class the two into a single, ethno-scientific disease category. Illustrating from the foregoing examples, Figure 2 provides a graphic representation of the taxonomic process involved.

In brief, for the disease selected for the Kaloleni study, the disease names volunteered by informants appeared to fall into three normative, ethnoscientific categories that can be taken as generally corresponding to the Western-scientific definition of theileriosis. The three categories are: *ngai*, a KiMijikenda term that

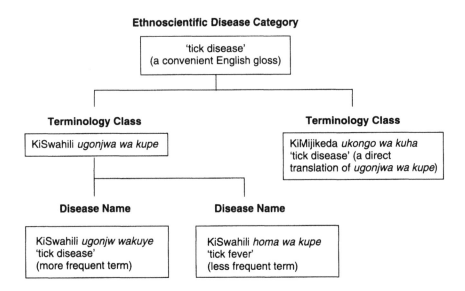

Figure 2. *'Tick disease' as an example of the construction of an ethnoscientific category of livestock disease*

also occurs in other languages; the KiSwahili and KiMijikenda equivalents for 'tick disease' described in the preceding paragraph; and the English loan-phrase 'East Coast Fever'. These categories are still somewhat fluid, however. There is considerable malleability and overlap in local disease terminology. For example, *ngai* usually signifies calf theileriosis; but some farmers also apply this word to other diseases with similar clinical signs. Nor can it be assumed without clinical verification that *ugonjwa wa kupe* and *ukongo wa kuha* always refer to theileriosis, as distinct from some other tick-borne disease. *Homa* is not properly a theileriosis cognate[4] since it can be applied to any fever. But, farmers sometimes class mild theileriosis cases as *homa*, so the term cannot be ignored as an occasional reference to theileriosis. Similarly, the diarrhoea and helminthosis clusters of disease names are included in Table 2 because of a few informants' applied these terms to some cases of theileriosis, which can be accompanied by diarrhoea and dysentery (bloody diarrhoea). Also, one informant thought 'tick disease' might be caused by intestinal worms. Table 2 suggests the kind of on-the-ground complexity that faces the ethnoveterinary researcher in analysing even a single Western disease in ethnoscientific terms.

Three categories signifying theileriosis

Theileriosis is a prominent disease of cattle in much of eastern and southern Africa. It is also one of the most economically damaging (Mukhebi 1991). It is caused by the protozoan parasite *Theileria parva*, transmitted by the tick *Rhipicephalus appendiculatus*. Detailed information on the life cycle and pathogenesis of the parasite is available in Irvin and Mwamachi (1983), who summarize the clinical and diagnostic features of the disease as follows.

> . . . the severity of the disease and the outcome are closely related to the parasite load which develops in the host. [Susceptibility, course and outcome] . . . can also be altered by host factors, such as breed, age and state of health. Young animals or those that are debilitated normally die more quickly than older, healthy animals. Similarly, animals of *Bos indicus* (zebu) stock appear more resistant than those of *Bos taurus* origin. These factors, however, tend to be irrelevant in practical terms, since morbidity and mortality rates in all susceptible stock will approach 100 per cent in those animals which receive a potentially lethal challenge.
> [Initial symptoms] . . . are rather vague and similar to those associated with any pyrexic [feverish] condition. Animals appear dull and listless, appetite begins to wane and bodily condition and milk production deteriorate. There is enlargement of the lymph nodes draining the site of parasite entry . . . This hyperplasia becomes generalized and external nodes, such as parotids, pre-scapulars and precrurals become noticeably and palpably enlarged and hot . . . (Irvin and Mwamachi 1983:193–4)

As the disease progresses, the following clinical signs are observed. Appetite and rumination cease and bodily condition degenerates rapidly. Lethargy and weakness increase, and the animals are reluctant to move; they may stand with their heads hung down or may even become recumbent. Diarrhoea and dysentery may develop. Blood may be seen in the faeces. Urine may darken as a result of dehydration. Lacrimation is common, sometimes accompanied by photophobia. In the terminal stages, severe respiratory distress develops, with a watery cough, frothy secretions from the mouth and nostrils, and build-up of fluid in the lungs and trachea. Cattle may die before these respiratory signs appear; but once these symptoms develop, death is highly likely (ibid.).

In Western veterinary practice, theileriosis control relies mainly on dipping or washing cattle with acaricides. Public dip tanks exist in Kaloleni, but most are unusable. Thus, farmers who desire and can afford acaricides tend to rely on sprays or topical applications. For treatment, (typically injectible) drugs such as oxytetracycline can be used; but such drugs are most efficacious when the disease is diagnosed early, which often means before it is clinically evident. The drugs' cost and farmers' poor access to veterinary services limit local familiarity with such therapies.

Tables 3 and 4 (see below) present findings specific to the three major ethnoscientific categories that roughly correspond to theileriosis. Table 3 gives reporting rates overall and by various baseline characteristics of the sample population. These disaggregated rates must be interpreted cautiously given the small sample sizes involved. For the same reason, only arithmetic rates are presented in Table 3, and not percentages. Table 4 numerically summarizes informants' descriptions of *ngai*, 'tick disease', and East Coast Fever.

Ngai
Ngai was reported by 58 of the 158 informants. It occurred in all three agro-ecozones and affected all breeds of cattle, but it was considered almost exclusively a disease of calves. It was more frequently reported in the semi-arid and

Table 3. Reporting rates by subpopulations of informants for *ngai*, 'tick disease' and East Coast Fever

	Number of farmers reporting		
	Ngai	'Tick disease'	ECF
By agro-ecozone			
semi-humid	21/67	7/67	10/67
transitional	27/67	2/67	6/67
semi-arid	10/24	6/24	2/24
By cattle breeds kept			
grade cattle only	15/48	3/48	8/48
mixed herds	25/63	5/63	8/63
local cattle only	18/47	7/47	2/47
By herd size			
1–5 cattle	12/41	3/41	7/41
6–20 cattle	19/58	5/58	7/58
21+ cattle	27/59	7/59	4/59
By tick control			
controls ticks	47/123	9/123	17/123
does not control	11/35	6/35	1/35
By NDDP membership			
member	9/30	3/30	6/30
non-member	49/128	12/128	12/128
Overall	58/158	15/158	18/158

Table 4. Summary of informants' detailed descriptions of *ngai*, 'tick disease' and East Coast Fever

	Ngai	'Tick disease'	ECF
Total No. of detailed descriptions	14	10	10
Cattle normally affected			
calves only	13/14	2/10	2/10
cows only	1/10		
all cattle	1/14	7/10	8/10
Main production effect			
death of calves	8/14		
death of cattle	1/10	3/10	
reduced milk output	1/14	9/10	7/10
none noted	5/14		
Most commonly noted signs			
swollen glands in neck	11/14	4/10	3/10
swollen glands on shoulders	10/14	2/10	2/10
rough haircoat	2/14	4/10	6/10
no appetite	5/14	4/10	8/10
dripping saliva	1/14	1/10	8/10
swelling on hindquarters	4/14		
bleating/crying	4/14	1/10	
diarrhoea	3/14	2/10	2/10
blood in faeces (dysentary)	3/10		
Perceived cause			
ticks	2/14	9/10	10/10
calf suckles too much	4/14		
dam gives insufficient milk	1/14		
black water in glands	1/14		
intestinal worms	1/10		
unknown	6/14		
Traditional treatments			
hot iron applied to glands	5/14	3/10	
acidic botanicals to glands	5/14	1/10	
none noted	4/14	7.10	9/10
Modern treatments			
injection by vet	6/14	6/10	8/10
oral medicine by vet	1/10		
informant says none exists	7/14		
none noted	1/14	3/10	2/10

transitional zones, and by farmers owning large (>20) herds (Table 3). These two trends may be related, since average herd size increases towards the drylands. Again, though, because of small sample size, these data can suggest only a moderate relationship between *ngai* and dryland production systems.

The clinical signs reported for *ngai* (Table 4) are largely consistent with clinical theileriosis: fever (rough haircoat) and lack of appetite, followed most notably by lymphatic swelling. In prolonged cases, the diarrhoea and dysentery reported in Table 4 often are observed. A few informants noted several additional common manifestations of acute theileriosis not shown in the table: listlessness, constipation, photophobia and respiratory distress. However, the key factor in ethnodiagnosis of *ngai* appears to be swollen lymph nodes in calves, particularly the parotid node. While other infections can also produce lymphadenitis, this is by far the most readily observable sign of acute theileriosis. Thus it is entirely reasonable to assume that *ngai* is usually (though not always) theileriosis.

Thirteen of the 14 farmers offering detailed descriptions of *ngai* said it affects calves only. Classic production effects of theileriosis are loss of weight and vigour, depressed milk output and, in acute cases, death. But Kaloleni stockraisers were nearly unanimous in citing calf death as the major production effect of *ngai*.

Six of the 14 farmers who offered detailed accounts of *ngai* were unwilling to speculate as to its etiology. Only two suggested that it might be 'caused' by ticks. Four believed it is caused by over-consumption of milk or overly vigorous suckling. Traditional cures are widely known. They involve cauterizing the parotid lymph node with a hot iron or with highly acidic botanicals. Some informants have complete confidence in these cures, and almost half reported using traditional methods to treat their most recent cases. Others expressed scepticism about these practices. A few believed that Western injections were available, but none had any experience with such drugs.

'Tick disease'

'Tick disease', reported by 15 of 158 informants, is seen as a malady of both calves and mature cattle. Only two of the 10 informants who provided detailed descriptions of this ailment linked it with calves alone. 'Tick disease' was reported across all of Kaloleni, albeit less often than *ngai* or East Coast Fever. But like *ngai*, reports were most frequent in the semi-arid zone and they increased with herd size and the proportion of zebus in the herd. In addition, farmers who do not dip, spray or hand-wash for ticks were more likely to mention 'tick disease'.

Informants enumerated fewer clinical signs than for *ngai*. Those they did give were entirely consistent with theileriosis, although they were also broad enough to incorporate fevers and acute infections of various, unknown provenance. Unlike *ngai*, mortality was not a prominent feature in farmers' descriptions. Most said the chief production effect of 'tick disease' is reduced milk yields from affected cows. In sum, this disease category appears to reference, at least in part, clinical theileriosis (including relatively mild cases) in cattle of all ages.

Not surprisingly, 90 per cent of informants identified ticks as the cause (or vector) of 'tick disease', and tick control as the principal prophylaxis. Thirty per cent indicated knowledge of a traditional cauterization treatment for this ill; 70 per cent thought there was a Western commercial treatment; and 30 per cent had recently used such a treatment on the recommendation of a veterinarian or a dip-tank operator. But their assessments of its efficacy were mixed.

East Coast Fever

'East Coast Fever' was reported by 18 of the 158 informants. Like 'tick disease', it is perceived as a malady of both young and mature animals. It was most commonly reported in two locations, Rabai and Kaloleni, where grade cattle are common and NDDP membership is widespread. Overall, the characteristics of farmers using this phrase are the opposite of those who cited *ngai* and 'tick disease'. East Coast Fever was most often mentioned in the semi-humid zone, among keepers of small herds and/or grade stock, and by those who regularly control for ticks or who are NDDP members. In sum, farmers citing East Coast Fever were mainly men who had adopted recent livestock innovations or who lived close to others who had done so.

Informants were generally vague about the presentation of East Coast Fever, and they were apt to attribute serious maladies of all sorts to this term. Only three of the 10 farmers who offered clinical details mentioned swollen parotid lymph nodes, and only two cited swollen prescapular nodes. Yet these are typical and obvious (though not quite universal) signs of acute theileriosis. Certainly they are likely to be observed in animals that die eventually of theileriosis; and a number of mortalities *were* reported.

All those reporting East Coast Fever knew the role of the tick vector, however; and all indicated that the key to prevention was tick control. Only one informant mentioned the traditional cauterization treatment, but eight of the 10 believed there was a Western injection to cure East Coast Fever. Seven reported that a veterinarian had injected their sick animals when the disease was last contracted in their herds. However, four of these seven observed that their animals died anyway.

Analysis and implications for veterinary extension in Kaloleni

Of the total number of stockraisers interviewed, 58 per cent volunteered a disease name clearly falling within the semantic domain of *ngai*, 'tick disease' or East Coast Fever. This figure does not include additional possible cases of theileriosis referenced as fevers, helminthosis or diarrhoea. In sum, theileriosis appears to be a widely acknowledged threat to cattle production throughout Kaloleni Division, with recognition of the disease approaching 100 per cent.

The native KiMijikenda term *ngai* appears to be a long-standing theileriosis description that applies almost exclusively to calves. It suggests that calf theileriosis has been, and remains, a significant health problem in the division. In fact, under conditions of endemic stability—when infected ticks continuously challenge local cattle—theileriosis is likely to manifest itself most acutely in a susceptible population such as calves (Barnett 1968).

Moreover, the greater frequency of *ngai* usage among keepers of large herds in the drylands accords well with recent serological studies suggesting high theileriosis risk to calves in this zone (Maloo 1990). Mature animals may suffer subclinical theileriosis and occasional acute breakthroughs, but most will have attained some degree of immunity. Serological surveys indicate that Kaloleni calves in fact do face relatively high risks of clinical theileriosis. Zebu calves in the semi-arid zone show especially low antibody prevalence (ibid.). This finding most likely relates to the distinctly seasonal challenge of ticks in the semi-arid zone. During the rainy season, challenge is heavy, but the rest of the year it is light. Calves born during the dry season may thus be unable to mount an effective immune response when they are abruptly exposed to heavy challenge during the following rainy season. Serological data suggest that, in contrast, most calves in the wetter zones face a modest challenge from birth and attain resistance gradually.

Such correspondences between ethnoveterinary data and laboratory diagnostic data have immediate relevance for saving on scarce veterinary diagnostic and extension resources. For targeting extension services to the areas or problems where they are most needed, ethnoveterinary information may offer a cheap, useful and 'rough-cut' alternative to more precise but costly laboratory measures of variable disease risk.

A further test of this proposition would have been possible given comparative serological data on the prevalence of other tick-borne diseases that are likely also present in Kaloleni, such as babesiosis, anaplasmosis and heartwater disease. In the Kaloleni ethnoveterinary study, informants gave no specific terms for these diseases, and they rarely reported their major clinical signs: red urine in babesiosis, jaundice in anaplasmosis, and nervous behaviour in heartwater. These findings suggest that clinical cases of these three ills are rare and/or that they have reached endemic stability in Kaloleni. While stockraisers may occasionally class acute cases of these diseases as *ngai*, 'tick disease', or East Coast Fever, semantic overlap of this sort and the apparent lack of specific names for these other tick-borne diseases suggest that they may not be major problems or merit significant extension attention. It would be instructive to learn whether this prediction from the ethnoveterinary data is borne out by other measures.

'Tick disease' probably emerged as a theileriosis descriptor with the advent of early colonial campaigns to control ticks via dipping with acaricides. This ethno-scientific category may be widespread because, along with infusions of exotic stock, dipping probably increased the incidence of acute non-calf theileriosis by blocking the acquisition of natural resistance in regularly or sporadically dipped stock. Thus, stockowners would require a disease name other than the calf-specific *ngai* in order to refer to this 'new' disease of adult cattle.

The distinction between 'tick disease' and *ngai* is a good illustration of overlaps in local terminological systems. For example, of the 58 informants who identified *ngai*, five also mentioned 'tick disease'. Conversely, of the 18 who cited East Coast Fever, two also mentioned *ngai*. In other words, people tend to assign two or more names to a disease when it manifests itself differently in different livestock populations. Such findings have obvious implications for communication between stockraisers and extensionists and for the success of disease-control campaigns.

The term 'East Cost Fever' was most popular among 'progressive' cattle keepers (especially those with grade stock) in the semi-humid zone. These farmers exhibit a good understanding of the role of ticks in vectoring theileriosis and of the susceptibility of animals of all ages and sexes (Table 4). Paradoxi-cally, however, this group described the clinical signs of the disease less precisely than did farmers who employ a more traditional nomenclature. There are two possible explanations. In the semi-humid zone, cattle appear more readily to acquire some natural immunity to theileriosis (Maloo 1990). Also, many stockraisers in this zone control ticks assiduously and thus may encounter acute theileriosis very rarely. Alternatively or additionally, they may employ the English term as either a sign or a product of their greater sophistication in Western veterinary matters or of their general 'progressiveness'. But they apparently do not always fully understand this term. They fail to connect it with every presentation of the disease, and sometimes they incorrectly connect it with other maladies. Veterinary extension among such farmers would therefore be wise to build upon their terminological preference for East Coast Fever, but to work to instil a better understanding of the disease's presentation.

This study also found marked differences in the ethno-etiologies of the various theileriosis-related disease categories. Kaloleni farmers appear to have a poor understanding of the root cause of *ngai*. Many associate it with suckling behaviour. On the other hand, the role of the tick vector seemed manifestly clear to farmers reporting 'tick disease' and East Coast Fever. Thus an essential first step in any campaign to implement a theileriosis control programme in Kaloleni should be to bridge the various theileriosis cognates by pointing out their etiological relatedness.

In veterinary extension efforts, it might be tempting to choose or devise and then promote a single term for theileriosis to replace the many local names currently in use. Certainly this approach would be preferable to everywhere promulgating the English term 'East Coast Fever' since knowledge of English is not widespread. Moreover, the foreign phrase introduces an inappropriate abstraction and a sense that diseases are only the domain of professionally trained experts. If a single-descriptor approach were taken, then the best choice might be a direct KiMijikenda or KiSwahili translation of East Coast Fever, accompanied by a thorough campaign to outline the etiology of the disease, identifying it where appropriate with other local disease names, including *ngai*, *ugonjwa wa kupe* or *homa wa kupe*, *ukongo wa kuha* and some cases of *homa*. A more practical solution, however, is for veterinary workers to adjust to farmers' own terms by adopting local theileriosis cognates, explaining their interrelatedness, and then using the local lexicon to educate stockraisers about the causality, prevention and cure of theileriosis.

Lessons for and from ethnoveterinary R&D

The Kaloleni study offers a number of telling lessons for both the conduct of ethnoveterinary research and the application of ethnoveterinary findings to development and extension efforts worldwide.

First, the study furnishes a semi-quantitative method for handling several difficulties inherent in research on local technical knowledge generally, and specifically on disease classification. One frustration familiar to all who have conducted ethnoveterinary investigations is the lack of correspondence between local and Western disease categories (Grandin 1985, McCorkle 1989). In the field, the researcher typically obtains accounts of several uniquely named animal-health problems whose ethno-etiologies and clinical signs suggest they may in fact be the same disease. This is especially true where the acute manifestations of a disease vary dramatically by breed, age and sex. People often assign separate names to what, in their eyes, appear to be separate afflictions. Where more than one language and/or dialect group is involved, this complication is compounded.

Conversely, certain local terms encompass a variety of diseases as defined by Western veterinary science. Especially where the clinical signs of one disease resemble closely those of another, people are unlikely to distinguish the two in their ethno-scientific taxonomies. Stockraisers everywhere tend to read clinical signs and to assign disease names on that basis alone (McCorkle 1986, McCorkle and Mathias-Mundy 1990, Wolfgang and Sollod 1986). This tendency introduces further confusions in that many terms elicited from local people are merely clinical signs rather than disease names; that is, they do not gloss culturally encoded disease entities. Examples from the larger ethnoveterinary study in

Kaloleni include 'coughing', 'refuses to graze', 'avoids the sun', 'crazy', 'drips saliva', 'too much blood in the heart' and 'fever' (Delehanty 1990).

The approach followed here was to accept, record and code all disease names as given by informants. Ethnoetiologies were collected even for ills that were scientifically indefinite or questionable. In this respect, the approach was more or less standard for classificatory work in ethnosemantics (Grandin 1985, ITDG 1989). In such work on ethnoveterinary medicine to date, however, data manipulation and analysis have seldom gone beyond hand-tabulated vocabulary lists and ethno-etiological summaries for seemingly important animal health problems. The Kaloleni study shows how a more quantitative approach, beginning with computerized data entry, can ease the organization and analysis of inherently untidy ethnoveterinary information. Case designation of each instance of a local disease name assures accurate replication of local descriptive nuance in the data base; and it facilitates production of a lexicon that accurately reflects local classificatory knowledge. Meanwhile, cross-tabulations and other automated procedures speed the task of tentatively or experimentally collapsing possibly-related terms for more refined analysis.

Second, there is reason to believe that—perhaps with some modifications and refinements—the methodology described here could be useful in estimating variable disease risk, in lieu of more accurate but expensive laboratory diagnostic surveys. Of course, key to any such effort is selection of the major variables on which epidemiological variance is likely to hinge, plus careful collection of baseline as well as lexical and ethno-diagnostic/clinical data from each informant. In addition, however, more rigorous sampling frames and larger sample sizes than were possible in the Kaloleni study would be advisable. It might also be useful to obtain progeny histories in conjunction with this work, especially to gauge mortality. Ideally, too, targeted clinical observations or laboratory diagnostics should be done to confirm presumed associations between ethnoscientific and scientific disease categories. Under field conditions in the developing world, however, laboratory facilities are not always available. Actual clinical or laboratory-diagnostic data were not collected in the Kaloleni study because its research focus was local veterinary knowledge and not current ailments in an informant's herd. Furthermore, for the purposes of the Kaloleni study, recall data were used. But this approach gives prominence to health problems the informant has seen or heard of in the recent past. Thus, serious maladies that occur only rarely or sporadically could be over- or underestimated.

Despite these caveats, it was possible to draw some tentative conclusions from Kaloleni informants' reporting rates about differences in the incidence of disease across population subgroups. Certainly, the general methods followed here merit further testing and refinement for their potential as a cost-effective way to estimate variable disease risk. Especially useful would be trials in regions where ethnoveterinary knowledge is more highly developed than it is in Kaloleni, and where patterns of disease incidence are more diverse.

Third and finally, the Kaloleni study suggests how ethnoveterinary research on the concordance, or lack thereof, between local and Western disease concepts and on the semantic interpenetration of clinical signs and diseases can help veterinary extensionists to communicate more effectively with their clientele—in turn, making for more effective programmes of disease control. Ethnoveterinary research can furnish veterinary extensionists, researchers and decision-makers with a more accurate picture of local terminology, concepts and knowledge of livestock disease than the anecdotal information commonly available at the outset of veterinary campaigns in the developing world. Several general principles emerge from the Kaloleni research in this respect.

o Any campaign to control a given disease should be identified to the general public as being aimed at the entire range of locally named and defined ailments likely to correspond to the disease in question.
o Labels in every relevant language should be used.
o When there is doubt whether a local term X corresponds, or sometimes corresponds, to the scientificaly defined disease in question, it should be explained to the public that the latter *could* be X.
o As far as possible, a campaign should elucidate the clinical signs of the disease in question, since some stockraisers will not have precise ethno-scientific definitions beyond the most obvious clinical manifestations.

Ethnoveterinary research is especially important when a campaign is targeted at relatively inexperienced stockraisers. Pastoralists and others with a long history of animal husbandry typically possess a well-codified lexicon of livestock disease, challenging in its subtlety and complexity, but amenable to translation precisely because of its richness and more uniform usage within the society (see Fraudin and Young, this volume). But less experienced stockraisers like those of Kaloleni often display many conceptual gaps and considerable uncertainty about livestock diseases. They share no universal or common culture of animal health and husbandry, so their veterinary vocabulary is much more varied. It would be satisfying to be able to identify every local disease name with a Western-scientific equivalent. However, the independence of local disease construction is precisely the point of an exercise such as the Kaloleni study. The lineaments of local disease classification, for all its ambiguity and variability, must be factored into the planning and implementation of disease control campaigns and other veterinary interventions if these are to be successful and sustainable.

Notes

1. The author wishes to thank the following persons for their contributions to this work: Dr Barbara Grandin, formerly of the International Laboratory for Research on Animal Diseases (ILRAD), who helped design and supervise the project during its initial phases; Mr Mohammed Salim Baya, who carried out the bulk of the fieldwork; Dr Brian Perry of ILRAD, who provided veterinary epidemiological support; Dr Adrian Mukhebi of ILRAD, who commented on early findings and subsequent drafts; Mr John Young of the Intermediate Technology Development Group, and the volume editors, all of whom made many valuable comments on drafts of this chapter; and Dr Bill Thorpe of ILCA, who facilitated fieldwork in Kaloleni. The work was completed under a collaborative research agreement between ILRAD and the Kenya Agricultural Research Institute (KARI), and is published with the kind permission of the Director of KARI.
2. The infection-and-treatment method involved infecting cattle with the sporozoite form of parasite stocks while at the same time treating the animals with an antibiotic to lessen the severity of the infection. Ethnoveterinary research was conducted under the auspices of the Epidemiology and Socioeconomics Program (ESEP) in ILRAD, Nairobi. As part of a collaborative research agreement between ILRAD and the Veterinary Division of KARI, the ESEP agreed to provide background epidemiolo-gical and socio-economic studies in support of KARI's infection-and-treatment trials in Kaloleni. The research reported here was carried out in partial fulfilment of that agreement.

3. For complete detail on sampling procedures and subjects, the survey instrument, issues of language use in interviewing, and so forth, consult Delehanty (1990). This report also provides much more extensive tabular data, from which the tables presented here have been abstracted.
4. Here, 'cognate' is employed in the third dictionary definition of 'allied or similar in nature or quality', rather than in its strict etymological sense.

21. Veterinary science and savvy among Ferlo Fulße[1]

ANGELO-MALIKI BONFIGLIOLI AND YERO D. DIALLO
WITH SONJA FAGERBERG-DIALLO

THIS CHAPTER PROVIDES a brief overview of traditional knowledge and practice pertaining to cattle health among Fulße (Fulani) herders of the Ferlo region of northern Senegal. The chapter draws in part upon the authors' work with the Oxfam—UK Pastoralist Programme in Senegal.[2] One of the objectives of this programme was to study local technical knowledge, cultural values and social and economic organization—all in the native Pulaar language (also known as Fulfulde).[3] The material thus obtained was used in development activities such as training local herders in selected animal husbandry practices and mounting local literacy campaigns in Pulaar-speaking regions of Senegal.

The emphasis here is on description of the ethnoveterinary system as seen from an insider's point of view. The information presented is based on several research and training activities. First is a lifetime of 'insider' research by the second author, a well-known Fulße writer and a member of a prestigious Ferlo family that is renowned for its ethnomedical knowledge, both veterinary and human. Working in his native Pulaar, he systematically collected and recorded extensive information on animal husbandry and the daily life of Fulße agro-pastoralists. With Oxfam support and in conjunction with the first author, this information was then brought together and published in book form (Diallo 1989a, 1989b) during a summer's field study in the second author's home village and the surrounding areas. During this time, the authors also conducted additional field research on Fulße veterinary knowledge and practice (Bonfiglioli et al. 1988).

The Ferlo and the Fulße

In French, 'Ferlo' refers to the whole of central Senegal's sylvo-pastoral zone. In Pulaar, however, the name delimits specifically the region south of Matam and east of Linguère. The Ferlo is flat and sandy, its topography unrelieved by mountains, hills or major rivers or streams. Local people define the region by its distinctive geomorphology and vegetation. Ferlo soils are 'black' (*leydi ɓaleeri*) and mineral-poor, in contrast to the 'white' soils (*leydi ndaneeri*) in neighbouring regions. The black soil gives rise to a characteristic vegetation dominated by *geelooki*, *ɗooki* and *kojolo* trees (respectively, *Guiera senegalensis*, *Combretum glutinosum* and *Anogeisus leocarpus*).

The Ferlo is bounded socio-politically by three important states: Jolof in the west, Bunndu in the east, and Fuuta Tooro in the north. In all four areas, Pulaar speakers are dominant. But the Ferlo never had a centralized state structure. It is instead organized around major local lineages. Today, the area is dominated by Fulße lineages that have traditionally held large herds of cattle. In recent years, rainfed agriculture has become more important, with millet as the staple food-crop. Today, every Ferlo family farms. However, the millet a family produces generally lasts only a couple of months. To obtain grain during the rest of the year, livestock are marketed or exchanged in a system known as *jiggoore*. This includes relatively little milk or milk products, however, because almost all Fulße families in the Ferlo produce their own milk and consume most of it; also, markets where fresh milk is in demand are too far for them to transport and sell their surpluses of fresh milk.

Herders in the Ferlo maintain a precarious existence in an annual cycle of changing seasons. Moreover, their larger ecological, economic, demographic and socio-political situation is currently in a state of flux. But whether individually or collectively, they have a major stake in maintaining a human–animal–environment equilibrium that allows both themselves and their livestock to survive (Bonfiglioli 1990). In this context, wealth is neither the accumulation of capital nor the production of surplus. Rather, it is the capacity to maintain a basic standard of living even during difficult seasons and bad years. A successful herder is one who can properly feed the family all year round. Likewise, a good herder is not necessarily one who has a highly productive herd; rather, it is one who can surmount seasonal and other fluctuations that impact on the herd, as well as occasional epidemics. These values and perceptions are reflected in the way Fulße conceptualize, classify and respond to livestock health problems.

Concepts of animal health problems

Ferlo herds are subject to numerous health problems. Diallo (1989b) has identified 35 emically recognized 'diseases' (*ñawu*, pl. *ñabbuuji*) plus some 26 other conditions that are specific to given sexes or ages of animals or that result from accidents or other misfortunes. For each of these health problems, herder interviewees could identify their contagiousness, characteristic symptoms, seasonal prevalence and causes or predisposing factors. The following sections offer a sampling of this vast body of knowledge, grouped and classified emically.

Contagious diseases

Fulße are at once very concerned and very knowledgeable about the contagious diseases of their cattle—including the speed with which such diseases strike (*jaawgol*, lit. 'to occur rapidly'), their mode and rate of spread and their severity. Herders classify six diseases as contagious: pleuro-pneumonia (*jofe* or *yeedi*), foot-and-mouth disease (*safo*), blackleg (*bernal*, *laañel*, or *kurel*), anthrax (* δaasu* or *δaaso*), rinderpest (*caaru*) and a form of chronic botulism (*lacce*).

Herders say these diseases are mainly spread by infected animals' mixing with healthy ones at watering places (*tufnde*, pl. *tufle*), along cattle routes (*lappol*, pl. *lappi*), in pastures (*durngol*, pl. *durδe*), and in the cattle camps (*jofnde*, pl. *jofle*) at night. These modes of transmission are of particular concern because they can introduce unfamiliar contagious diseases from other regions or countries; Ferlo herders may therefore not recognize or know how to cure these diseases. People are also aware that, as much as a year later, the carcasses of animals who died of certain contagious diseases can still infect healthy stock that come into contact with the remains.

Fulße recognize that wild animals, insects and birds can carry contagion, too. Herders say infection can also be spread by wind (*henndu*) and certain odours (*uurngol*) borne on the wind. (See also Brisebarre, this volume and Schillhorn van Veen, this volume.) For example, people believe that wind is both a predisposing and a causative factor in the spread of blackleg. They also consider that the steam from cooking the meat of an animal that has died of an infectious disease is contagious. In addition, they note that touching such meat and then handling a healthy animal without washing properly can transmit the disease.

Non-contagious diseases

Ferlo herders class non-contagious diseases into six broad categories, as follows.

Fevers A number of ills that Fulße do not consider contagious nor especially life-threatening are termed simply 'fever' (*paawnooji*). A complex of such fevers is identified by symptoms like aches and pains, general fatigue, and the inability to stand or walk. An example is *becce*, which is identified by pains in the side or rib-cage. Other fevers include *birgo boofel, birgo ծomka, paafu loɲel,* or *kofel,* and *paawle birgo*. These ailments can be fatal if they leave an animal unable to graze.

Swellings Another Fulße category of animal health problems is comprised of various forms of swelling (*ßuutoji*). These are identified and named according to the part of the body affected. For example, *bakkaaծe, ծaծol* (phlebitis) and *njokto* affect the legs and joints, causing swelling, lameness and sometimes even complete loss of mobility. *Haande* affects the neck, where it can inhibit drinking or eating. *Jappo* or *nofal* (ear myiasis) affects the head and face of the animal, causing the ears and eyes to become swollen and painful.

Diseases attributed to environmental causes The Pulaar word for 'environment', *falnde*, refers to natural resources such as grasses, trees, shrubs, water, soils and wildlife (including non-mammalian species). In the cultures of the Ferlo, *falnde* is the source of all life. A good environment promotes good livestock production. However, *falnde* can also be the source of livestock diseases and disorders, whether via grazing sites and forages, seasonal changes or wildlife.

For instance, certain grazing sites and habits, often combined with a given season of the year, are said to cause different types of intoxication (generically termed *filto*). Examples include: grazing cattle on sandy pastures (*seeno*) or dunes during the rainy season; grazing for long periods on dry puncture vine (*Tribulus terrestris,* Pulaar *tuppere hokkunde*); and grazing late into the evening toward the end of the rainy season. Herders note that intoxication from such sources can also sometimes cause abortions (*woppere* or *werlere*). The common practice of *ñaayngol*, or grazing cattle on millet residues, has both benefits and dangers. Fulße believe it protects livestock against anthrax but predisposes them to foot-and-mouth disease (FMD).

Fulße also attribute various types of *kifu* 'bloat' to the fodder or other items that animals ingest. For example, eating the *ñendiko* variety of millet when it is in flower causes *kifu njuumaan. Kifu ßoorol* results from ingestion of such unhealthy substances as snake skins and plastic bags. *Kifu dengo* is associated with *dengo* grass. If this forage is in flower when consumed, it can cause death; if dry, it is believed to cause night-blindness (*bompel*). However, the latter condition is alleviated when the rains come (see Stem, this volume). Poor grazing habits can also cause *cartu* 'diarrhoea' (see also Schillhorn van Veen, this volume). Herders know diarrhoea can be fatal, especially when it leads to dehydration.

Seasonal changes greatly influence pastoral production in the Ferlo. They radically transform the environment and thus alter human–livestock–environment relationships. Ferlo herders attribute various ailments to animals' poor adaptation to seasonal changes. Fulße recognize seven seasons (*dumunnaaji*): *demminaare* in June marks the beginning of the rainy season; *korse* is a transitional period in July that leads into *ndunngu*, the rainy season proper; *kawle*, the end of the rains in October, precedes *dabbunde*, the long cold season from November to February; *ceeδu* is the hot dry season from March to April; and *ceeδ-ceeδle* marks the end of the hot season in May.

Health problems associated with the hot dry season include mastitis (*felwere, gañangel* or *summmilde*) and FMD. Rinderpest is also said to be worst at this time. Herders of course know that conditions such as night-blindness or extreme weight loss and malnutrition (*wofaare*) are related directly to the inadequate pasture of the dry season. Fulße also recognize that the cold season and the preceding, transitional season bring particular veterinary problems, too. Chronic botulism, anthrax, contagious bovine pleuro-pneumonia (CBPP) and internal parasitism leading to intestinal disorders (e.g., *diimol, fiδo beeli*, and 'coccidiosis' *kumol*) are said to be more prevalent at this time.

With regard to wildlife, birds—especially *cerwaali* 'oxpeckers' (*Buphagus africanus*)—are believed to cause, infect or at least exacerbate chronic sores. They may also facilitate the spread of botulism. Warthogs (*bamδi girji*) are thought to contaminate pastures and spread rinderpest and other diseases. Ticks (*kooti*)—which preferentially attack young animals—flies (*buubi*) and worms (*gilδi*) cause various well-known problems, too.

Malnutrition Fulße consider all clinical syndromes involving malnutrition and general weakness very important. They realize that most animals are subject to seasonal or annual cycles of malnutrition that can prejudice growth, reproductive capacity, milk production and disease resistance. Herders in the Ferlo distinguish many forms and degrees of malnutrition (generic *heege*) depending on the quantity and quality of forage available, the season of the year, the types of animals affected and their clinical signs. Fulße also generally link malnutrition to lack of salt (see also Schillhorn van Veen, this volume).

Herders say malnutrition is a problem not only during the difficult dry season when forage is scarce but also during transitional seasons, when the quality of pasturage is poor. For example, they know that severe malnutrition can occur at the end of the rainy season or in years of exceptionally abundant rainfall, when the grass is *huδo heewi ndiyam* 'full of water'. People note that animals display a particular craving for salt (*yooytinde*) at such times. Cattle may wander about looking for anything salty to eat: rags, bones, garbage, dirt, even excrement. This is an apt observation on herders' part, because grass that receives too much moisture is low in proteins, minerals and other critical nutrients. Under such conditions, herders search for *kudol daneewol* 'white grasses', which they consider to have the needed nutrients, especially salt.

Wofaare describes a state of malnourishment and complete exhaustion, immobility, and even recumbancy that often occurs at the end of the long dry season. Undernourishment that affects the growth of young animals is called *δakku. Yooyre* or *soymo* refers to severe and progressive weight loss in livestock at any time of the year, even when sufficient feed is available. Herders consider this the worst form of malnutrition. Again, they attribute it to lack of salt in the diet.

Fulße also associate certain illnesses with the weakened condition brought on by poor nutrition. In effect, herders are aware that cattle without sufficient salt cannot properly metabolize their feed and thus become vulnerable to many diseases. People say that malnourished stock are especially susceptible to anthrax. They also blame poor nutrition at the end of the dry season for one type of night-blindness that can be accompanied by an itching rash known as *nduwaaki* and/or a skin condition called *yaynde* in which sores do not heal properly. Cows thus affected give little milk, and their milk is said to sicken anyone who drinks it. Finally, malnourished animals are more easily and seriously affected by intestinal parasites.

Health problems associated with sex or age

All Ferlo herders recognize that a number of health problems affect only or mainly specific sex or age groups. Cows may have abortions, calving problems (*faloreede* or *jahreede*), mastitis, infertility (*enδi*), prolapse of the uterus (*seere* or *saare*) or impaired milk production (*jaaδo enndu*). These problems are important since they affect herd reproduction and productivity directly and hence the well-being of herders and their families.

New-born calves are particularly susceptible to severe and often fatal diarrhoea and to intestinal parasitism, which can lead to a potentially fatal condition called *δeeδu*. Calves suffer from problems such as the following: a swollen tongue (*δesngu*), which prevents proper nursing; a condition known as *fiδo kanndi* that is caused by over-consumption of colostrum (*kannde*) and sometimes leads to fevers; a swollen and inflamed navel (*gulli* 'navel ill') contaminated by dirt or insects—a condition that can block urination and eventually kill the calf; a frothy cough (*δojjo*)—thought to be due to ingestion of the dam's hair while suckling—that is most common among calves whose mothers are poor milkers; and *ñiiye* 'teeth', (calves born with teeth—that is, which prevent proper and sufficient suckling).

Two genital disorders commonly afflict mature bulls. One, *ŋeeco kaladi*, produces infertility (though not impotence) as a result of severed *δaδel* 'nerves' in the scrotum. In *piδal ngaari*, a venereal infection, the penis may fail to retract, causing urinary difficulties.

Accidents and sorcery

Significantly, Pulaar has no word or concept for 'accident'. Yet animals frequently suffer broken legs, intestinal obstructions, repeated snake bites, falls and other unpredictable problems. Fulβe believe that some animals, and even whole herds, are 'fated' to be especially vulnerable or prone to accident and disease. Animals subjected to sorcery (*dabare*) also share this condition, known as *parwugol*. *Parwugol* accounts for animal health problems that find no other explanation.

Animal healthcare practices

Ferlo herders have access to local healers (*ñeeñδuβe* or *gannduβe*), most of whom specialize in treating certain unusual or complex livestock diseases. But even ordinary Fulβe herders know many ways to prevent, control and cure common animal health problems themselves. Some of the most common techniques and treatments are outlined below.

Preventive care

For certain diseases (for example, rinderpest and chronic botulism), quarantine may be instituted. The carcasses of animals that succumb to infectious disease are buried so as to forestall further contagion. If contaminated bones were left lying on the ground, for example, cattle in search of salt would be tempted to lick or chew them. To dispel or repel contagion, herders may also fumigate (*cuur-kingol*) their kraals by burning medicinal leaves, roots or barks. At the same time, incantations may be uttered to provide added protection. These techniques are used to ward off blackleg, for example. Branding (*cumooδe*) is done to prevent a number of contagious diseases that are said to be 'afraid' of fire.

However, most preventive measures are simply a normal part of judicious herding and grazing strategies. Chief among these is herd movement, which is Fulße's main strategy for providing their animals with the best and most varied diet, and therefore with greater resistance to disease in general. A number of such moves can be distinguished.

First is the daily movement between pastures, watering points, and the camps outside the village where stock are milked and kraaled at night. Camps are always kept clean and safe. Second is the monthly movement (*costingol*) of the camp in order to provide the herd with fresh, clean quarters. Third are seasonal movements designed to maximize grazing and good nutrition. The most important of such moves, *ruumoyde*, scatters herds during the rainy season so they can search out the best pasture while water is available in temporary pools and also so they can locate the 'white grasses' that combat the acute mineral deficiencies of the rainy season. *Mooδtinoyde* is movement specifically to find such grasses in areas of 'white soil'. *Kawnoore* is the movement at the end of the rains, to keep herds away from ripening fields. Next comes the cold-season *dabboore*, a move intended to satisfy cattle's craving for salt. Dry-season moves (*seeδoore*) are made in search of adequate water and pasture in this most difficult time of the year. The move called *korsol* corresponds with the end of the long dry season when livestock malnutrition and weakness are greatest and herders set out to follow the first rains that fall.

As part of their preventive healthcare regime, Fulße add minerals to their herds' diet whenever undernourishment threatens. The type of supplement varies with the season and with animal health and age. Salt is given in a number of ways, but never alone. In a large bowl or a hole in the ground (*tuppal*), salt may be mixed with water and a mash of bitter (*haaδi*) or salty (*lammi*) leaves from trees such as the baobab (*δokki*) and the *gelooki*, *keekeeli kelli*, and *duuki* (respectively, *Heeria insignis*, *Grewia bicolor* and *Cordylla pinnata*), and with *Combretum* spp. and other plants such as okra (*kañnje*). Called *mooδnde*, these mixtures are fed especially towards the end of the rainy season. Cattle also receive them once or twice during the rains in order to prevent *yooyre*.

For CBPP and some other diseases, Fulße practise a form of vaccination known as *coodgol*, which builds resistance by exposing animals to a mild case of the disease in question. Herders prepare the vaccine by removing a small piece of lung from an animal who has died of CBPP and steeping the tissue overnight in milk or a millet mixture (*saaño suuna*). This procedure is said to 'reduce the toxicity'. The next morning the piece of lung is placed in a small incision made on the nose in such a way that the animal cannot lick it. The vaccinated stock usually run a fever for two or three days and then recover. Occasionally, though, if the lung tissue is 'too hot' (i.e., virulent), an animal may contract a full-blown case of CBPP and die.

To prevent or combat sorcery against animals, herders often hire a special type of traditional healer (*bileejo*) to prepare and/or administer protective medicines, fetishes and incantations (*ñawndugol*). These may consist of a mixture of herbs, a liquid to put on the ground in the cattle camp, or an amulet made of a cord knotted while reciting protective formulae (*cefi*).

Curative care

Herders in the Ferlo use a variety of curative treatments called *cafrugo* (pl. *cafruδi*, from the verb *safrude* 'to treat, cure, heal'). Some involve the administration of drenches or ointments prepared from roots or leaves; others require physical manipulation; still others make extensive use of fire (*jaynge*) or water (*ndiyam*). Treatments may be applied simultaneously or successively. And since Fulße do not draw a sharp distinction between the natural and the supernatural world, medical interventions are often mixed with ritual acts and incantations. Thus science and ceremony reinforce each other to promote herd health, well-being and security. (See also Brisebarre, this volume and Lawrence, this volume.)

Fulße generally administer medicines in one of two ways: orally (*safaara*) or externally. *Njarnugol* is the term for drenching, while *koygol* refers to the force-feeding of non-liquids designed to make the animal vomit. Some examples include: for diarrhoea or FMD, drenching with *gawde*, a millet mixture; to relieve bloat, feeding fresh milk or a sugar mixture; or to induce vomiting, forcing the animal to drink soap suds using the locally-made black soap.

External treatments take various forms involving massage or rubbing, sometimes with medicaments and sometimes without. *Moomgol lekki* is the application of a sort of plaster of butter and leaves or roots. Administering a pomade or thick liquid to wounds or sores is called *gujgol*. *Coccugol* refers to vigorous massage with unguents or pomades in order to bring down swelling or relieve pain. *ɓoosgol* is deep massage. Medicaments typically administered in these ways include, for example, butter (*nebbam keccam*), cream (*kettungol*), herbal mixtures of leaves, ash (*kaata*) and dirt or mud (especially the earth from termite hills). In the case of *δakku*—a spinal problem that causes extreme weight loss—herders may massage butter or cream into the area of the backbone.

Common surgical techniques include bloodletting to remove *ŷiiŷam*[4] *ßalejam* 'black blood' or *ŷiiŷam maayδam* 'dead blood', and piercing or incising the skin. The latter techniques are used to treat bloat and blackleg, and sometimes an itching skin condition called *nduwaaki*. Cutting or piercing the skin is always accompanied by other treatments, however. For example, the *δakku* treatment described above may be supplemented by piercing the hide, inserting a reed or straw, and blowing air between the skin and the muscles. Finally, wounds (*gaañannde*) and abscesses (*lawre*) are often opened (*pesgol*), cauterized (*uppol*), and/or anointed. Ferlo herders are also adept at setting bones and adjusting dislocations. In the case of a fracture (*kelol*), the limb is wrapped and tied (*kaɓɓol*), usually in a mat (*leeso*). In dislocations (*fokkitere*), the limb is pulled and reset in its proper place (*pokkugol*).

As noted earlier, fire is used for branding or scarring, cauterizing and fumigating. Again, these techniques are usually accompanied by other treatments or medications. Numerous health problems call for branding with parallel marks (*cumooδe caawndiiδe*) or cross marks (*gallaaδi ɓurgal*) on designated parts of the body. Selection of the proper marks is considered essential to the success of the treatment. Branding is used for a variety of conditions, including anthrax, FMD, fevers, myiasis, phlebitis, hoof diseases (*fecco*) and inflamed tick bites. Finally, water has particular uses in healing, especially for fevers. Just pouring water over the animal's body is often considered sufficient treatment for fever. Water is also used to treat a certain type of night-blindness believed to be caused by a snail (*guje*) that thrives in rainy-season puddles.

Putting principles of ethnoveterinary R&D into practice

Whether in conceptualizing, classifying, preventing, controlling, or treating livestock health problems, veterinary concerns among Fulße herders inhabiting the difficult and fluctuating environment of the Ferlo focus on the practical implications for human well-being and food security. Herders judge the severity of a problem mainly in terms of its effects on live weight, milk yields, fertility and reproduction in their animals. They have a vast array of strategies and treatments—ecological, nutritional, ethnopharmacological, manipulative, immunological, surgical and magico-religious—to counter health problems in their herds. In short, their veterinary science and savvy span every domain of animal healthcare recognized by Western medicine.

This chapter has sought to illustrate the breadth of Fulße veterinary knowledge and practice, but not to evaluate them systematically for accuracy or efficacy. (However, see Schillhorn van Veen, this volume.) The authors' objectives in collecting and organizing this information instead embodied a different kind of research–development relaticnship. The goal was to share the findings with herders themselves, allowing them to examine and analyse their own knowledge and beliefs, practices and habits, and to judge for and among themselves what works and what doesn't.

In collaboration with the Senegalese Groupe d'Initiative pour le Promotion du Livre en Langues Nationales (GIPLLN), this was achieved by supplying herders in literacy classes with the Pulaar-language books that resulted from the authors' research (Figure 21.1). Two important development principles were thereby put into practice: seeing that research results are shared with the people from whom they were derived; and using literacy not only for transmitting messages from outside experts but also for promoting a participatory process of self-discovery in which people learn to analyse, value, and perhaps modify what they already know.

One of the advantages of this approach was demonstrated clearly during Oxfam training of veterinary auxiliaries, when the same herders who had served as research interviewees used the resulting written materials as texts. The Pulaar-speaking veterinarian who delivered the training based his course on the information in these books. He was thus able to establish a common body of knowledge with trainees about the diagnosis and treatment of livestock disease. Then, taking what herders already knew as the starting-point for naming and diagnosing diseases, it was easy for the instructor to teach them about new medicines and dosages (also see Grandin and Young, this volume).

This corpus of ethnoveterinary data was also uscd in designing local post-literacy classes, where participants learned to keep records on the frequency and incidence of specific diseases among the herds in their zone. This application made learning to read and write a more relevant, meaningful and interesting task for herders. At the same time, it afforded a further forum for the exchange and validation of ethno-scientific information and opinion. In sum, along with Ibrahim and Abdu (this volume), the present authors have found that the results of research on local knowledge systems can play an important role in educational as well as agricultural development.

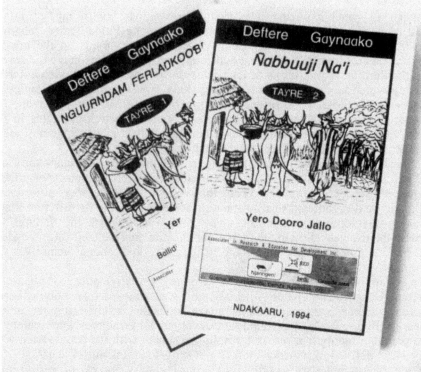

Figure 1. *Pulaar-language books on Fulße ethnovetinary medicine used in functional literacy training for herders. (The book covers are displayed above, and a sample of the text is shown below.)*

Notes

1. The authors are grateful to the editors of this volume and especially to Karla Schillhorn van Veen for her assistance in translating the chapter from the French.
2. For further information on this programme, contact Oxfam, BP 3475, Dakar, Senegal, or consult Bonfiglioli and Diallo (1988).
3. All Pulaar terms are transcribed using the UNESCO system, which has also been adopted officially in Senegal, but see note 4 below.
4. Readers should note that the normal right-hooked 'y' symbol in Pulaar has been replaced in this chapter with 'ŷ' due to printer problems.

22. Traditional and re-applied veterinary medicine in East Africa[1]

DEAN A. ROEPKE

THIS CHAPTER REVIEWS selected field experiences of the author, a veterinarian who worked for five years with Heifer Project International (HPI) on smallholder dairy development in Tanzania and other East African countries. The genetically improved milk cattle on which HPI concentrated were presumed to require more sophisticated husbandry and healthcare technology than the traditional stock-raising system could provide. The veterinarian's assignment was thus to prioritize the choice of commercial drugs *vis-à-vis* the economic value of these dairy animals and the losses of productivity resulting from disease. In the course of performing this task, the author learned a number of important lessons.

First is that local people have many traditional veterinary treatments of their own that parallel Western techniques. This fact was highlighted by the author's initial encounter with ethnoveterinary medicine, when smallholders were observed injecting the milk of unripe coconuts subcutaneously as a fluid- and electrolyte-replacement therapy for young stock suffering from scours, much as humans may be given a drip to offset the dehydration of acute diarrhoea.

The second lesson is that some ethnoveterinary practices appear to be just as effective as their Western commercial equivalents; moreover, they may be far more accessible. This lesson is illustrated by field experiences with treating bovine dermatophilosis, which can reduce productivity in lactating cows. One task of the project veterinarian was to inject cows thus afflicted with large quantities of antibiotics, and then to disinfect and poultice the skin lesions, so as to keep off flying insects. However, antibiotics were available only through the HPI project; and all in all, this costly treatment resulted in a long-term nursing rigour of only marginal success. As healing began, a new rainy season opened and so did the old lesions, along with fresh ones as well. Meanwhile, WaSwahili villagers in southern coastal Tanzania were observed to have achieved equal if not greater success in combating dermatophilosis with topical applications of a certain seed oil.

The third lesson is that much of this kind of valuable ethnoveterinary knowledge is in danger of being lost or suppressed. To continue with the foregoing example, the seed oil just mentioned derives from the *chalmoogra* tree (*Hydnocarpus wightiana* Blume). This tree used to be cultivated in leper colonies of the 1930s in the tropics, where its kern oil was applied topically to combat leprosy (Trease and Evans 1983). Seeing this, WaSwahili who lived in the vicinity of a leper colony experimented with using the oil to cure skin diseases in their livestock. They found that it worked very well, indeed. Yet the Western pharmacopoeia has relegated this remedy to the dustbin of history. Likewise for many other therapies and prophylaxes recorded in the rich colonial literature on East Africa between the 1920s and the 1950s.

The fourth and final lesson is that, given the foregoing considerations, ethnoveterinary medicine can offer a much-needed alternative or complement to Western-style treatments. Taken together, these lessons led the author to modify his original assignment to include: learning about local drugs and practices—whether from stockraisers themselves or from nineteenth- and early twentieth-century veterinary literature; then confirming the findings with villagers; and finally, applying promising ethnotherapies and -prophylaxes in the field, whether alone or together with commercial drugs. This was done with a number of the local remedies described below that were observed to be effective.

The following description of East African veterinary practices is organized by types of local drugs and focuses mainly on medicinal plants. In each section, firsthand field experiences and observations are supplemented with supporting or related information from scientific studies on both human and animal, past and present, Western and non-Western ethnobotanicals. The goal is to suggest the usefulness of rescuing and re-applying local veterinary knowledge and resources to the field-level healthcare of livestock in developing countries.

Field experiences and findings from the literature

Antimicrobials

Fieldwork in Tanzania revealed the widespread application of natural ascorbic acids as antimicrobials, whether for livestock or humans. Stockraisers made both internal and topical use of acidic compounds derived from, for example, citrus fruits and tea leaves. In addition, various East African societies employ *Solanum incanum* L. for bacterial infections. The author observed its use especially in arid areas of East and North Africa. But villagers in the Pare Mountains of Tanzania—a region characterized by high humidity—also reported that they used the juice of *S. incanum* berries to treat wounds, ringworm and fevers in ruminants. For example, one farmer demonstrated how he squeezed the juice of *Solanum* berries into the mucus-filled nostrils of a heifer suffering from shipping fever. When the author returned two days later, the condition of the heifer had improved remarkably—without the use of any Western antibiotics. This plant has proved effective against both Gram-positive and Gram-negative bacteria *in vitro* (Beaman-Mbaya and Muhammed 1976); it is also a confirmed antifungal (see below).

East Africans know and use numerous plants to treat infectious diseases and festering wounds, as evidenced in lengthy compilations of ethno-medical plants from Tanzania and East Africa (for example, Riley and Brokensha 1988, Haerdi 1964, Kokwaro 1976). In testing the extracts of 76 plants traditionally employed in East Africa to treat infectious diseases in humans, approximately 97 per cent showed antimicrobial activity against one or more micro-organisms *in vitro* (Chhabra *et al.* 1981, 1983). Tables 1 and 2 list the most active of such plants, all of which could be used to treat animal diseases as well.

Table 1. Plants found in East Africa with proven antimicrobial activity[a]

Family	Genus and species	Test organisms[b]
Caesalpiniaceae	*Brachystegia utilis*	1,2,4
	Tamarindus indica	2,5,6
Combretaceae	*Terminalia mollis*	1,2,3,4,6
Mimosaceae	*Terminalia sambesica*	1,2,4,6
	Acacia kirkii	4
	Albizia schimperana	1,2,3,4,5

[a] Source: Chhabra *et al.* 1981.
[b] 1. *Salmonella typhi*, 2. *Shigella duysenteriae*, 3. *Escherichia coli*, 4. *Staphlococcus aureus*, 5. *Klebsiella pneumoniae*, 6. *Pseudomonas aeruginosa*.

258   *Ethnoveterinary Research and Development*

Table 2. Plants found in East Africa that inhibit bacterial growth[9]

Family	Genus and species	Test organisms[b] and zone of inhibition[c]
Agavaceae	*Dracaena deremensis*	1.(+++) 3.(+) 4.(+++)
Anacardiaceae	*Lannea schimperi*	1.(+++) 3.(++)
Celastraceae	*Maytenus senefaensis*	1.(+++) 2.(+++) 3.(+)
Compositae	*Senecio* spp.	1.(+++)
	Vernonia spp.	1.(+++)
Mimosaceae	*Acacia nilotica*	1.(+++) 2.(+) 3.(++)
	Acacia xanthophloea	1.(+++) 2.(++) 4.(++)

[a] Source: Chhabra *et al.* 1983.
[b] 1. *Staphylococcus aureus*, 2. *Escherichia coli*, 3. *Neisseria gonorrhoeae*, and 4. *Shigella boydii*.
[c] (+++) = > 20 mm, (++) = 15–20 mm, (+) = 10–15 mm. For the reader's information, the zone of inhibition is an area within a bacterial colony that shows no growth of bacteria because of the presence of an inhibitor—in this case, the plant extract tested.

Antifungals

The antifungal efficacy of *S. incanum* L., noted above, is due to its saponine content (Wolters 1964 cited in Hegnauer 1973:429). Two other plants used throughout East Africa for fungal skin lesions of animals are *Fagara chalybea* and *Zanha africana*. Near Songea in southern Tanzania, villagers were observed to soak the root bark of *Z. africana* in cold water for two to three days, and then apply either the root bark or the infusion to skin lesions of their cattle. The same villagers reported that they similarly prepared and used *Fagara* spp.

According to Hegnauer (1973), *Fagara* contains methyl-n-undecylketone, a chemical precursor of undecylenic acid still listed in Western *materia medica* as a topical antifungal (Budavari *et al.* 1989). In a study of *Fagara* spp., *Z. africana*, and four other East African plants whose root or root bark are traditionally used for such lesions, Chhabra *et al.* (1982) tested the inhibitory effect of the plants on the *in vitro* growth of five fungal species that are pathogenic for domestic livestock. All but one of the six plants were found to inhibit the growth of *Trichophyton mentagrophytes* and *T. rubrum*, with *Z. africana* being especially effective. Two of the plants also inhibited other fungi (Table 3).

Another plant with a widespread antifungal reputation among East Africans is *Thelypteris dentata*. WaSwahili of Mafia Island, for example, cover fungal skin

Table 3. Plants found in East Africa with antifungal activity[a]

Plant species	Fungi inhibited
Fagara spp.	*Trichophuton rubrum, T. mentagrophytes*
Harrisonia abyssinica	*T. rubrum, T. mentagrophytes, Asperigillis niger, A. flavus*
Plumbago zeylanica	*T. rubrum, T. mentagrophytes, Candida albicans*
Rhoicissus revoilii	*T. rubrum, T. mentagrophytes*
Zanha africana	*T. rubrum, T. mentagrophytes*

[a] Source: Chhabra *et al.* 1982.

lesions and infected wounds with crushed leaves of this species (Chhabra *et al.* 1984). Other East African plants with known fungicidal properties include *Allophylus abyssinicus* and *Cardiospermum grandiflorum* (Kokwaro 1976).

Finally, a traditional antifungal of non-plant origin is sulphur. In areas of volcanic alteration or geothermal activity, like the Great Rift Valley, people seek sulphur-rich water and mud for bathing or packing fungal skin lesions of live-stock. These practices were also observed among WaSafwa cattle raisers of Mbeya-Rukwa, in the southern Rift Valley.

Antivirals

According to Bally 1938 (cited in Watt and Breyer-Brandwijk 1962), cattle raisers in southern and eastern Africa apply *Microglossa oblongifolia* for opthalmic diseases and buccal sores; and they use a relative of this plant, *M. pyrifolia*, for coryza. Field observations confirmed the use of a concoction of *M. oblongifolia* for pink eye in cattle. Also, Maasai in Kenya and Tanzania prepare a decoction of *Crassocephalum vitellinum* to treat buccal sores accompanied by fever and sometimes profuse sweating. These clinical signs are indicative of foot-and-mouth disease, vesicular stomatitis and possibly other viral diseases, which are difficult to differentiate without laboratory analysis. For such condi-tions, Maasai herders indicated that they cook the roots and leaves of *C. vitellinum* in milk, then sour the milk to a yoghurt-like paste and either apply it directly to the sores or drench their cattle with it. Informants regarded this treatment as effective. According to Hedberg *et al.* (1982), Tanzanians also use this plant to cure buccal sores in humans.

East Africans have many remedies for colds and influenza in humans (Haerdi 1964, Kokwaro 1976, Watt and Breyer-Brandwijk 1962), and a number of these remedies are employed for fevers in cattle, as well. HPI fieldworkers from several areas in Tanzania reported that farmers drenched feverish ruminants with decoctions of cardamon, garlic, onions or *Philodendron* leaves. All these plants contain flavonoids (Hegnauer 1963), and the antiviral activity of a number of flavonoids has been scientifically proven (Hudson 1990).

Anthelmintics

Two plant preparations are commonly used as endoparasiticides by Sukumu, a semi-nomadic group in north and central Tanzania. One involves seeds of the baobab tree (*Adansonia digitata*). Sometimes called 'cream of tartar' and listed in old Western veterinary pharmacopoeias as a vermicide (for example, Milks 1917), this preparation contains potassium bitartrate (Watt and Breyer-Brand-wijk 1962). The other involves the betel palm (*Areca catechu* L.), the nut of which contains the taeniacide arecoline (Budavari *et al.* 1989). Based on dosages specified in Milks (1917) and other early veterinary texts, preparations of both plants were administered to clients' cattle, goats and dogs. Both treatments met with reasonable success, although faecal examinations about two weeks after treatment often indicated the need for follow-up drenchings.

Another natural anthelmintic noted during fieldwork among the peoples of Tanzania's Mbeya, Tukuyu and Njombe Districts is the dried flower of *Hagenia abyssinica*, also known as *brayera* or *kuosso*. This plant contains kosotoxin, volatile oils and tannin, and it has been used to control tapeworms in livestock (Budavari *et al.* 1989). Moreover, faecal samples collected in the field suggested that it works against *all* intestinal worms. Likewise for the rhizome of the male shield fern (*Dryopteris filix-mas* Schott),[2] which contains oleoresin of Aspidium (ibid.). In Tukuyu, the author introduced this old Western remedy to a group of 35 dairy farmers. They treated their animals with the fern's pulped root at a dosage adapted from early Western pharmacopoeias. Faecal samples indicated that the treatment was effective against tapeworms and other intestinal worms, with no side-effects.

Fieldwork also revealed that Zanzibari stockowners feed the chopped bark or root of the *Cinnamomum cassia* tree to cattle to combat intestinal worms. One or two handfuls are given to the infested animal twice a day for a week. The bark contains volatile oils and is rich in tannin (Tyler *et al.* 1988). In early Western veterinary medicine, cinnamon was used as a carminative and antidiarrhoeal (Budavari *et al.* 1989).

Inhabitants of mountainous areas in East Africa, where pine and juniper trees grow, boil the sap of these species to make oil of turpentine or tar pitches to feed to livestock to combat intestinal worms in general. By boiling the sap or other parts of the tree in a confined space, farmers in Tukuyu and Mbeya districts also administer pine and juniper as an inhalant for lungworms. The latter treatment was observed to improve the clinical condition of affected animals. In central Tanzania, people treat lungworms by feeding their stock raw onions and garlic, gauging the dosage by the animals' breath. Among farmers of Tanzania's Iringa region, the preferred treatment for lungworm consists of slowly burning the dried root, bark and leaf of *Steganotaenia araliacea* Hochst in the shed of the afflicted cow. In addition, the animal is drenched with an infusion of the root. This drench is also used to prevent liver parasites. Kokwaro (1976) confirms *S. araliacea* as a popular cure for lung and liver disease in cattle throughout East Africa.

Treatments for blood parasites

East Coast Fever (ECF) is a threat to cattle throughout East Africa (Delehanty, this volume). Ethnoveterinary remedies for this disease are similar to those used for the blood parasite that causes malaria in humans. Treatments draw upon a wealth of plant material containing quinine, an alkaloid found in certain species of the Rubiaceae family (Trease and Evans 1983). One such ECF treatment was observed to be quite effective. It consists of heating 20g of the root bark of a vine (*Pavetta schummaniana* F. Hoffman) for four minutes, then adding 15 to 20 vine leaves to the broth and boiling for another minute. This produces enough for one drench. Drenching is repeated two or three times daily for several days. Derived directly from indigenous practice, this remedy was widely adopted by early settlers and missionaries. Now, however, it is remembered by only a few elderly settlers and monks who have outlived their African counterparts. Currently, widespread use of this treatment is constrained by the limited availability of the vine, although possibly it could be transplanted and protected or multiplied in home gardens or other locales.

ECF is often complicated by pulmonary and occasionally pericardial oedema. In addition to administering the antibiotic prescribed by Western veterinary medicine, the author encouraged stockowners living in coffee- and tea-growing areas to prepare a strong one-litre brew of either drink and give it cooled as a supplemental drench three times daily. The cardiac stimulation and diuresis from the caffeine or theophylline found in coffee and tea often assist considerably in recovery.

Ectoparasiticides
As the vectors of blood parasites, ticks cause great economic losses in East African livestock in terms of both herd numbers and productivity. All efforts at tick eradication in Africa have failed so far, and most authorities do not believe eradication is feasible. In principle, public control measures in the form of dips are one alternative. However, their effects are short-lived; so constant, costly repeat dipping is required. Moreover, dips present a number of environmental problems;[3] and in general, they are difficult to maintain in the long run because of myriad economic, political and technical constraints (see also Shanklin, this volume).

Partly paralleling current scientific research,[4] East Africans have long used a number of plant substances to ward against ticks (Table 4). Many rely on saps, resins and washes from woody species common in their environment (ICRAF 1986). Others derive from the plants that provide the poisons used in fishing, hunting, or other activities (also see Ibrahim, this volume). An example is *Tephrosia vogelii* Hook, a leguminous bush common throughout much of East Africa. Tanzanian farmers cultivate it around villages and use it as a fish poison (Watt and Breyer-Brandwijk 1962); the active ingredient is tephrosin. Several societies prepare an ectoparasiticidal wash by soaking the crushed leaves of *T. vogelii* in an equal volume of water for 24 hours. Based on fieldwork in various regions of Tanzania, in the Western Provinces of Zimbabwe, and among the Taposa people of southern Sudan, this preparation appeared highly effective against ticks, lice and mites in both animals and humans.

Table 4. Traditional East African ectoparasiticides for livestock[a]

Plant species	Application
Carolina kola Heckel	Sap rubbed on animal
Mammea africana G. Don	Sap rubbed on animal
Ptaeroxlyon obliquum Radlk.	Sap rubbed on animal
Ptaeroxlyon utile	Leaf decoction as wash
Sclerocarya caffra Sond.	Fruit emulsion as wash
Selaginella scandens spring	Cattle boys burn fronds where cattle are tethered
Symphonia globulifera L.	Resin rubbed on animal
Tephrosia vogelii Hook[b]	Leaf infusion as wash (also used as a fish poison)

[a] Source: ICRAF 1986, except where otherwise indicated.
[b] Author's fieldwork.

Styptics
East Africans employ a number of effective techniques to halt bleeding in livestock. For example, in coastal areas of Tanzania such as Mafia Island and the Rufiji Delta region, stockowners apply gelatins derived from marine vegetation. A widespread styptic whose use was observed in Kenya, Sudan, Uganda and Zimbabwe is ash prepared from various plant species and parts. The ash may be applied glowing, warm or cold. Nilotic people in southern Sudan, for example, press the ash-covered yet still-glowing end of a stick on venisecture wounds. Both gelatin and ash serve as a mechanical barrier on

which a clot can quickly form. Moreover, ash that is still hot or glowing can cause a mild to severe burn, thus inducing granulation and stimulating the formation of scar tissue.

Preparations from *Geranium* and *Pelargonium* root (personal observation) and *Achyranthes aspera* (Kokwaro 1976) constitute three other styptics widely used throughout East Africa. *Geranium* contains tannin and gallic acid; the Merck Index lists the former as a hemostatic and the latter as a styptic (Budavari *et al.* 1989).

Cathartics and laxatives

East African stockowners often use purges for maladies they cannot readily explain. Such ills include, among others, poisoning and worm infestation. The list of local remedies identified during fieldwork is long: the gelatins described above, gum arabica extracted from various *Acacia* spp., aloes, oils of various beans and seeds, roughage like bran and methyl cellulose prepared from wood pulps, tannins from barks and roots, and vegetable oils. During a farm call near Mbeya, for example, the author expected to find worm infestation and intended to collect a faecal sample and return later with a commercial de-wormer. But the farmer said that he would rather drench his cow with latex from the leaves of aloe plants growing around his house. Aloe is rich in volatile oils and emodine, and the latter is a cathartic (ibid.).

Another especially effective and widely applied cathartic observed in the field and also documented in the literature is latex from *Euphorbia candelabrum* (Haerdi 1964). Most of the substances just mentioned were—and some still are—common ingredients in Western pharmacopoeia (cf. ibid. and Milks 1917).

Antivenins

WaSwahili stockowners on Mafia Island described their use of tourniquets, wound-site excision, and botanicals to treat snake bite. Many of the plants employed as antivenins also serve other functions such as arrow or fish poisons. An example is the latex of *Euphorbia candelabrum* (Watt and Breyer-Brandwijk 1962). The following four treatments for snake bite in live-stock were observed in Tanzania. Coastal WaSwahili pound the seeds of *Achyranthes aspera* to a paste, which they then pack into the snake bite wound after first opening and cleaning the wound. WaSwahili and Makonde of the southern coastal area similarly employ a mash of *Tamarindus indica* leaves as a poultice; the mash is prepared by the stockraisers' chewing the leaves without swallowing the juices. WaSwahili of the southern coast and Makonde of Mafia Island also use the root bark of *Diplorrhynchus condylocarpon mossambicensis* to treat snake bite. The bark is pounded with water and stored in a vessel until needed. Then, the bite wound is opened a bit, cleaned, and washed with this fluid. The same groups employ an infusion of the pounded root of *Cissampelos pareira* L., which is given as a drench.

Watt and Breyer-Brandwijk (1962) note that all four of these plants are used in antivenins for humans; Kokowaro (1976) provides an additional reference to this use for *Diplorrhynchus*. All four also have known pharmacological effects in humans. *Achyranthes apsera* has a positive inotropic effect, dilating the blood vessels and stimulating respiration; it also acts as a spasmolytic on smooth muscle (Kapoor and Singh 1967), as a hypotensive (Gupta *et al.* 1972), and a head-ache cure (Kokwaro 1976). Tamarind works as a purgative, diaphoretic and anthelmintic (Watt and Breyer-Brandwijk 1962) while *Diplorrhynchus* is a hypotensive (Goutarel *et al.* 1962, Stauffacher 1961) and sympatholytic (Raymond-Hamet 1969). *Cissampelos* increases blood pressure, respiration, salivation, lacrimation and pupil dilation (Sur and Pradham 1964).

Curiously, though, based on the literature reviewed here, none of the plants used in snake bite remedies in East Africa seems to evidence antiserum activity, although some do contain alkaloids of various subgroups. Examples include, again, *Cissampelos pareira* L. (Manske and Holmes 1950:60, cited in Watt and Breyer-Brandwijk 1962) and *Securinega virosa* (Paris *et al.* 1955, cited in Perry 1980). In fact, the alkaloids' effects on the nervous and circulatory systems may resemble the symptoms provoked by certain snake venoms. This similarity might explain these plants' folk use as antivenins, as per the law of signatures in which 'like affects like' (Brisebarre, this volume, Mathias-Mundy and McCorkle 1989).

Galactogagues
Insufficient lactation in cattle is a major concern of East African stockowners. During fieldwork, the following techniques were observed to stimulate lactation. Sukumu brew a beer from the seeds of the sausage tree (*Kigelia pinnata*) and give it to their cattle as a galactogogue. Farmers in Tanzania's Tanga District pound the fresh root of *Lanchocarpus bussei* Harms, let it stand a while in water, and then drench their dairy cows with the mixture; they may also drench with a decoction of the root. Stockraisers in Lushoto District prepare a drench from the root of *Vernonialesiopus*, while Tukuyu in the southern highlands feed the nut of *Telfairia pedata* Hook ('oyster nut') to their cows. Both *L. bussei* (Watt and Breyer-Brandwijk 1962) and oyster nut (Kokwaro 1976) are also known and used in East Africa as galactagogues for women.

The future of ethnoveterinary medicine in East Africa

This brief overview of 'lessons from the field' demonstrates that East Africa is rich in medicinal plants presently or potentially suitable for the treatment of livestock diseases. Moreover, this overview suggests that, based on observations of their current use and efficacy plus a search of the literature and perhaps also some modest field trials, a number of traditional botanicals can be readily rescued, 're-applied' and more broadly extended in order to help meet animal healthcare needs among contemporary African stockraisers. Fieldwork revealed that many elderly stockowners still know which medicinal plants to use and how to prepare and administer them. However, it also revealed that this knowledge base is gradually being eroded by (among other things) the introduction of Western technologies and commercial drugs. Yet such drugs and technologies are very expensive for the average stockowner, and their regular supply is uncertain in many areas. Thus, stockraisers may be left with neither traditional nor modern weapons to combat livestock disease. Where economic or infrastructural conditions conspire against the use of expensive Western drugs, the promotion of effective, locally available plant remedies would certainly benefit stockowners, veterinarians, and all these concerned with the delivery of animal healthcare.

However, at least two conditions would have to be met for the significantly increased use or widespread re-application of many such remedies to become feasible. First is scientific validation, via controlled experiments, of the efficacy of plant medicines on which the literature is silent or uncertain. Many medicinal plants have not yet been reported or analysed. Their study using modern botanical, pharmacological and chemical methods would not only identify their active ingredients; it would also suggest new directions for future pharmaceutical developments.

The second condition is the recognition of the value of traditional veterinary medicine by both national scientists and professional veterinarians. During fieldwork in East Africa, an attempt was made to form an interdisciplinary ethnovetinary study group of Tanzanian scholars, veterinarians, pharmacists and other professionals concerned with animal health. The attempt failed because, in addition to many Westerners, Africans with a Western education often scoff at traditional ways. Even when their country's economic situation makes modern pharmaceuticals difficult or impossible to obtain, they feel embarrassed to be digging up old remedies instead of prescribing the drugs they learned of in their sophisticated training. They are often inordinately proud of their foreign-style education, despite the fact that they may be unable to exercise it because of the lack of tools, instruments and supplies. Ultimately, for the widespread re-application of ethnoveterinary drugs and skills really to be of benefit, in addition to international researchers and developers, scientists and practitioners in the national veterinary community need to recognize and work to validate traditional treatments as a pragmatic alternative to commercial drugs. Fortunately, however, as many chapters in this volume attest, this is now occurring.

Notes

1. The author would like to thank the many individuals who assisted in various phases of fieldwork, research and manuscript preparation: Mrs F. C. Uiso of the Traditional Medicine Research Unit in Dar es Salaam, for her help in obtaining research reports; Drs Kagaruki and Weenen of the University of Dar es Salaam Chemistry Department, for locating literature on woody plants containing pherones and pheromones; Mr Kibuwe, Curator of the Tanzania National Herbarium, for assistance in plant identifications; Mr Gillet of the Royal Botanic Gardens in Kew, for country-specific references; Dr M.M.J. Minja at the Animal Disease Research Institute in Dar es Salaam, for his continuing dedication to this area of research; and Mr H. R. Wildbolz, Swiss coffee planter and settler in Tanzania, for providing a wealth of information on traditional plant usage and for introducing the author to individuals knowledgeable on this subject.
2. The shield fern should not be confused with the bracken fern (*Pteridium aquilinum* Kuhn), which causes poisoning and photosensitization.
3. Dip tanks are commonly built with easy access to fresh water. Draining and cleaning the tanks can cause contamination of the sole source of drinking-water for villagers and their animals.
4. For example, researchers are currently experimenting with suffocating ticks by saponifying the wax in their spiracles (breathing tubes). There are many anionic and nonionic emulsifying surfactants available from vegetable sources that would be cheap, renewable and non-toxic—or at the very least, less toxic than current agrochemicals.

23 Field trials in ethnoveterinary R&D: lessons from the Andes[1]

CONSTANCE M. McCORKLE AND HERNANDO BAZALAR

To DATE, most efforts in ethnoveterinary research and development (ER&D) have been of an exploratory, descriptive, bibliographic, or conceptual nature. The literature abounds with prescriptions for traditional veterinary remedies, anecdotal reports of their success, sometimes laboratory analyses of their active ingredients, and considerable discussion of their potentials. But actual field trials to validate specific ethnoveterinary treatments and techniques for immediate use in practical development work have so far been rare. (However, see Roepke's and Stem's chapters.) Rarer still has been field-level validation that takes full advantage of participatory approaches and that is readily 'do-able' using national-level R&D resources. Yet such approaches are less expensive relative to on-station trials; and they generally are carried out in the context of smallholders' often harsh ecologies and resource-poor management regimes (see Mathias *et al.*, this volume).

As noted in the introduction to this volume, validation of ethno-medical technologies and practices is important from all the foregoing perspectives as well as for ethical and other reasons. It serves to establish the general reliability, safety, efficacy, cost-effectiveness and practicality of treatments. It also suggests the possible applicability of a given treatment (or treatment model) to broader contexts, beyond those in which tests are conducted. Furthermore validation trials may reveal ways that, with modest inputs of Western-scientific information or (both biomedical and sociological), useful ethnoveterinary practices can be made even more effective or accessible. Moreover, validation can be an empowering experience for producer participants when they see their ethno-scientific knowledge and their active participation being taken seriously by what are usually high-status outsiders. This is especially true where for decades or (as in the Andes) even centuries, powerful outsiders have denigrated or ridiculed local know-how, leading to people's loss of confidence in and abandonment of often valuable practices.

This chapter reports on one ethnoveterinary validation effort implemented in the Andes mountains of Peru under the aegis of the Small Ruminant Collaborative Research Support Program (SR–CRSP) within its Project for the Validation of Technologies in Communities (PVTC). Drawing mainly upon findings detailed in Bazalar and McCorkle 1989, the PVTC experiences recounted below should prove instructive for future R&D aimed at validating and/or enhancing ethnoveterinary alternatives.

The research context

The SR-CRSP programme formally collaborated with scientists of the National Agricultural Research Institute and of the Universidad Nacional Mayor de San Marcos' Veterinary Institute for Tropical and High-Altitude Research (IVITA).[2]

Baseline field research in the SR–CRSP/Peru began in 1980 (see next section). Targeted unidisciplinary and community case studies on various

aspects of smallholder stockraising in different agro-ecological and socio-organizational contexts started a year or so later. By 1983, however, there was a need
to ensure increased unidisciplinary integration; to stimulate more direct,
dynamic and systematic producer input into R&D agendas; and to furnish a
real-world venue to test technologies under smallholders' day-to-day healthcare
and husbandry regimes and resources. Thus the PVTC was initiated, continuing
until 1988 when the SR–CRSP was forced to withdraw from Peru due to
terrorists' and murder of two PVTC team members (a Peruvian veterinarian
and a US economist) on the trail down the mountainside from one of the PVTC
research sites (Aramachay).

Situated in representative clusters of *comunidades campesinas* 'peasant communities' of Peru's central and southern sierras, the PVTC featured the following
key elements.

o Establishment of a resident interdisciplinary team of researchers at each field
  site, so as to provide for tight co-ordination across disciplines[3] as well as for
  the intensive 'insider/outsider' interface that is imperative for generating truly
  appropriate technology (Mathias *et al.*, this volume).
o Involvement of mainly national researchers, both at the field and country
  level. Resident PVTC researchers[4] were backstopped in fieldwork by
  national scientists such as IVITA's. US counterpart scientists also provided
  support and input, but less frequently and directly.
o Adoption of a participatory–action–research methodology that engaged producers in every phase of the R&D process: problem definition, trial design,
  trial implementation and the recording and, especially, evaluation of results.
o Relatedly, at each research site, elaboration of a formal accord negotiated
  equally between the PVTC and the Community Assembly, which is the local
  governing body for legally incorporated peasant communities in Peru. This
  accord laid out the general research thrusts and organizational arrangements
  that both parties agreed to, along with their relative R&D rights and responsibilities. The latter might include community contributions in the form of
  committees or subcommittees of producers to participate in different PVTC
  activities, of experimental animals, of land for agronomic field trials, and so
  forth, plus PVTC agreement to shoulder any undue risks that might accrue to
  producers as a result of on-farm testing. Any other matters identified by
  community members as important were also included in such accords.[5]

The development problem

In 1980, as part of its baseline research into every aspect of Andean smallholder
production systems and their associated social structures, the SR–CRSP also
made its first investigations into local veterinary knowledge, practices, beliefs,
service access and needs.[6] Conducted initially by an expatriate anthropologist
(McCorkle 1982). Preliminary analysis of the resulting data highlighted where
local knowledge, practice and services appeared sufficient for meeting the
animal healthcare needs of community-based stockraisers. Conversely, analysis
also suggested areas where, in the scientists' and/or the producers' view, additional information or technical assistance from the 'outside' might be beneficial.
In all cases, research underscored producers' profound concern over their
animals' health and well-being. At the same time, it also revealed difficulties

for remote and often roadless communities of the high Andes in gaining any access to outside veterinary services and inputs.

For one thing, agro-supply stores are few and far between in the Andes. Western-trained veterinarians, zootechnicians or livestock extensionists. Moreover, such individuals are usually unwilling to travel to remote smallholdings. It is equally difficult for stockraisers to travel to where such help can be found in time to deal with an immediate animal health problem. From most highland villages, it takes at least a day to trek down and back up a mountainside to the nearest town. Moreover, the traveller may well well arrive only to discover that the necessary help or medicines are not available. Government agents often are absent from their posts; and throughtout the 1980s, provisioning of regional and rural towns with drugs and other manufactured items—most of which must make the rugged overland trip from the coast—was uncertain and irregular. Travel routes and communication networks were often severed by rains or terrorist bombings of bridges, rail lines and power stations; and terrorists and bandits prowled the roads.

For another thing, most Western-commercial drugs and services were too expensive for smallholders, especially when their travel and opportunity costs are considered. Worse, the price of all manufactured goods, professional services and transport soared as Peru passed through periods in which annual inflation rates rocketed as high as 10 000 per cent. Stockraisers interviewed in various communities throughout the Andes emphasized an additional economic consideration. They noted that even if they *could* afford commercial drugs or (hypothetically) visits from veterinarians, these would not often prove cost-ineffective. Particularly for small stock like sheep, such healthcare options could easily outstrip the value of the ailing animals.

Producers catalogued still other problems with store-bought pharamaceuticals. Interviewees reported that although they had occasionally attempted using such drugs—mostly for camelids or for the high-risk investment that cattle represent in the Andes—usually their money was wasted. They said that the medicines worked only for a week or two, or not at all; that they cured some animals but not others; or even that they hastened the ailing creatures' demise! ER&D revealed that such outcomes were sometimes due to stockraisers' and/or storekeepers' poor knowledge of commercial drug selection and application (see also Grandin and Young or Heffernan *et al.*, this volume). In addition, storekeepers of the dominant, *misti* (mestizo) ethnicity habitually took advantage of Amerind clients or other illiterate rural consumers to foist off the oldest, shoddiest or slowest-moving merchandise. Consequently, the few veterinary pharmaceuticals that stockraisers might buy were often past their effective shelf-life or were even inappropriate to the health problem for which they were intended.

Ethnoveterinary medicine in the form of home remedies prepared from locally available materials appeared to offer a solution to the foregoing problems for a number of the diseases plaguing Andean smallholders' herds. As scientists and producers alike agreed, the paramount healthcare needs centred on parasitism.[7] Along with many other ethnomedicines, SR–CRSP research had turned up quite a few Andean treatments for both ecto- and endoparasitism, comprised mainly of botanicals. Some were known only to a few people through recall or hearsay, or they were referenced briefly in a scattered corpus of folk medical and/or historical literature. Others, however, were still employed in various parts of the Andes. And a few had received some positive attention in Latin American veterinary or pharmacological publications.

Based on all these sources of information plus additional literature review of the plants in question, several ethnoveterinary treatments appeared to be 'good bets' as viable alternatives to Western-commercial parasiticides. Thus, in collaboration with interested stockraisers, the PVTC initiated on-farm trials to validate (or invalidate) their usefulness. Trials on four such treatments were completed before the SR–CRSP was forced to withdraw from Peru.

The field trials

The trials reported here all took place within one PVTC site. It embraced a cluster of 14 mixed-farming communities in the Aramachay district of Peru's central sierra, in the Department of Junin. The study villages—which consisted of one central community and 13 outlying hamlets—are located between 3 500 and 4 000m on the western slopes of the Mantaro Valley. The inhabitants are of largely Amerind ancestry, descendants of the Incas. Although today they practise Catholicism, wear mostly Western-style clothing and speak only Spanish, they retain considerable indigenous agro-ecological knowledge. The principal livestock species in the area are *criollo* (rustic mixed-breed) sheep and, to a lesser extent, cattle. Poultry, swine, donkeys and guineapigs are also important. The sheep are raised for their wool, manure, and sale of meat and hides. All household ruminants graze freely on communal range lands; any village animals may also freely graze privately-owned fields after harvest. The cropping system centres on native Andean tubers (potatoes, *mashua*, *uqa*, *ulluqu*) and introduced cereals (barley, oats, wheat).

In Andean agro-pastoral communities, women generally have principal responsibility for most aspects of livestock care, while men see mainly to the plant crops. This gendered division of labour, knowledge and decision-making meant that women should be the major community actors in most PVTC work on animal agriculture. Initially, however, Community Assemblies in the Aramachay area appointed only male farmers to work with the PVTC, even though the men evinced interest primarily only in agronomic research. To overcome this bottleneck, the PVTC team began to hold weekly informal gatherings with village women in order to identify what *they* deemed to be priority agricultural development needs, whether for livestock or crops. Significantly, women's top three concerns centred on livestock; and foremost among these was control of parasites.

Gratified that someone had finally consulted their interests, within a month after the meetings were initiated, nearly a third of the women in every village were attending. At that point, the women requested and obtained what was a 'first' in the Aramachay area: formal Assembly recognition of the establishment of village associations specifically for women. These became the Women's Agricultural Production Committees (WAPCs) which participated in the PVTC research reported here (after Fernández 1991:83). (For greater detail on the WAPCs, the research site and participants in general, and on local knowledge and production systems and social organization, also see Fernández 1992, Fernández and Huaylinos 1986 and McCorkle 1990).

Besides focusing on parasitism and working mainly with women, the trials described below shared the following methodological features (enumerated here to save repetition). All were conducted on-farm with local sheep. The participating PVTC families to whom the sheep belonged were matched for similarity in socio-economic status and husbandry regimes (such as grazing areas and habits, livestock housing and inputs). Treatment and non-treatment control groups of animals were also systematically matched for sex, age and reproductive status (for example, no pregnant animals were included). Throughout the trials, all the animals involved continued to be managed under the normal husbandry routine, by day grazing together with the rest of the herd and with other families' flocks on the same lands, and at night being corraled with their herdmates (see McCorkle 1987 on grazing regimes in Andean agro-pastoral communities). This meant that trial animals were constantly exposed to reinfection by the parasites being treated against. In all trials, careful pre-, interim- and post-measurements were made of parasite burdens and of all trial animals' weight. In addition, treatment groups were monitored closely for adverse side-effects; but none appeared at any time during any of the trials. To encourage participants to permit both treatment and non-treatment animals to be culled for necropsy, the PVTC replaced such culls with the same number and sex but younger (ewes) and/or improved (rams) stock. However, the proper economic analysis envisioned for each trial (see Mathias *et al.*, this volume) was forestalled by the murders that terminated both the PVTC and the SR–CRSP/Peru. Thus only very crude cost comparisons of ethnoveterinary versus corresponding Western-commercial treatments can be presented here.

A dip against ectoparasites of sheep

To control ovine ectoparasitism, for the past two decades or so Aramachay farmers had purchased commercial sheep-dipping compounds, as per the urging of agricultural extensionists (see also Shanklin, this volume). But by the 1980s these chemicals had become too expensive for all but a few families. Also, unscrupulous storekeepers were know to adulterate the dips sold to villagers, and this practice was doubtless exacerbated by the inflationary environment.[8] As a result, ectoparasites had returned in force to plague Aramachay flocks.

In their weekly committee meeting and in other discussions and surveys, the women of Aramachay's central community identified the sheep ked *Melophagus ovinus*, known locally as *kerolina*, as their primary parasite problem, specifically citing losses in wool production and their flocks' overall 'debilitation'.

In one meeting between Aramachay farmers and PVTC team members, when the subject of *kerolinas* arose, a young man happened to mention an all-but-forgotten home remedy that his grandmother had regularly used to get rid of lice in cattle, donkeys and horses. The treatment consisted of strong black soap and the crushed, fresh leaves of a plant known locally as *utashayli*, which grew wild on communal land. According to the young man, when his grandmother rubbed these materials into the hides of affected animals, within a matter of seconds lice could be observed dropping off their victims. Meeting attendees wondered if this treatment could work on sheep and keds, too. The farmers decided to collect samples of the *utshayli* for PVTC researchers to have identified botanically. The plant in question turned out to be a native tobacco (*Nicotiana paniculata* L.). The ectoparasiticidal properties of the powerful alkaloids in tobacco have long been known and used around the world, including in twentieth-century Europe. Aware of these properties, the PVTC proposed a simple initial test of the tobacco treatment's effect on sheep keds. With WAPC members participating, they simply rubbed the crushed leaves into the hides of heavily infested local sheep, as in the traditional therapy. The result? The treatment indeed worked much as described by the young man.

The next question was, could this therapy somehow be used as an effective and convenient substitute for the commercial dips, which served mainly a prophylactic and control purpose? Traditionally, the tobacco remedy was applied topically. But even for an average-size Andean flock (around 30 animals), this is a time-consuming process; and it is harder to practise effectively on fleece-bearing species than on bovines and equines, who have only hair coats. Indeed, dips were invented as a faster and more thorough alternative to topical applications. Since community members were already familiar with this technique, they hoped the traditional therapy could be reformulated for use in this form.

Working together, the WAPC of Aramachay's central community, the resident PVTC team and IVITA veterinarians mounted an on-farm trial to test out this idea. First, they modified the traditional prescription for bovines and equines so as to make an aqueous solution, taking into account the smaller size of sheep. This yielded a formula of 500g of ground fresh leaves in 6.25l of water per animal.[9] The flocks of two families were designated as experimental versus non-treated control groups. Within each flock, 25 animals of mixed sex roughly matched for age were included in the trial. On the day of the dipping, men, women and children all helped to gather the plant materials. The women then weighed out the leaves and ground them to a paste, which they mixed with the stipulated amount of water. Village men performed the actual dipping. And many families observed the procedures and helped to evaluate the results.

Evaluation was done by making iterative counts of parasite mortality, averaged across animals and calculated against pre-treatment counts. The counts were consistently taken in an approximately 6-inch-square area at stipulated anatomical sites preferred by the keds' (for example, the throat, axilla and britch). The formula tested caused an average reduction in adult parasites of 89 per cent at the knock-down point on the third day after dipping. This figure rose to 90 per cent on day 7. With a follow-up dip on day 15, parasite mortality rates on days 3 and 7 thereafter reached 97 and 98 per cent, respectively (Table 1). Scientists would have preferred to administer the follow-up treatment on day 30 instead, so as to attack the full reproductive cycle of the ked. However, this was not possible because sufficient fresh *utashayli* leaves would not have been

Table 1. Counts and per cent reduction of keds in the tobacco trial

Treatment group	(0)[a, b]	Number of days post-treatment							
		(1)	(3)	(7)	(15)[a]	(18)	(22)	(30)	(60)
Tobacco dip (n=25)									
Total parasites counted[c]	619	101	67	61	178	18	15	38	45
Mean count per sheep	25	5	3	2	7	1	1	1	2
Per cent mortality	–	84	89	90	71	97	98	94	93
Non-treated controls (n=25)									
Total parasites counted[c]	454	404	420	371	375	347	331	320	262
Mean count per sheep	18	16	17	15	15	14	13	12	11
Per cent mortality	–	11	8	18	18	24	27	30	42

[a] Days on which dipping treatments were administered.
[b] These figures represent the pre-treatment situation, against which the other figures are calculated.
[c] As counted at stipulated anatomical sites (see text). Total parasite burdens were likely much larger.

available by then, due to the onset of the dry season. In the final evaluation, 60 days after the dipping regimen had been initiated, parasite mortality rates in the treated sheep stood at 93 per cent (Table 1). A further finding of interest was that, at the conclusion of the trial, the treated animals averaged nearly a kilogram more weight-gain than the non-treated controls. (For greater experimental detail, consult Bazalar and Arévalo 1989.)

The participating families plus many other farmers who assisted in or monitored the experiment concluded that the two-step home-made dip was just as, or even more, effective than the store-bought agrochemicals they had formerly used. Certainly it was cheaper. The equivalent organophosphates (Cooper D60, Fosmet, Butox) recommended by Ministry of Agriculture extensionists cost about US$0.30 per animal per treatment.[10] But the tobacco dip cost nothing more than the time and labour to gather and prepare the materials. Based on the field trial, for an averaged-sized family flock, preparation would require approximately four hours. This is far less than the time needed to travel to and from the agro-supply shops in the valley market-town, not to mention transport costs and dangers. Moreover, by comparison with the organophosphate compounds available in the area, the home-made dip is probably safer all around— whether in terms of people's handling of the the dipping solution, in terms of possible toxic effects on the animals, or in terms of bioaccumulation of dip residues either in the dipped animals' bodies or in the environment. Above all, however, farmers know they could rely on the quality of their home-made dip.

Based on all these findings and especially on their community co-researchers' positive evaluation of the tobacco dip, collaborating SR–CRSP institutions like IVITA went on to extend the practice widely throughout the Mantaro Valley. Meanwhile, the next steps in a combined biological/sociological R&D agenda, approved by the participating community, focused on ways to: ensure an environmentally sustainable supply of the wild plant in question, whether through controlled harvesting or semi-domestication; provide socio-economically equitable access to this resource; and establish socio-organizational and juridical mechanisms for financing and maintaining dipping structures and for universally enforcing the treatment, so as to reduce constant reinfestation across flocks. Also, further trials were envisioned using dried leaves instead of fresh ones. Fresh leaves are available mainly during the rainy season. Although that is when parasitism of all sorts is greatest, keds are a problem year-round. An effective formula based on dried leaves would provide stockraisers continual access to dipping materials; would save time spent in gathering trips; and would facilitate the sustainable management of this valuable native plant resource.

A drench for gastrointestinal parasites
The same WAPC went on to test other promising ethnoveterinary remedies with PVTC researchers. Besides ectoparasites, the women also worried about *gusanera del estómago y de las tripas* 'stomach and gut worms' in their flocks. They had repeatedly observed massive infestations upon slaughter and while cleaning the viscera. Indeed, helminthosis is an important and universal affliction of smallholder flocks throughout the Andes, especially during the rainy season. Laboratory analysis of faecal samples from local sheep confirmed the women's assessment that their flocks were parasitized. For the parasitic species identified (see below), common effects in sheep are anaemia, diarrhoea, depressed milk production, sometimes inappetence and submandibular oedema (bottle jaw), and

other variable signs of poor condition (progressive weight loss, weakness, rough coat, anorexia). Regular dosing with commercial anthelmintics is the usual response to gastrointestinal parasitism. But this option was economically out of the question for Aramachay's peasant farmers. However, villagers had heard that elsewhere in the region, a preparation made from seeds of the giant pumpkin *Cucurbita maxima* Duch (Spanish *zapallo*) was used to combat gastrointestinal worms in both livestock and humans.

Following up on this fragment of ethnoveterinary intelligence, PVTC social scientists consulted a respected expert on Andean ethnomedicine, who provided them a pumpkin-seed prescription known to work as an effective vermicide in human patients.[11] The veterinary scientists then modified the recipe to arrive at a likely dosage for an average-sized (25kg) *crillo* sheep. The resulting preparation consisted of toasting 50 dried squash seeds and then removing and grinding the kernals into a paste (yielding on average 11g of kern material) to be mixed with 100 cc of water and, after straining, administered as a drench.

All WAPC members of the central community participated in preparing the squash-seed anthelmintic, contributing the labour to collect wood and water and bringing their own tools (buckets, grinding stones or hand-mills) to the task. The trial was conducted on two members' flocks, using 30 sheep of mixed sex and aged 15 to 18 months. Half the sheep were randomly assigned to an experimental group, while the other half served as non-treated controls. Seven days after drenching, three sheep from each group were sacrificed in order to determine whether the squash-seed treatment had reduced adult parasites in the treatment group. *Vis-à-vis* the non-treated controls, necropsy revealed reductions of between 79 per cent and 89 per cent in each of four categories of helminths detected (Table 2). Using a variant of the McMaster method, faecal egg counts were taken for two of the four categories of helminths among the remaining 24 animals at seven, 14, 21 and 28 days after drenching (Table 3). Counts showed significant drops in the number of eggs per gram of faeces on day 7 (75 per cent), peaking at 81 per cent on day 14, and climbing again thereafter.

Overall, the findings presented in Tables 2 and 3 indicate that the pumpkin-seed formula significantly reduces worm burdens and produces a transient reduction in egg counts for the species examined. Drug preparation time for an average-sized family flock was calculated at approximately three hours. Administration time was perhaps twice that for equivalent commercial drugs sold in the region because of the bulkiness of the pumpkin-seed extract. The least

Table 2. Counts and per cent reduction of gastrointestinal worms for necropsied sheep in the pumpkin-seed trial

Type of parasite	Mean number of worms per necropsied animal, and per cent reduction in treated sheep	
	Non-treated control group (n=3)	Squash-seed treatment group (n=3)
Nematodirus spp.[a]	649 (–)	133 (80%)
Ostertagia spp.	976 (–)	112 (89%)
Trichostrongylus axei	1 332 (–)	266 (80%)
Other *Trichostrongylus* spp.[b]	633 (–)	133 (79%)

[a] Includes mostly *N. spathinger*.
[b] Includes *T. vitrinus* and *T. columbriformis*.

Table 3. Counts[a] and per cent reduction of eggs of selected gastrointestinal parasites in the pumpkin-seed trial

	Number of days post-treatment[b]									
	(0)		*(7)*		*(14)*		*(21)*		*(28)*	
Treatment group	S	N	S	N	S	N	S	N	S	N
Pumpkin-seed drench (n=12)										
Mean egg counts	347	53	89	11	78	0	100	27	133	33
Overall reduction	–		75%		81%		68%		59%	
Non-treated controls (n=12)										
Mean egg counts	320	40	291	18	310	30	260	36	292	25
Overall reduction	–		14%		6%		18%		12%	

[a] Counts represent mean number of eggs per gram of faeces.
[b] Day 0 represents pre-treatment counts. S = eggs of *Strongylus* spp., N = eggs of *Nematodirus* spp.

expensive commercial product that can most often be found in the area (Ripercol^{TM}) costs US\$0.20 per dose per animal. In contrast, dried seeds are readily and cheaply available in all the local markets, and seeds store well. Although precluded by the PVTC's untimely termination, further research had been planned in order to discover an even more effective posology and treatment schedule for this promising indigenous remedy. (For greater detail on this experiment, consult Arévalo and Bazalar 1989a.)

Two treatments for liverfluke disease
In one of the outlying hamlets of Aramachay, still other treatments were tested with the WAPC there. These women pointed to fasciolosis or liverfluke disease (local name *alicuya*) as one of their major concerns (see also Perezgrovas, this volume). A zoonoses endemic to the Andes, fasciolosis is also prevalent among the human population, especially in rural areas.

In this hamlet, one well-known and still-popular local treatment against this destructive trematode in both sheep and cattle relied on artichoke (*Cynara scolymus*) leaves. Although it is an Old World perennial, the artichoke thrives well on the lower, warmer slopes of the Andes, and it has a good market in many Peruvian cities. People usually obtained the leaves free, as refuse in regional markets. Aramachay's artichoke treatment for sheep consisted of drenching with a decoction of fairly fresh leaves combined with salt and mineral or cooking oil. As observed by PVTC researchers, preparation consisted of boiling approximately 250g of leaves in 5l of water until the liquid was reduced by a fifth, and then straining it. To the resulting extract were added 250cc of oil and 100g of common table salt. Farmers administered this mixture as a drench in the amount of 5cc/kg of body weight. Informants felt that this remedy was particularly powerful. They cited reports that, in other regions where cattle fed regularly on artichoke leaves, the animals seldom contracted *alicuya*. Informed by the botanical and pharmacognastic literature of the artichoke plant's high cyanide content, IVITA veterinary scientists' *ex ante* assessment was that the artichoke treatment might well work as informants indicated.

When artichoke leaves were unavailable, hamlet residents said some people employed another drench prepared from the leaves of a perennial shrub known as *jaya-shipita*. Taxonomically unidentified but reported in fugitive literature on

Table 4. Counts[a] and per cent reduction of liverfluke eggs in the artichoke and jaya-shipita trials

| Treatment Group | (0) | Number of Days post-treatment[b] | | | |
		(7)[c]	(14)[c]	(21)	(28)
Artichoke Drench	7 (–)	2 (72%)	2 (72%)	3 (57%)	4 (43%)
Jaya-shipita Drench	6 (–)	2 (67%)	2 (67%)	3 (50%)	4 (33%)
Non-treated Controls	7 (–)	6 (14%)	6 (14%)	7 (0%)	8 (+14%)

[a] Counts represent mean number of eggs per gram of faeces.
[b] Day 0 represents pre-treatment counts.
[c] For days 7 and 14, differences between treatment and control groups are statistically significant at the p < .05 level. Differences between treatment groups were not statistically significant.

human ethnomedicine in the Andes (Carlier 1981), this plant grows wild in the southern reaches of the province to which Aramachay belongs; and the leaves are sold regularly in regional markets. According to hamlet informants, for preparation as a flukicide for livestock, the extract from a cold infusion (24 hours) of the leaves is mixed with mineral or cooking oil. Although informants were unsure of the precise quantities of ingredients, they recalled having seen a write-up of the recipe in an agricultural development magazine for Andean farmers. (Córdova 1981) People interpreted the fact that the remedy had been printed as meaning that it, too, was a good one. It turned out to deal with cattle, for which it recommended using 1kg of *jaya-shipita* leaves to one gallon of water and then mixing the extract in a ratio of 2:3 with mineral oil.

PVTC/WAPC trials were mounted on both these ethnoveterinary treatments. For the artichoke remedy, the women simply prepared it according to their traditional prescription. For the *jaya-shipita*, an equivalent dosage for sheep was calculated from the information in Córdova's article. Three hamlet families lent their flocks for this experiment. Within each flock, a random sample of 45 mixed-sex sheep aged 18 to 24 months was selected. One group of 15 served as non-treatment controls while the second received the artichoke treatment and the third the *jaya-shipita*.

Five days after treatment, two sheep from each group were sacrificed and the adult flukes in their livers were counted.[12] Results revealed fluke reductions of 89 per cent (14 flukes) and 84 per cent respectively, in the artichoke and *jaya-shipita* treatment groups versus the baseline of 125 flukes discovered in the necropsied controls. Using the methods described by Dennis *et al.* (1954), faecal egg counts were conducted on the remaining 39 sheep at seven, 14, 21 and 23 days post-treatment (Table 4). As the necropsy and egg-count data suggest, both remedies alleviate burdens of adult flukes and produce a transient reduction in parasite eggs. However, the artichoke treatment consistently performed slightly better than the *jaya-shipita*. Also, animals in the artichoke treatment group gained on average 1kg of weight across the trial period. In contrast, for the *jaya-shipita* and control groups, this figure was −0.28kg.

In sum, results suggest that the treatments may be fairly effective against adult flukes, but are less so against immature forms. (However, the same is true for many commercial flukicides commonly available in the developing world.) Nevertheless, hamlet participants were so enthused over the outcome that they decided to conduct additional tests of the artichoke remedy with the PVTC. This time, they offered the whole of their communal flock—herded in turns by all the women of the hamlet—as experimental animals. Based on the findings from the first trial, the decision was also taken to try out stronger, more frequent and more carefully timed drenchings in hopes of increasing treatment efficacy. (For greater detail about all these trials, consult Arévalo and Bazalar 1989b.)

Lessons learned

Many lessons are to be learned for the conduct of future ER&D from the PVTC experiences sketched above. The first and foremost lesson reflects the overarching goal of ER&D (and indeed, of the study of local knowledge generaly): its potentials for identifying effective, inexpensive, and readily accessible local solutions to problems. Such solutions are workable precisely *because* they are grounded locally. Aramachay and other Andean stockraisers with whom PVTC trial findings have been shared know now that, when they cannot afford to access outside options, they can nevertheless take useful action to address certain of their livestock health problems. For the treatments tested, they can do so with new-found confidence in and understanding of their quality and reliability, unlike non-validated local remedies or the often adulterated or outright fradulent commercial veterinary products sold in the area.

A second lesson is the virtue of 'techno-blending'. Techno-blending can be defined briefly as combining information and skills derived from different knowledge bases (for example, ethno- and Western science, human and veterinary medicine) to achieve more powerful yet still readily-accessible solutions to development problems. As in the tobacco trial, through techno-blending, new uses for old remedies may be discovered—for ovines as well as bovines and equines, for prophylaxis as well as therapy. Or a more efficient route of administration may be found—for example, dipping versus topical application. Or, as with the artichoke-leaf drench, a more effective treatment regimen may be devised (see also Roepke this volume).

As attested by the presence of the Old World artichoke in the Andean pharmacopoeia, a third lesson is that not all ethnoveterinary savvy is 'indigenous' in any strict sense of the word (McCorkle 1989b). This observation might constitute only a minor semantic point were it not that scholarly abuse of the term has all too often left the impression that local knowledge is static, invariably site-specific and possibly even of a different cognitive order from other bodies of human knowledge (see the discussion in Agrawal 1995). But in truth, as people cast about for solutions to their development problems in an ever-more rapidly changing world, local know-how is constantly evolving, being borrowed and techno-blended among producers themselves, and even generated *de novo* (for example, Chambers *et al.* 1989, McCorkle 1994). Though not reported in this chapter, this fact was clearly evidenced in the SR–CRSP's baseline investigations in Andean ethnoveterinary medicine.[13] A corollary of this lesson is that overly zealous researchers of 'indigenous' knowledge must beware of ignoring valuable local treatments or practices merely because they do not conform to some preconceived unicultural or historical source criteria.

Of course, it is equally important to rescue ethnoveterinary knowledge that may be in the process of disappearing—as seemed to be the case in the Aramachay area with all the treatments discussed here except the artichoke drench. In this regard, a fourth PVTC lesson is that there may be more ways to effect such rescues besides conducting recall surveys and discussions with stockraisers or traditional healers in the study area. Sometimes local knowledge of a particular treatment or practice may be so eroded or fragmentary that, in order to reconstruct it, recourse to other individuals and sources external to the immediate community or region is necessary—as with the *jaya-shipita* and squash-seed prescriptions. As the PVTC found, regional experts and literature on human ethnomedicine may yield clues to lost veterinary arts (see also Roepke, this volume).

Fifth, a major set of lessons pertains to issues of empowerment and participation. Even where stockraisers still cling to ethnoveterinary treatments, often they do so out of economic necessity while yet believing their traditional ways to be uniformly inferior. But participatory R&D like that in the PVTC—which makes men and women producers true R&D partners and validates own-culture know-how—can liberate people from such intellectual imperialism, engendering a fresh sense of confidence in themselves and in their capacity to take greater and more direct control over their development needs. In part, this is because new research and socio-organizational skills and concepts are transferred, or existing ones strengthened, by participatory approaches. At the very least, the process enhances people's ability to assess critically other research and extension information offered to them, and to take joint development action. At best, it encourages them in experiments of their own. In illustration of these lessons, note that the PVTC's participatory approach recognized and reinforced local authority structures via the research accords drawn up with each Community Assembly. It also led to the first-time formation in the study area of women's organizations concerned with agricultural development. Testimony to the potential development impacts of such localized, self-help groups is the decision of the WAPC in the hamlet where the artichoke trial was conducted to continue tests on this remedy, extending it to their communal flock. Moreover, it is likely that even after the withdrawal of the outsider researchers, some PVTC farmer-researchers used their strengthened R&D skills to continue experimenting on their own to improve the performance of the squash-seed drench.

So obvious a lesson that perhaps it hardly requires repeating is the importance of making room for the participation of both female and male producers in the integrated, holistic approach to ER&D espoused here. One or the other gender, or both, may have unique or key insights and expertise to contribute to the R&D effort—as in the young man's recollection of his grandmother's lice remedy, or as in Aramachay women's generally superior knowledge of animal health and disease by contrast to village men, who are more concerned with cropping. This gender lesson is particularly clear in animal production systems like those of Andean or Mayan (Perezgrovas, this volume) agropastoralists, where women play major roles in multiple arenas of livestock production, and in the transformation, distribution/marketing and consumption of animal products. But in virtually every rural stockraising society, along with men, women are responsible for tasks that have implications for the management of animal health and/or zoonoses.[14]

The many virtues of empowering, gender-sensitive participatory R&D approaches have been expounded elsewhere, and need not be reiterated here. (See, e.g., Fals-Borda and Rahman 1991, Farrington and Martin 1990, Haverkort *et al.* 1991, Hiemstra *et al.* 1992, Okali *et al.* 1994, and for some recent self-critical commentary, IIED 1995. For greater detail on the application of the PVTC's participatory action research methodology, consult Fernández 1986, 1989, 1991, Grupo Yanapai 1989 and McCorkle 1990.) It perhaps merits mention, however, that such approaches can be empowering in another sense that is less often remarked. To wit, by providing national researchers of all levels with significant firsthand experience of their clients' real-world stockraising situation and of clients' existing healthcare and husbandry savvy, and by adding considerable R&D effort and *materiél* in the form of local human resources and experimental herds (see below), participatory approaches also empower the national agricultural science system to act more responsively and dynamically on behalf of its clientele.

In this process, there is participation across disciplines as well as between outsider scientists and producers *cum* ethnoscientists. Such polyvalent approaches as the PVTC's make for a more holistic appreciation of, and thus successful attack on, development needs. The trials described here are illustrative. Community members provided the critical initial inputs, in the form of problem definition plus local knowledge of possible solutions. Botanists identified the plants in question. Veterinary scientists then searched the pharmcological literature and added their insights into the plants' likely medicinal action; in consultation with Aramachay farmers, they also provided the general trial designs. Community members put forward individuals willing to lend their animals to the experiments; in addition they contributed their labour tools, and, more importantly, their end-user assessments of experimental outcomes. In the case of the tobacco dip, after farmer-participants and community observers judged it effective and workable, the PVTC team then made available their sociological, environmental, agronomic and animal production expertise to assist the community in deciding how best to protect and use the valuable plant resources on which this techno-blended treatment depended.

This brings us to a sixth lesson implicit in the PVTC experience. That is, ER&D can yield bonuses in other development sectors, such as environment or human health. For example, to the extent that—as with the Andean tobacco—disappearing local knowledge of the medicinal and economic value of wild or domesticated plant and animal species is rescued, confirmed and disseminated, greater impetus may be given to the protection of biodiversity.

A seventh set of lessons pertains to trial design and analysis. In retrospect, the PVTC trials embody several methodological peculiarities or shortcomings. A few examples are given below for the benefit of future such work in ethnoveterinary R&D.

For one thing, PVTC sample sizes were too small. Sample size is important for accurate herd-level analysis of treatment effect on those parasites (like gastrointestinal nematodes and flukes) that have an over-dispersed distribution; that is, a small group of animals may host a disproportionately large part of the parasite population while other animals carry a relatively low burden. For another thing, double-blind procedures were not followed in any of the trials. Nor, where appropriate, were control groups established for treatment only with carrier materials (for example, the water, mineral oil, and salt of the liver-fluke trials). Yet this would have ruled out these substances as the possible cause of observed effects. If determination of the relative efficacy of specific ethnoveterinary treatments *vis-à-vis* equivalent Western-commercial drugs under real-world husbandry conditions had been an additional trial goal (which it was not for the PVTC), then control groups given only those drugs should also have been constructed. Finally, no steps were taken to prevent reinfection of treated animals by untreated ones. Wherever household herds are grazed together on communal grazing grounds, control of reinfestation is an especial methodological challenge if the research goal is to determine the absolute effects of a given remedy. Again, however, this was not an initial PVTC goal, given producers' pressing need for something they could afford in order to alleviate parasitism in their livestock.

Many of the foregoing considerations—such as small sample size and limited types of treatment groups—in part reflect the limited holdings of resource-poor stockraisers, their initial doubts about participating in trials, and relatedly, their unfamiliarity with researchers and research methods. With regard to sample size, however, as the PVTC trials described here hint, there are methodological ways to overcome this problem by amalgamating statistically smallholder herds that are carefully matched for relevant household husbandry and socio-economic variables. With regard to treatment groups, as Stem (this volume) suggests, it may take some time to garner sufficient stockraiser confidence and understanding before more sophisticated trial designs can be implemented on-farm. Most participants will want their animals to be included in the experimental (or Western-drug) treatment group, for instance: they may resist the idea of carrier treatments or placebos. As Stem also points out, however, when stockraisers are included as full partners in the R&D enterprise, acquiring increased research skills of their own in the process, they soon come to appreciate more complex trial designs. They also become more open to other kinds of R&D. For instance; based on their positive experiences with the ethnoveterinary experiments, Aramachay women later agreed to participate in a PVTC-proposed programme of selective breeding.

Examples of imperfections, for whatever reasons, in trial design or analysis include the following. In the fluke trials, no reference point for gauging treatment efficacy on-farm was first determined via on-station trials with fluke-free animals artificially infected. And no matter what, carrier treatment groups should have been established. In all the on-farm trials, perhaps measures might have been taken over a longer period so as to be sure to capture the full span and uniqueness of different parasites' life cycles. Also, in interpreting results, more explicit attention should have been paid to normal fluxes in parasite life cycles and host burdens by rainy versus dry season. Greater attention to environmental epidemiology might have suggested more strategic treatment regimens (see also Schillhorn van Veen, this volume and Stem, this volume). A further shortcoming included sometimes less-than-precise documentation of each step taken in the R&D process—a not uncommon feature of participatory action research, in which researchers become so caught up in the 'action' that scientific reporting suffers.

Doubtless readers will envision still further ways in which the PVTC trials might have been improved or might have been re-designed to meet other goals. Certainly, their results can be considered as only preliminary and indicative, not definitive, of the efficacy of the ethnoveterinary remedies tested. However, as one of the pioneering efforts at systematic on-farm ER&D, they point to the eighth lesson: the potential cost-effectiveness and feasibility for national agricultural science systems of conducting certain kinds of R&D on-farm. Discounting general expenses entailed by the SR–CRSP's larger mandate to develop and test methodologies (of which the PVTC concept was one) for arriving at appropriate agricultural technologies for smallholder stockraisers, and assuming a national agricultural science system that has at least some extensionists *in situ* and that provides its scientists with salaries and basic equipment like microscopes and scales, it is estimated that each trial cost only some US$2 500 to US$3 000. These figures take into account such expenditures as local travel and daily expenses for one veterinary and social scientist, miscellaneous laboratory expendibles (reagents, slides, preservatives, collection bags and so forth), photo-copying of literature, communications, and in the case of the higher figure, the replacement cost of necropsied animals. But by comparison with the expense of maintaining experimental herds on-station, this seems a small price to pay for the many advantages that ethnoveterinary alternatives offer.[15]

PVTC experiences with obtaining cull animals for necropsy suggest some further cost, methodological, and also ethical lessons for on-farm R&D, whether in ethno- or conventional veterinary medicine. These centre on the need to build culturally appropriate assurances and reasonable incentives for producer co-researchers into on-farm trial design, as well as strategies to cushion resource-poor smallholders against any undue losses or risks entailed by trials. Aramachay farmers were wary about selling the PVTC any experimental animals for necropsy. Like most smallholders of Amerind ancestry in the Andes, they had bitter memories of being cheated and exploited in livestock transactions with powerful outsiders of oppressor ethnicities. Direct replacement of culled animals with younger and/or improved stock allayed suspicions that the PVTC's expressed interest in R&D might be but a thin veneer for further such exploita-tion. For local people, this strategy engendered greater trust in the national researchers on the team, setting them apart from other *mistis*. It also saved on unfair opportunity costs to participating farmers, who would otherwise have had to expend considerable time and effort seeking suitable replacement stock. Moreover, if farmers had had to go outside of the community to do so, they would again have been exposed to the negative reciprocity of transactions with outsider groups.

With regard to potential losses and risks, it goes almost without saying that producer participants should be fully informed of these. And for poor small-holders who live near the edge of survival, adequate provision should be made to recompense them for any losses resulting from their participation in on-farm trials with technologies that are still largely experimental, as versus trials conducted for purely adaptive or demonstration purposes.[16] This is where the line between experimentation and validation blurs. For example, given the well-known and long-standing use of tobacco-based compounds as insecticides, PVTC work with this local treatment lay more towards the adaptive end of the R&D continuum. In contrast, the trials on Andean remedies for endoparasitism were less well established in Western scientific literature.

To conclude, relative to human ethno-medicine, little validation in the form of clinical trials using animal subjects under real-world conditions has been done for ethnoveterinary treatments and techniques. While this absence results from a variety of reasons (including some of the methodological challenges just men-tioned) one in particular merits comment. This is the view, espoused by some students and native proponents of local knowledge, that applying etic/scientific standards to emic/ethnoscientific phenomena is not legitimate. This school of thought holds that translating local knowledge and practices into Western-scientific referents—whether for validation or other purposes—deprecates eth-noscientific understandings and does injury to cultural and/or religious integrity. (Ironically, a few dyed-in-the-wool Western veterinary academicians have made much the same complaint to the first author about subjecting their professional canons and dogma to scrutiny from an ethnoveterinary perspective.)

Yet for local knowledge to be broadly and responsibly put to use, it is imperative to sort the wheat from the chaff, as it were. Indeed, producers themselves often second this motion. This was evidenced in the PVTC, for example, in a set of agronomic trials conducted at the insistence of one Aramachay community as a condition of the project's continuing in this community. Specifically, farmers charged the research team with helping them determine whether their traditional potato-planting methods, keyed to certain lunar phases, were mere superstition (as they had so often been told by Western-trained agricultural experts) or whether they in fact had some validity.[17] When people express such concerns over potatoes, how much more vital must be validation of ethnomedical interventions that are to be applied directly to living sentient beings such as farm animals? Biomedical ethics and humane considerations alone would demand validation before any attempt at widespread dissemination of ethnomedical alternatives.

Moreover, validation ultimately must be grounded in trial designs that are scientifically sound and credible. To do otherwise is to shortchange producers. That said, however, the usefulness of less rigorous research protocols as a starting point for winning producer interest and participation should not be discounted. In any case, had terrorism not forced the PVTC to withdraw when it did, the next steps in its ER&D would have been to institute more sophisticated trial designs as well as rigorous economic analyses of ethnoveterinary alternatives.

There is not space in the present chapter to engage fully in the science/ethnoscience debate (see Agrawal 1995 and McCorkle 1995 for further discussion). Suffice it to reiterate that, as in the PVTC, proper ER&D trials should seek to integrate fully biological/technical and social-scientific understandings and expertise, with inputs coming from insiders (emic) as much as from outsiders (etic) in a highly participatory paradigm. This approach need in no way deny the validity of either local/traditional or conventional medical, ideological, or other realities. Quite the contrary, in fact—as the Andean farmer/co-researchers of Aramachay would firmly agree.

Notes

1. The research reported here was funded by the SR–CRSP under the US International Development and Food Assistance Act of 1975 and its Title XII amendment, the Famine Prevention and Freedom from Hunger Act. During the time covered in the present chapter (1980 to 1989), the funds were administered under Grants No. AID/DSAN/XII-G-0049 and AID/DAN/1328-G-SS-4093-00. Additional support was provided by the University of Missouri–Columbia and Colorado State University, which respectively housed the SR–CRSP's Sociology Project and a unit of its Veterinary Medicine Project. Acknowledgements are due the PVTC field team plus the late Dr Francisco Arévalo of IVITA for their many contributions to the ER&D effort. The authors are also grateful to veterinary colleagues John Claxton, Jørgen Hansen, Peter Roeder and Tjaart Schillhorn van Veen for their critical comments on trial design and implementation.

2. However, more than 30 other governmental and non-governmental agencies as well as regional universities also participated actively in the SR–CRSP/Peru. For an overview of SR–CRSP work in Peru and of its endeavours worldwide see, respectively, McCorkle (1990) and Blond (n.d.).

3. The disciplines represented in the PVTC varied across the years and across sites. But typically they included veterinary medicine, rural sociology or anthropology, range management, animal production, agricultural economics, agronomy and occasionally forestry. All researchers at a given PVTC site were expected to help with all ongoing research, regardless of discipline. Thus, veterinarians often found themselves

administering sociological as well as animal health surveys, so as to take advantage of their visits to outlying households. Meanwhile, especially when experimental timing was of the essence, sociologists (and stockraisers) might assist in taking faecal samples or doing parasite egg counts.

4. Numbering between three and six at each site, resident researchers were comprised mainly of Peruvian nationals with the equivalent of BA or MA degrees. In the Aramachay site, however, several expatriate MA or PhD students were also involved at various times, as per SR–CRSP field-training mandates.

5. For example, in the central Aramachay community reported on here, the Assembly insisted that, even though the SR–CRSP was devoted to research in animal agriculture, it also include cropping experiments of special interest to the community (see the concluding section on Lessons Learned). Given the intimacy of crop-livestock interactions in the Andes—as, indeed, in most mixed farming systems (McCorkle 1992)—this turned out to be a very astute input into research programming on the part of the community.

6. Before this time, livestock development projects had largely ignored the existence and potentials of traditional veterinary know-how. Subsequently, the SR–CRSP/ Indonesia also conducted considerable research into ethnoveterinary medicine (see the various Mathias-Mundy and Wahyuni references cited in Chapter 1).

7. Of course, 'parasitism' was not a familiar term to most Andean peasant producers. Some of the parasitic problems they pointed to were conceptualized by them in other terms as is true in many ethnomedical systems.

8. As verified by the second author, storekeepers diluted these commercial products with substances such as iodine and creosote.

9. All metric figures given in the text were calculated by PVTC researchers from local measures observed by or reported to them. Of course, in conducting on-farm trials with farmers and in thereafter establishing prescriptions for farmer use, all quantities were couched in terms of familiar local measures.

10. All monetary figures are calculated on the basis of 3 000 Intis to US$1.00, which was the official exchange rate on the day that the calculations were originally made (22 June 1989).

11. This individual was César Náquira, MD and Principal Professor of the College of Medicine of the Universidad Nacional Mayor de San Marcos. He also provided some experimental and pharmacological literature on the remedy indicating that its active ingredients reside in the kern resins.

12. Immature flukes were not counted because so few were encountered.

13. For one example involving a desperate stockowner's efforts to save his camelids, see McCorkle 1982. Also see Vondal (this volume) on Indonesian farmers' techno-blending of duck rations. The present chapter is not the place for an exegesis on the sociology of knowledge, the fundaments of human cognition, or the universality of the scientific method, however. Suffice it to note that the Western-scientific 'etic' is really but another emic, and that cognitive anthropology has repeatedly demonstrated the basic structural similarity in all types of human knowledge. Moreover, at least since the domestication of plants and animals some 12 000 to 15 000 years ago, farmers and stockraisers have been conducting empirical agricultural experiments and exchanging their findings. Interestingly, the historiography of agricultural inventions and recommendations at IARCs (the global system of international agricultural research centres) reveals that a large percentage of the technologies they promote derives from producer knowledge and practice. Certainly, in the authors' not inconsiderable experience, stockraisers care little what is the source of useful knowledge and techniques. They are interested mainly in whether a given intervention makes sense to them and works to their satisfaction (and then, or course, whether it is available, affordable, convenient, and so forth)—no matter what its source.

14. Such activities include, at a minimum, product handling and processing. But they also often span care of ailing, pregnant, neonate and settlement animals and/or of

small stock such as poultry, rabbits, and guineapigs. Davis (1995) offers an exemplary case study on gendered roles in ethnoveterinary medicine in one society. Also see the the chapters in this volume by Grandin and Young, Heffernan *et al.*, Ibrahim and Abdu, and Stem.

15. The comparison with the R&D investments that an international pharmaceutical firm may incur in bringing even a single, simple drug to market is even more dramatic. Of course, it must be borne in mind that ethnoveterinary medicine is not a panacea, and cannot effectively address every kind of disease. See again Mathias *et al.* (this volume).

16. In the present authors' opinion, even with risk-compensating mechanisms in place, as per the first principle of good medicine ('Do no harm'), producers should not be urged to participate in trials on any ethnoveterinary treatments that they and scientists do not first jointly agree constitute 'good bets' from the outset. Otherwise, preliminary trials should be done on-station before moving to the field.

17. As it turned out, the test plots that the PVTC agronomist laid out and planted according to traditional methods did much better than the plots he established alongside and planted according to conventional agronomic dictates (Fernández and Huaylinos 1989).

References

1. Introduction

Agrawal, A. (1995), 'Dismantling the Divide Between Indigenous and Scientific Knowledge'. *Development and Change* 26, pp. 413–39.

Baïracli Levy, J. de (1991), *Herbal Handbook for Farm and Stable* (4th edition). London, Faber and Faber.

Bannerman, R.H., J. Burton and C. Wen-Chieh (eds.) (1983), *Traditional Medicine and Health Care Coverage*. Geneva, World Health Organization.

Bazalar, H. and C.M. McCorkle (eds.) (1989), *Estudios Etnoveterinarios en Comunidades Altoandinas del Perú*. Lima, Perú, Lluvia Editores.

Bierer, B.W. (1955), *A Short History of Veterinary Medicine*. East Lansing, Michigan State University Press.

Bizimana, N. (1994), *Traditional Veterinary Practice in Africa*. Eschborn (Germany), GTZ.

Bodeker, G. (1994), 'Traditional Health Knowledge and Public Policy'. *Nature and Resources* 30, pp. 5–16.

Brokensha, D., D.M. Warren and O. Werner (eds.) (1980), *Indigenous Knowledge Systems and Development*. Lanham, University Press of America.

Cheneau, Y. (1985), 'The Organization of Veterinary Services in Africa'. *Revue Scientifique et Technique de l'Office International des Épizooties* 5, pp. 107–54.

Chesworth, J. (ed.) (in press), *Alternative Perspectives on Health: An Ecological Approach*. Thousand Oaks, Sage Publications.

Cox, P.A. and M.J. Balick (1994), 'The Ethnobotanical Approach to Drug Discovery'. *Scientific American* 271, pp. 82–7.

CTA/GTZ/IEMVT (1985), *A New Policy for the Development of Livestock Production in Africa [sic] South of the Sahara: Primary Animal Health Care Structure. Summary Report of a Seminar on a Primary Animal Health Care Structure, Bujumbura (Rep. of Burundi), 24–6 October 1984*. Bujumbura, Technical Centre for Agricultural and Rural Cooperation, The Netherlands; Deutsche Gesellschaft für Technische Zusammenarbeit, F.R. Germany; and Institut d'Élevage et de Médecine Vétérinarie des Pays Tropicaux, France.

Daly, D.C. (1983), The National Cancer Institute's Plant Collections Program: Update and Implications for Tropical Forests. In *Sustainable Harvest and Marketing of Rain Forest Products*. M. Plotkin and L. Famolare (eds.), pp. 224–30. Covelo and Washington, Island Press for Conservation International.

Daniels, P.W., S. Holden, E. Lewin and S. Dadi (1993), *Livestock Services for Smallholders: A Critical Evaluation of the Delivery of Animal Health and Production Services to the Small-scale Farmer in the Developing World. Proceedings of an International Seminar held in Yogyakarta, Indonesia, 15–21 November 1992*. Bogor, Indonesia International Animal Science Research and Development Foundation.

DeMaar, T. (1992), 'Ask What's in Those Bottles'. *Ceres: The FAO Review* 24, pp. 40–45.

Dolan, T.T. and D.J. McKeever (1992), Current and Future Vaccines against Theileriosis. In *Veterinary Vaccines*. R. Pandey, S. Höglund and G. Prasad (eds.), pp. 318–37. New York, Springer Verlag.

Duke, J.A. (1992), Tropical Botanical Extractives. In *Sustainable Harvest and Marketing of Rain Forest Products*. M. Plotkin and L. Famolare (eds.), pp. 53–62. Covelo and Washington, Island Press for Conservation International.

Eisenberg, D.N., C.C. Kessler, C. Foster, et al. (1993), 'Unconventional Medicine in the

United States: Prevalence, Costs and Pattern of Use'. *New England Journal of Medicine* 328, pp. 246–52.

FAO (Food and Agriculture Organization) (1991), Report: Expert Consultation on Food Losses due to Non-infectious and Production Diseases in Developing Countries. Rome, FAO.

FAO–RAPA (Regional Office for Asia and the Pacific) (1980), *Preliminary Study of Traditional Systems of Veterinary Medicine*. Bangkok, FAO–RAPA.

——— (1984a), *Traditional (Indigenous) Systems of Veterinary Medicine for Small Farmers in India*. Bangkok, FAO–RAPA.

——— (1984b), *Traditional (Indigenous) Systems of Veterinary Medicine for Small Farmers in Thailand*. Bangkok, FAO–RAPA.

——— (1984c), *Traditional (Indigenous) Systems of Veterinary Medicine for Small Farmers in Nepal*. Bangkok, FAO–RAPA. [Reprinted in 1991.]

——— (1986), *Traditional (Indigenous) Systems of Veterinary Medicine for Small Farmers in Pakistan*. Bangkok, FAO–RAPA.

——— (1991a), *Traditional Veterinary Medicine in Sri Lanka*. Bangkok, FAO–RAPA.

——— (1991b), *Traditional Veterinary Medicine in Indonesia*. Bangkok, FAO–RAPA.

——— (1992) *Traditional Veterinary Medicine in the Philippines*. Bangkok, FAO–RAPA.

Fox, M.J. and C.M. McCorkle (1995), Animal Uses and Values, Past and Present. Paper presented to the Hastings Center Conference on the Ethics of Creating Transgenic Animals, New York.

Haan, C. de and S. Bekure (1991), *Animal Health Services in Sub-Saharan Africa: Initial Experiences with Alternative Approaches*. Washington, DC, World Bank.

Haan, C. de and N. Nissen (1985), 'Animal Health Services in Sub-Saharan Africa'. World Bank Technical Paper No. 44. Washington, DC, World Bank.

IIRR (International Institute of Rural Reconstruction) (1994), *Ethnoveterinary Medicine in Asia: An Information Kit on Traditional Animal Health Care Practices (4 volumes)*. Silang, Cavite, Philippines, IIRR.

——— (1996), A Manual for the Recovery and Use of Indigenous Knowledge in Sustainable Development. Silang, Cavite, Philippines, IIRR.

Jacobs, J.J. (1993), Alternative Medicine. In *Doing more Harm than Good: The Evaluation of Health Care Interventions*. K.S. Warren and F.S. Mosteller (eds.). Annals of the New York Academy of Science 703, pp. 304–09.

Kasonia, K. and M. Ansay (eds.) (1994), *Métissages en Santé Animale de Madagascar à Haïti: Actes du Séminaire d'Ethnopharmacopée Vétérinaire ' KAGALA', un Partage de Savoirs BURKINA-FASO, Ouagadougou, 15–22 Avril 1993*. Namur (Belgium), Presses Universitaires de Namur.

Kirsopp-Reed, K. and F. Hinchcliffe (1994), *RRA Notes: Special Issue on Livestock*. London, International Institute for Environment and Development with ITDG, Oxfam and VetAid.

Lalonde, A. and G. Morin-Labatut (n.d.), Indigenous Knowledge, Innovation and Sustainable Development: An Information Sciences Perspective. Unpublished ms. International Development Research Centre, Ottawa.

Last, M. (1990), Professionalization of Indigenous Healers. In *Medical Anthropology: Contemporary Theory and Method*. T.M. Johnson and C.F. Sargent (eds.), pp. 349–66. New York, Westport, CN, and London, Praeger.

Leonard, D.K. (1987), 'The Supply of Veterinary Services: Kenyan Lessons'. *Agricultural Administration and Extension* 26, pp. 219–36.

——— (1993), 'Structural Reform of the Veterinary Profession in Africa and the New Institutional Economics'. *Development and Change* 24, pp. 227–67.

Lin, J.H. and R. Panzer (1994), 'Use of Chinese Herbal Medicine in Veterinary Science: History and Perspectives'. *Revue Scientifique et Technique de l'Office International des Épizooties* 13, pp. 425–32.

McCorkle, C.M. (1982), Management of Animal Health and Disease in an Indigenous

Andean Community. SR-CRSP Publication No. 4. Columbia, MO, Department of Rural Sociology.

McCorkle, C.M. (1986), 'An Introduction to Ethnoveterinary Research and Development'. *Journal of Ethnobiology* 6, pp. 129–49.

—— (1989a), 'Toward a Knowledge of Local Knowledge and its Importance for Agricultural R&D'. *Agriculture and Human Values* 6, pp. 412.

—— (1989b), 'Veterinary Anthropology'. *Human Organization* 48, pp. 156–62.

—— (1992), Agropastoral Systems Research in the SR-CRSP Sociology Project. In *Plants, Animals & People: Agropastoral Systems Research.* C.M. McCorkle (ed.), pp. 31–9. Boulder, CO, Westview Press.

—— (1994a), 'A Framework for Analysis of Gender and other Socioeconomic Variables in Ag&NRM'. Working Papers on Women and International Development No. 241. East Lansing, MI, Women in Development Program, Center for International Programs, Michigan State University.

—— (1994b), *Ethnoveterinary R&D and Gender in the ITDG/Kenya RAPP (Rural Agricultural and Pastoral Development Programme).* Nairobi, ITDG.

—— (1994c), 'The "Cattle Battle" in Cross-Cultural Context'. *Culture & Agriculture* 50, pp. 2–4.

—— (1994d), The Role of Animals in Cultural, Social and Agroeconomic Systems. In *Animal Agriculture and Natural Resources in Central America: Strategies for Sustainability—Proceedings of a Symposium/Workshop Held in San Jos, Costa Rica, October 7–12, 1991,* pp. 105–23. San José, CATIE, UGIAAG and AID–RODCAP. USAID/ROCAP/UGIAAG/CATIE symposium on Natural Resources and Animal Agriculture in Central America: Strategies for Sustainability. San José, Costa Rica.

—— (1995), 'Back to the Future: Lessons from Ethnoveterinary RD&E for Studying and Applying Local Knowledge'. *Agricultural and Human Values* 12, pp. 52–80.

—— (in press–a), Intersectoral Healthcare Delivery. In *Alternative Perspectives on Health: An Ecological Approach.* J. Chesworth (ed.). Thousand Oaks, CA, Sage Publications.

—— (in press–b), The Roles of Animals in Cultural, Social and Agroeconomic Systems. In *Sustainable Development in Third World Countries: Applied & Theoretical Perspectives.* V. James (ed.), Westport, CN, Greenwood Publishing.

McCorkle, C.M. and E. Mathias-Mundy (1992) 'Ethnoveterinary Medicine in Africa'. *Africa: Journal of the International African Institute* 62, pp. 59–93.

Mathias, E. (1995), 'Framework for Enhancing the Use of Indigenous Knowledge'. *Indigenous Knowledge and Development Monitor* 3, pp. 17–18.

Mathias, E. and C.M. McCorkle (in press), Ethnoveterinary Medicine. In *Rural People's Biotechnology.* W. Hiemstra *et al.* (eds.). The Netherlands, Information Centre for Low External Input Agriculture.

Mathias-Mundy, E. and C.M. McCorkle (1989), *Ethnoveterinary Medicine: An Annotated Bibliography.* Bibliographies in Technology and Social Change No. 6. Center for Indigenous Knowledge and Agricultural and Rural Development (CIKARD). Ames, Iowa State University Research Foundation.

—— (1995), Ethnoveterinary Medicine and Development—A Review of the Literature. In *The Cultural Dimension of Development: Indigenous Knowledge Systems.* D.M. Warren, L.J. Slikkerveer and D. Brokensha (eds.), pp. 488–98. London, Intermediate Technology Publications.

Mathias-Mundy, E. and T.B. Murdiati (eds.) (1991), *Traditional Veterinary Medicine for Small Ruminants in Java.* Bogor, Indonesia, Indonesian Small Ruminant Network.

Mathias-Mundy, E., S. Wahyuni, T.B. Murdiati, A. Suparyanto (1992), 'Traditional Animal Health Care for Goats and Sheep in West Java: A Comparison of Three Villages'. Working Paper No. 139 of the Small Ruminant Collaborative Research Program/Indonesia. Bogor, SR–CRSP and Balai Penelitian Ternak.

Matzigkeit, U. (1990), *Natural Veterinary Medicine: Ectoparasites in the Tropics.* Weikersheim, Germany: Verlag Josef Margraf Scientific Books for AGRECOL.

Mez-Mengold, L. (1971), *A History of Drugs.* Totowa, NJ, Parthenon Publishing.

NIH (National Institutes of Health) (1994), 'Alternative Medicine: Expanding Medical Horizons'. NIH Publication No. 94–066. Washington, DC, NIH.

NIH (National Institutes of Health) (1995), 'Reflections'. *Alternative Medicine at the NIH* 2(3–4): p. 1.

Nuwanyakpa, M., J. De Vries, C. Ndi and S. Django (1990), *Traditional Veterinary Medicine in Cameroon: A Renaissance in an Ancient Indigenous Technology.* Little Rock, AR, Heifer Project International.

OIE (1994), 'Anciennes méthodes de prophylaxie des maladies animales—Early methods of animal disease control—Los antiguos Métodos de profilaxis de las enfermedades animales'. *Revue Scientifique et Technique de l'Office International des Épizooties* 13, Issue 2. Paris, Office International des Épizooties.

Okali, C., J. Sumberg and J. Farrington (1994), *Farmer Participatory Research: Rhetoric and Reality.* London, Intermediate Technology Publications for the Overseas Development Institute.

Plotkin, M.J. (1988), 'Conservation, Ethnobotany, and the Search for New Jungle Medicines: Pharmacognosy Comes of Age . . . Again'. *Pharmacotherapy* 8, pp. 257–62.

Salih, M.A.M. (1992), *Pastoralists and Planners: Local Knowledge and Resource Management in Gidan Magajia Grazing Reserve, Northern Nigeria.* Dryland Networks Programme Paper No. 32. London, International Institute for Environment and Development.

Sansoucy, R. (1994), Livestock: A Driving Force for Food Security and Sustainable Development. Working paper. Rome, Animal Production and Health Division (AGA) of FAO.

Schillhorn van Veen, T.W. (1993), 'The Present and Future Veterinary Practitioners in the Tropics'. *The Veterinary Quarterly* 15, pp. 43–7.

––––––– (1994), Changing Paradigms in the Delivery of Livestock Services. Paper presented to the Pan-American Health Organization's Animal Health Workshop on Alternative Models for Delivery of Official Livestock Services, Acapulco, 8–10 October 1994.

Schillhorn van Veen, T.W. and C. de Haan (1995), 'Trends in the Organization and Financing of Livestock and Animal Health Services'. *Preventive vetinary medicine*, 56, pp. 225–40.

Schillhorn van Veen, T.W. and I.K. Loeffler (1990), 'Mineral Deficiency in Ruminants in Subsaharan Africa: A Review'. *Tropical Animal Health and Production* 22, pp. 197–205.

Schoen, A.M. (ed.) (1994), *Veterinary Acupuncture: Ancient Art to Modern Medicine.* Goleta, CA, American Veterinary Publications, Inc.

––––––– (in progress), *Veterinary Alternative and Complementary Medicine* (working title). St. Louis, MO, The C.V. Mosby Co.

Schwabe, C.W. (1993), Interaction between Human and Veterinary Medicine: Past, Present and Future. *Advancement of Veterinary Science: The Bicentenary Symposium 1991*, pp. 119–33. Oxford, CAB International.

Shirlaw, L.H. (1940), 'A Short History of Ayurvedic Veterinary Literature'. *Indian Journal of Veterinary Science* 10, pp. 1–39.

Stoufer, K. and N. Ohja (1993), 'An Animal Health Programme in Nepal'. *Appropriate Technology* 19, pp. 13–16.

Swanson, T.M. (ed.) (1995), *Intellectual Property Rights and Biodiversity Conservation: A Multidisciplinary Analysis of the Values of Medicinal Plants.* New York, Cambridge University Press.

Thompson, J. and I. Scoones (1994), 'Challenging the Populist Perspective: Rural People's 'Knowledge, Agricultural Research and Extension Practice'. *Agriculture and Human Values* 11, pp. 58–76.

Thrupp, L. (1989), 'Legitimizing Local Knowledge: From Displacement to Empowerment for Third World People'. *Agriculture and Human Values* 6, pp. 13–24.

Umali, D.L., G. Feder and C. de Haan (1992), 'The Balance between Public and Private

Sector Activities in the Delivery of Livestock Services'. World Bank Discussion Paper No. 162. Washington, DC, World Bank.

Van Puyvelde, L. (1994), Importance sur le Plan Biomédical des Produits Naturels en Matière de Sant: le CURPHAMETRA à Butare—Recherche et Développement de Nouveaux Médicaments. In *Métissages en Santé Animale de Madagascar à Haïti: Actes du Séminaire d'Ethnopharmacopée Vétérinaire 'KAGALA', un Partage de Savoirs BURKINA-FASO, Ouagadougou, 15–22 Avril 1993*. K. Kasonia and M. Ansay (eds.), pp. 101–10. Namur (Belgium), Presses Universitaires de Namur.

Wahyuni, S., T.B. Murdiati, Beriajaya, H. Sangat-Roemantyo (1991), 'The Sociology of Animal Health: Traditional Veterinary Knowledge in Cinangka, West Java, Indonesia—A Case Study'. CRSP Working Paper No. 127. Bogor, Indonesia, Small Ruminant Collaborative Research Support Programme, Balai Penelitian Ternak, Pusat Penelitian dan Pengembangan Peternakan.

Wanyama, J. (1995), 'Animal Health Options for the Poor'. *Appropriate Technology* 21, pp. 14–16.

Ward, D.E., R. Ruppaner, P.J. Marcho and J.W. Hansen (1993), 'One Medicine— Practical Application for Non-sedentary Pastoral Populations'. *Nomadic Peoples* 32, pp. 55–63.

Warren, D.M. (ed.) (1991a), 'Indigenous Agricultural Knowledge Systems and Development'. *Agriculture and Human Values* Volume 8, Issues 1–2.

——— (1991b), 'Using Indigenous Knowledge in Agricultural Development'. World Bank Discussion Paper No. 127. Washington, DC, World Bank.

Warren, D.M., L.J. Slikkerveer and D. Brokensha (eds.) (1995), *The Cultural Dimension of Development: Indigenous Knowledge Systems*. London, Intermediate Technology Publications.

WHO (World Health Organization) (1991a), *Guidelines for the Assessment of Herbal Medicines*. Geneva, World Health Organization.

WHO (World Health Organization) (1991b), *Report of the Consultation to Review the Draft Guidelines for the Assessment of Herbal Medicines*. Munich, World Health Organization.

WIIAD (Winrock International Institute for Agricultural Development) (1992), *Assessment of Animal Agriculture in Sub-Saharan Africa*. Morrilton, AR, WIIAD.

Zeutzius, I. (1990), *Ethnobotanische Veterinärmedizin: Literaturrecherchen—konventionell und online—zur ethnobotanischen Veterinärmedizin. Aufbau einer strukturierten Bibliographie*. Diplomarbeit im Studiengang Biowissenschaftliche Dokumentation an der Fachhochschule Hannover, Federal Republic Germany.

2. Sense or nonsense? Traditional methods of animal disease prevention and control in the African Savannah

Ajayi, F. (1990), 'How to Raise Better Poultry: Violet Chicks and Other Tips'. *African Farmer* 5, pp. 52–3.

Albers, G.A.A. and G.D. Gray (1987), 'Breeding for Worm Resistance: A Perspective'. *International Journal of Parasitology* 17, pp. 559–68.

Allan, W. (1965), *The African Husbandman*. Westport, Greenwood Press.

Ba, A.S. (1982), 'L'Art vétérinaire des Pasteurs Sahéliens'. *Série Études et Recherche No. 73–82*. Dakar, ENDA.

Bah, M.S. (1983), *Observations on Disease Problems and Traditional Remedies Relating to the Use of Work Oxen in the Karina Area*. Freetown, Sierra Leone Work Oxen Project.

Benoit, M. (1982), 'Nature Peul du Yatenga: Remarques sur le Pastoralisme en Pays Mossi'. Travaux et Documents de l'ORSTOM No. 147. Paris, ORSTOM.

Bernus, E. (1969), 'Maladies Humaines et Animales chez les Touaregs Sahéliens'. *Journal de la Société des Africanistes* 34, pp. 111–37.

——— (1979), Le Contrôle du Milieu Naturel et du Troupeau par les Éleveurs Touaregs Sahéliens. In *Pastoral Production and Society. Proceedings of the International*

Meeting on Nomadic Pastoralism. L'Équipe Écologie et Anthropologie des Sociétés Pastorales (eds.), pp. 67–74. Cambridge and Paris, Cambridge University Press and Éditions de la Maison de Sciences de l'Homme.

——— (1981), 'Touaregs Nigériens: Unité Culturelle et Diversité Régionale d'un Peuple Pasteur'. Mémoires ORSTOM No. 94. Paris, ORSTOM.

Bizimana, N. (1994), *Traditional Veterinary Practice in Africa.* Eschborn (Germany), GTZ.

Bocquené, H. (1986), *Moi, un Mborobo: Ndoudi Oumarou, Peul Nomade du Cameroun.* Paris, Karthala.

Boutrais, J. (1988), 'Des Peul en Savanes Humides: Développement Pastoral dans l'Ouest Centrafriqain'. Études et Thèses Éditions de l'ORSTOM. Paris, ORSTOM.

Breman, H., A. Diallo, G. Traoré and M.M. Djiteye (1978), The Ecology of the Annual Migrations of Cattle in the Sahel. In *Proceedings of the First International Rangeland Congress.* D.N. Hyder (ed.), pp. 592–5. Denver, Society for Range Management.

Bruins, L.H. (1951), Leven en Werken van Geert Reinders, Grondlegger van de Immunologie. Thesis, University of Groningen, The Netherlands.

Chavunduka, D.M. (1976), 'Plants Regarded by Africans as Being of Medicinal Value to Animals'. *Rhodesian Veterinary Journal* 7, pp. 6–9.

Cuoq, J.M. (1975), *Recueil des Sources Arabes concernant l'Afrique Occidentale du VIIIe au XVIe Siècle.* Paris, Centre Nationale de la Recherche Scientifique.

Curasson, G. (1947), *Le Chameau et ses Maladies.* Paris, Vigot Frères.

Daubney, N. and J.R. Hudson (1936), 'Transmission Experiments with Bovine Malignant Catarrhal Fever'. *Journal of Comparative Pathology* 49, pp. 63–86.

Denham, D., H. Clapperton and W. Oudney (1826), *Narrative of Travels and Discoveries in Northern and Central Africa.* Murray, London.

Diallo, Y.D. (1989), *Nguurndam Ferlaŋkooɓe.* Ñabbuuji Na'i. Dakar, Goomu Winndiyankooße Demɗe Ngenndiije.

Dineen, J.K. and P.M. Outteridge (1984), *Immunogenic Approaches to the Control of Endoparasites.* East Melbourne, Australia Commonwealth Scientific and Industrial Research Organization.

Doutressoulle, G. (1947), *L'Élevage en Afrique Occidentale Française.* Paris, Larose.

Dupire, M. (1962), 'Peul Nomades: Étude Descriptive des Wodaaße du Sahel Nigérien'. Travaux et Mémoires No. 64. Paris, Institut d'Ethnologie.

Evans-Pritchard, E.E. (1938), 'Economic Life of the Nuer: Cattle'. *Sudan Notes and Records* 21, pp 31–77.

Ford, J. (1971), *The Trypanosomiases in African Ecology: A Study of the Tsetse Fly Problem.* London, Oxford University Press.

'Fulahn' (1933), The Savage as a Scientist. In *Tales from the Outpost XI, From Strange Places.* L.A. Bethell (ed.), pp. 121–39. Edinburgh, Blackwood.

Gillespie, I.A. (1966), 'The Nomads of the Sudan and their Livestock in the Twentieth Century'. *Sudan Journal of Veterinary Science and Animal Husbandry* 7, pp. 13–23.

Government of Nigeria (1929), *Annual Report of the Veterinary Department, Northern Provinces, for the Year 1928.* Lagos, Government Printer.

Hopkins, D.R. (1983), *Princes and Peasants: Smallpox in History.* Chicago, University of Chicago Press.

Ibrahim, M.A. (1986), Veterinary Traditional Practice in Nigeria. In *Livestock Systems Research in Nigeria's Subhumid Zone. Proceedings of the 2nd ILCA/NAPRI Symposium Held in Kaduna, Nigeria, 29 October–2 November 1984.* R. von Kaufmann, S. Chater and R. Blench (eds.), pp. 189–203. Addis Ababa, ILCA.

Ibrahim, M.A., N. Nwude, Y.O. Aliu and R.A. Ogunsusi (1983), 'Traditional Concepts of Animal Disease and Treatment among Fulani Herdsmen in Kaduna State of Nigeria'. Pastoral Development Network Paper No. 16c. London: Overseas Development Institute.

ILCA (International Livestock Centre for Africa) (1979), *Trypanotolerant Livestock in West and Central Africa. 2 Vols.* ILCA Monograph No. 2. Addis Ababa, ILCA.

Jousselin, M. (1950), 'Notes sur quelques Pâturages Camelins et la Cure de Sel dans l'Adras des Iforas et la Région de Tombouctou'. *Revue d'Élevage et de Médecine Vétérinaire des Pays Tropicaux* 4, pp. 209–11.

Knight, C.G. (1974), *Ecology and Change: Rural Modernization in an African Community*. New York, Academic Press.

Larrat, R. (1939), 'Médecine et Pharmacie Indigènes: Trypanosomiases et Piroplasmoses'. *Bulletin des Services Zootechniques et d'Épizootologie de l'Afrique Occidentale Francophone* 2, pp. 55–70.

—— (1940), 'Médecine et Hygiène Indigènes: Prévention Technique'. *Bulletin des Services Zootechniques et d'Épizootologie de l'Afrique Occidentale Francophone* 2, pp. 45–58.

Law, R. (1980), *The Horse in West African History*. London, Oxford University Press/ International African Institute.

McCorkle, C.M. and E. Mathias-Mundy (1992), 'Ethnoveterinary Medicine in Africa'. *Journal of the International African Institute* 62, pp. 59–93.

Maliki, A.B. (1981), 'Ngayaaka: L'Élevage selon les Wodaaße du Niger'. Discussion paper. Tahoua, Niger, Projet Gestion des Pâturages.

Mares, R.G. (1951), 'A Note on the Somali Method of Vaccination against Contagious Bovine Pleuropneumonia'. *Veterinary Record* 63, p. 166.

Mathias-Mundy, E. and C.M. McCorkle (1989), *Ethnoveterinary Medicine: An Annotated Bibliography*. Bibliographies in Technology and Social Change No. 6. Center for Indigenous Knowledge and Agricultural and Rural Development (CIKARD). Ames, Iowa State University Research Foundation.

Miller, N.N. (1980), 'Traditional Medicine in East Africa'. American University Field Staff Report No. 22 (Africa). Chicago, University of Chicago Press.

Monteil, V. (1952), *Essai sur le Chameau au Sahara Occidental*. St. Louis du Sénégal, Centre IFAN- Mauritanie.

Pélissier, P. (1966), *Les Paysans du Sénégal: Les Civilisations Agraires du Cayor à la Casamance*. Saint-Yrieix, Imprimerie Fabrègue.

Raikes, P.L. (1981), Livestock Development and Policy in Africa. Uppsala, Scandinavian Institute of African Studies.

Roberts, C.J. and A.R. Gray (1973), 'Studies on Trypanosome-resistant Cattle: The Breeding and Growth Performance of N'Dama, Muturu and Zebu Cattle Maintained under the Same Conditions of Husbandry'. *Tropical Animal Health and Production* 5, pp. 211–19.

St. Croix, F.W. de (1972), *The Fulani of Northern Nigeria (2nd edition)*. London, Gregg International Publishers.

Schillhorn van Veen, T.W. (1978), 'Epidemiological Aspects of Fascioliasis in the Nigerian Savanna'. Tropical and Geographical Medicine 30, p. 172.

Schillhorn van Veen, T.W. and I.K. Loeffler (1990), 'Mineral Deficiency in Ruminants in Subsaharan Africa: A Review'. *Tropical Animal Health and Production* 22, pp. 197–205.

Schinkel, H.G. (1970), *Haltung, Züchtung, Pflege des Viehs bei den Nomaden Ost- und Nordafrikas*. Berlin, Akademie Verlag.

Schwabe, C. (1978), *Cattle, Priests and Progress in Medicine*. Minneapolis, University of Minnesota Press.

Schwabe, C.W. and I.M. Kuojok (1981), 'Practices and Beliefs of the Traditional Dinka Healer in Relation to Provision of Modern Medical and Veterinary Services for the Southern Sudan'. *Human Organization* 40, pp. 231–8.

Scott, M.F. and Gormley, B. (1980), The Animal of Friendship (*Habbanaae*): An Indigenous Model of Sahelian Pastoral Development in Niger. In *Indigenous Knowledge Systems and Development*. D. Brokensha, D.M. Warren and O. Werner (eds.), pp. 92–110. Lanham, MD, University Press of America.

Serres, H. (1960), 'L'Engraissement des Zébus selon la Technique de "Boeufs de Fosse". *Revue d'Élevage et de Médecine Vétérinaire des Pays Tropicaux* 22, pp. 529–39.

Smith, L.P. and M.E. Hugh-Jones (1969), 'The Weather Factor in Foot and Mouth Disease Epidemics'. *Nature* (London) 223, pp. 713–15.

Stenning, D.J. (1959), *Savannah Nomads*. London, Oxford University Press.
Thys, E., B. Dineur and J. Hardouin (1986), 'Les "Boeufs de Case" ou l'Embouche Bovine Traditionnelle dans les Monts du Mandara (Nord Cameroun). I: Technique d'Élevage'. *Revue d'Élevage et de Médecine Vétérinaire des Pays Tropicaux* 39, pp. 113–17.
Wagner, G. (1970), *The Bantu of Western Kenya, with Special Reference to the Vugusu and Logoli. Vol. II: Economic Life*. London, Oxford University Press.
Weir, J.S. (1972), 'Spatial Distribution of Elephants in an African National Park in Relation to Environmental Sodium'. *Oikos* 23, pp. 1–13.

3. Ancient and modern veterinary beliefs, practices and practitioners among Nile Valley peoples

Adams, W. (1977), *Nubia: Corridor to Africa*. Princeton, NJ, Princeton University Press.
Aldred, C. (1965), *Egypt to the End of the Old Kingdom*. New York, McGraw-Hill.
Ater, J. Malou (1976), The Dinka Priesthood. Thesis, Near East School of Theology, Beirut.
Baumann, M. (1990), The Nomadic Animal Health Auxiliary System (NAHA-System) in Pastoral Areas of Central Somalia and its Usefulness in Epidemiological Surveillance. Thesis, University of California, Davis.
Buchheim, L. (1960), 'Die Verordnung von "lebendem" Fleisch in altaegyptischen Papyri'. *Sudhoffs Archiv für Geschichte der Medizin* 44 pp. 97–116.
Buxton, J. (1973), *Religion and Healing in Mandari*. Oxford, Oxford University Press.
Carlton, T. (1991), Geographical Analytical Epidemiology of Bovine Trypanosomiasis: Preliminary Results Using Desktop Mapping Software. Thesis, University of California, Davis.
——— (1992), Geographical Epidemiology: The Use of Geographical Information Systems (GIS) South of the Sahara and Geographical Analytical Epidemiology of Bovine Trypanosomiasis in the Southern Sudan. Thesis, University of California, Davis.
Childe, V.G. (1957), *New Light on the Most Ancient Near East*. New York, Grove Press.
Eggebrecht, E. (1973), Schlachtungsbräuche im alten Aegypten und ihre Wiedergabe im Flachbild bis zum Ende des mittleren Reiches. Thesis, Ludwig-Maximilians-Universität, Munich.
Ehret, C. (1982), Population Movement and Culture Contact in the Southern Sudan, c. 3000 BC and AD 1000: A Preliminary Linguistic Overview. In *Culture History in the Southern Sudan*. J. Mack and R. Robertshaw (eds.) [Page numbers not available.] Nairobi, British Institute in East Africa, Memoir No. 8.
Erman, A. and H. Grapow (1957), *Wörterbuch der ägyptischen Sprache (2nd edition)*. Berlin and Leipzig, Deutschen Akademien.
Evans-Pritchard, E.E. (1937), 'Economic Life of the Nuer: Cattle'. *Sudan Notes and Records* 20, pp. 209–45.
Frankfort, H. (1948), *Kingship and the Gods*. Chicago, University of Chicago Press.
Gardiner, A. (1947), *Ancient Egyptian Onomastica*. Oxford, Oxford University Press.
——— (1957), *Egyptian Grammar (3rd edition)*. Oxford, Griffith Institute.
Ghalioungui, P. (1973), *The House of Life, Per Ankh. Magic and Medical Science in Ancient Egypt*. Amsterdam, Israel Publishers.
——— (1983), *The Physicians of Pharaonic Egypt*. Cairo, Al-Ahram Center for Scientific Translations.
Gordon A.H. (1990), *Origins of Ancient Egyptian Medicine. Part 1: Some Egyptological Evidence*. KMT 1, pp. 26–9.
Gordon, A.H., and C.W. Schwabe (1989), 'The Ancient Egyptian *w3s*-scepter and its Modern Analogues: Uses as Symbols of (Divine) Power or Authority'. Agricultural History Center Working Paper No. 31. Davis, University of California.
Greenberg, J.H. (1963), 'The Languages of Africa'. Publication 25. Bloomington: Indiana University Research Center in Anthropology, Folklore and Linguistics.

Jonckheere, F. (1958), *Les Médecins de l'Egypte Pharaonique*. Bruxelles, Fondation Egyptologique Reine Elisabeth.

Kramer, C. (ed.) (1979), *Ethnoarcheology: Implications of Ethnography for Archeology*. New York, Columbia University Press.

Leca, A.-P. (1983), *La Médecine Égyptienne au Temps des Pharaons*. Paris, Roger Dacosta.

Lefebvre, G. (1956), *Essai sur la Médecine Égyptienne de l'Époque Pharaonique*. Paris, Presses Universitaires de France.

Lienhardt, G. (1961), *Divinity and Experience, the Religion of the Dinka*. London, Oxford University Press.

Majok, A.A. (1991), Pastoralism and Development: A New Veterinary Paradigm for Eastern Africa. Thesis, University of California, Davis.

Majok, A.A., and C.W. Schwabe (1992), Pastoralism and Development in Africa: A Practical Paradigm. In preparation.

Majok, A.A., H.-K. Zessin, M. Baumann and T. Farver (1991), 'Analyses of Baseline Survey Data on Rinderpest in Bahr el Ghazal Province, Southern Sudan'. *Tropical Animal Health and Production* 23, pp. 186–96.

Nanetti, O. (1942), 'Ippiatroi'. *Aegyptus* 22, pp. 49–54.

Pratt, D.J. and M.D. Gwynne (1977), *Rangeland Management and Ecology in East Africa*. Huntington, NY, R.E. Krieger.

Rawlinson, G. (translator) (1952), The History of Herodotus, Book II. In *Great Books of the Western World* 6, pp. 33–41. Chicago, Encyclopaedia Britannica.

Riggs, F.W. (1973), *Prismatic Society Revisited*. Morristown, General Learning Press.

Sauneron, S. (1960a), 'Le Germe dans les Os'. *Bulletin de l'Institut Français d'Archéologie Orientale* 60, pp. 19–27.

——— (1960b), *The Priests of Ancient Egypt*. London, Evergreen Books.

Schwabe, C.L. (1989), The ACCOMPLISH Joint Immunization Project—An Evaluation of Immunization Coverage, and Willingness to Pay for Vaccination. New York, UNICEF. Mimeographed report.

Schwabe, C.W. (1978), *Cattle, Priests and Progress in Medicine*. Minneapolis, University of Minnesota Press.

——— (1980), 'Animal Disease Control. Part II: Newer Methods, with Possibility for their Application in the Sudan'. *Sudan Journal of Veterinary Science and Animal Husbandry* 21, pp. 55–65.

——— (1981), 'Animal Diseases and Primary Health Care: Intersectoral Challenges'. *WHO Chronicle* 35: 227–232.

——— (1984a), 'A Unique Surgical Operation on the Horns of African Bulls in Ancient and Modern Times'. *Agricultural History* 58, pp. 138–56.

——— (1984b), *Veterinary Medicine and Human Health (3rd edition)*. Baltimore, Williams and Wilkins.

——— (1986a), 'Bull Semen and Muscle ATP: Some Evidence of the Dawn of Medical Science in Ancient Egypt'. *Canadian Journal of Veterinary Research* 50, pp. 145–53.

——— (1986b), 'The Male's Role in Reproduction and Bifurcated *Ankh*'. *Proceedings of the 29th International Congress on the History of Medicine, 1984 (Cairo)* 1, pp. 108–113.

——— (1987), 'Dinka "Spirits", Cattle and Communion'. *Journal of Cultural Geography* 7, pp. 117–26.

——— (1990a), 'Third World Odyssey'. *Intervet* 25, pp. 18–22.

——— (1991), Helminth Zoonoses in African Perspective. In *Parasitic Helminths and Zoonoses in Africa*. C.N.L. Macpherson and P.S. Craig, (eds.), pp. 1–24. London, Unwin Hyman.

Schwabe, C.W. (1994), Animals in the Ancient World. In *Animals and Human Society: Changing Perspectives*. A. Manning and J. Serpell (eds.), pp. 36–58. London, Routledge.

Schwabe, C.W., J. Adams and C.T. Hodge (1982), 'Egyptian Beliefs about the Bull's Spine: An Anatomical Origin for *Ankh*'. *Anthropological Linguistics* 24, pp. 445–79.

Schwabe, C.W. and A.H. Gordon (1988), 'The Ancient Egyptian *w3s*-scepter and its

Modern Analogues: Their Uses in Animal Husbandry, Agriculture and Surveying'. *Agricultural History* 62, pp. 61–39.

—— (1989), 'The Egyptian *w3s*-scepter: A Possible Biological Origin as a Dried Bull's Penis in Relation to an Ancient Theory on Bones as the Source of Semen'. Agricultural History Center Working Paper No. 53. Davis, University of California.

Schwabe, C.W., A.H. Gordon, C.R. Ashmore and H.B. Ortmayer (1989), '"Live Flesh": Rudiments of Muscle Physiology in Ancient Egypt'. Agricultural History Center Working Paper No. 54. Davis, University of California.

Schwabe, C.W. and I.M. Kuojok (1981), 'Practices and Beliefs of the Traditional Dinka Healer in Relation to Provision of Modern Medical and Veterinary Services for the Southern Sudan'. *Human Organization* 40, pp. 231–38.

Schwabe, C.W. and C.L. Schwabe (1990b), 'Veterinary Co-operation for Delivery of Primary Health Care to Pastoralists'. *Community Health Association of Southern Africa Journal of Comprehensive Health* 1, pp. 116–20.

Seligman, C.G. (1932), Egyptian Influence in Negro Africa. In *Studies presented to F.L. Griffith.* [Page numbers not available.] London, Egypt Exploration Society.

Waddell, W.G. (1971), *Manetho.* Cambridge, Harvard University Press.

Walker R.E. (1964), 'The Veterinary Papyrus of Kahun'. *Veterinary Record* 76, pp. 198–201.

World Bank (1978), Southern Sudan Crop and Livestock Project. Animal Diseases Control Program. Annex VI: Eastern Africa Region, Northern Agriculture Division. Washington, DC, World Bank.

WHO (World Health Organization) (1982), 'Report of the WHO Expert Committee on Bacterial and Viral Zoonoses'. WHO Technical Report Series 682. Geneva, WHO.

Yoyotte, J. (1962), 'Les Os et le Semence Masculine à Propos d'une Théorie Physiologique Égyptienne'. *Bulletin de l'Institut Français d'Archéologie Orientale* 61, pp. 139–46.

Zessin, H.-K. (1991), Ecology, Production and Health of Small Ruminant Flocks in Somalia: A Systems Approach. Thesis, University of California, Davis.

Zessin H.-K. and M. Baumann (1982), Report on the Livestock Disease Survey, Bahr el Ghazal Province, Sudan. Eschborn, F. R. German, Gesellschaft für technische Zusammenarbeit.

Zessin, H.-K., M. Baumann, C.W. Schwabe and M. Thorburn (1985), 'Analyses of Baseline Surveillance Data on Contagious Bovine Pleuropneumonia in the Southern Sudan'. *Preventive Veterinary Medicine* 3, pp. 371–89.

Zessin, H.-K. and T. Carpenter (1985), 'Benefit-cost Analysis of an Epidemiologic Approach to Provision of Veterinary Services in Sudan'. *Preventive Veterinary Medicine* 3, 323–37.

Zessin, H.-K., H.A. Nuux and M. Baumann (1988), *Livestock Disease Survey Central Rangelands of Somalia. Technical Report. Vol. I: Livestock Demographic Data of Flocks of Sheep and Goats. Vol. II: Disease Survey Data from Flocks of Sheep and Goats.* Mogadishu, Somalia, Central Rangelands Development Project–Veterinary Component.

4. Recourse to traditional versus modern medicine for cattle and people in Sidama, Ethiopia

Anonymous (1984), General Agriculture Survey, Preliminary Report 1983/84. Addis Ababa: Ministry of Agriculture Planning and Programming Department.

Ayele, G.M. (1975) *The Forgotten Aborigines.* Addis Ababa, Livestock and Meat Board.

Biasiutti, R. (1959) *Razze e Popoli della Terra. Vol III: Africa ed Oceania.* Torino, UTET.

Central Statistical Office (1971), *Local Names of Diseases and Pests in Farm Animals.* Addis Ababa, Statistical Bulletin of the Imperial Ethiopian Government.

Chavunduka, G.L. and M. Last (1986), African Medical Profession Today. In *The*

Professionalisation of African Medicine. M. Last and G.L. Chavunduka (eds.), pp. 259–69. Manchester, International African Institute and Manchester University Press.

Evans-Pritchard, E.E. (1940), *The Nuer: A Description of the Modes of Livelihood and Political Institutions of a Nilotic People.* London, Oxford University Press.

Foster, G. (1976), 'Disease Etiologies in Non-Western Medical Systems'. *American Anthropologist* 78, pp. 73–82.

Ghirotti, M. (1988), 'Farming Systems, Household Economics and Child Malnutrition in Sidama'. Report for the UNICEF/WHO Joint Nutritional Support Programme, Sidama. International Course for Primary Health Care Managers at District Level in Developing Countries. Rome, Istituto Superiore di Sanità.

Ibrahim, M.A. (1986), Veterinary Traditional Practice in Nigeria. In *Livestock Systems Research in Nigeria's Subhumid Zone. Proceedings of the 2nd ILCA/NAPRI Symposium held in Kaduna, Nigeria, 29 October–2 November 1984.* R. Von Kaufmann, S. Chater and R. Blench (eds.), pp. 189–203. Addis Ababa, ILCA.

Ibrahim, M.A., N. Nwude, R.A. Ogunsusi and Y.O. Aliu (1984), 'Screening of West African Plants for Anthelmintic Activity'. *ILCA Bulletin* 17, pp. 19–23.

ISS/ICU (1986), Programma PHC Regione Arsi-Etiopia: Project Proposal. Rome, Istituto Superiore di Sanità.

Last, M. and G.L. Chavunduka (eds.) (1986), *The Professionalisation of African Medicine.* Manchester, International African Institute and Manchester University Press.

Lewis, I.M. (1961), *A Pastoral Democracy.* London, Oxford University Press.

Oyebola, D.D.O. (1981), 'Professional Associations, Ethics and Discipline among Yoruba Traditional Healers of Nigeria'. *Social Science and Medicine* 15B, pp. 87–105.

Schwabe, C.W. (1978), *Cattle, Priests, and Progress in Medicine.* Minneapolis, University of Minnesota Press.

Slikkerveer, L.J. (1982), 'Rural Health Development in Ethiopia—Problems of Utilization of Traditional Healers'. *Social Science and Medicine* 16, pp. 1 859–72.

—— (1990), *Plural Medical Systems in the Horn of Africa.* London and New York, Kegan Paul International.

Sofowora, A. (1982), *Medicinal Plants and Traditional Medicine in Africa.* Chichester, John Wiley and Sons.

Wirsing, R. (1985), 'The Health of Traditional Societies and the Effects of Acculturation'. *Current Anthropology* 26, pp. 303–15.

Young, A. (1979), 'Why Amhara Get *Kureynya*: Sickness and Possession in an Ethiopian Zar Cult'. *American Ethnologist* 2, pp. 567–85.

5. Ethnotoxicology among Nigerian agropastoralists

Abraham, R.C. (1958), *Dictionary of the Hausa Language.* London, Hodder and Stoughton.

Baker, H.G. (1970), *Plants and Civilization (2nd edition).* London, Macmillan Press.

Bayer, W. and J.A. Maina (1984), 'Seasonal Pattern of Tick Load in Bunaji Cattle in the Subhumid Zone of Nigeria'. *Veterinary Parasitology* 17, pp. 301–06.

Dalziel, J.J. (1937), *The Useful Plants of West Tropical Africa.* London, Crown Agents.

Etkin, N.L. and P.J. Ross (1982), 'Food as Medicine and Medicine as Food'. *Social Science and Medicine* 16, pp. 1 559–73.

Fraser T.R. and A.T. Mackenzie (1910), '*Strophanthus sarmentosus*: Its Pharmacological Action and its Use as an Arrow-Poison'. *Transactions of the Royal Society in Edinburgh* 47, pp. 34–410.

Ibrahim, M.A. (1990), A Study of 'Gajimari', the Killer Rainbow Spirit of Hausaland. Unpublished manuscript.

Ibrahim, M.A. (n.d.), Human and Animal Toxicology according to Nigerian Hausa and Fulani Agropastoralists. Unpublished manuscript.

Ibrahim, M.A., N. Nwude, Y.O. Aliu and R.A. Ogunsusi (1983), 'Traditional Concepts of Animal Disease and Treatment among Fulani Herdsmen in Kaduna State of Nigeria'.

Pastoral Development Network Paper No. 16C. London, Overseas Development Institute.

Jensen, L.B. (1970), *Poisoning Misadventures*. Springfield, IL, Charles C. Thomas.

Keeler, R.F. (1975), 'Toxins and Teratogens of Higher Plants'. *Lloydia* 38, pp. 56–85.

Mathias-Mundy, E. and C.M. McCorkle (1989), *Ethnoveterinary Medicine: An Annotated Bibliography*. Bibliographies in Technology and Social Change No.6. Center for Indigenous Knowledge and Agricultural and Rural Development (CIKARD). Ames, Iowa State University Research Foundation.

Nwude, N. (1976), 'The Influence of Environment on the Toxicity of Plants'. *Student Veterinarian* 7, pp. 33–5.

——— (1981), 'Some Stock Poisoning Plants of Nigeria'. *Journal of Animal Production Research* 1, pp. 109–22.

——— (1982a), 'Plants Poisonous to Man in Nigeria'. *Journal of Animal Production Research* 2, pp. 100.

——— (1982b), *Tropical Veterinary Toxicology*. Zaria, Ahmadu Bello University Press.

Nwude, N. and C.N. Chineme (1980), 'Investigations into the Toxicity of the Leaves of *Erythrophleum guineense Don.* in Sheep'. *Research in Veterinary Science* 28, pp. 112–15.

Nwude, N. and M.A. Ibrahim (1980), 'Plants Used in Traditional Veterinary Medical Practice in Nigeria'. *Journal of Veterinary Pharmacology and Therapeutics* 3, pp. 261–73.

Nwude, N. and L.E. Parsons (1977), 'Nigerian Plants that May Cause Poisoning in Livestock'. *Veterinary Bulletin* 47, pp. 811–17.

Rosevear, D. (1976), 'Half a Century Ago'. *Nigerian Field* 41, pp. 24–31.

Singha, S.C. (1965), *Medicinal Plants of Nigeria*. Apapa, Nigerian National Press.

Trease, G.E. and W.C. Evans (1978), *Pharmacognosy (11th edition)*. London, Bailliere Tindall.

Watt, J.M. and M.G. Breyer-Brandwijk (1962), *Medicinal and Poisonous Plants of Southern and Eastern Africa (2nd edition)*. Edinburgh, E.& S. Livingstone.

6. *I stand for my horse*: equine husbandry and healthcare among some North American Indians

Allen, T.D. (1963), *Navahos Have Five Fingers*. Norman, University of Oklahoma Press.

Boller, H. (1972), *Among the Indians*. Lincoln, University of Nebraska Press.

Clark, L.H. (1966), *They Sang for Horses*. Tucson, University of Arizona Press.

Curtis, E.F. (1970), *The North American Indian. Vol. 4*. New York, Johnson Reprint Corporation.

Curtis, N. (1968), *The Indians' Book*. New York, Dover Publications.

DeMallie, R.J. and E.A. Jahner (1980), *James R. Walker. Lakota Belief and Ritual*. Lincoln, University of Nebraska Press.

Dobie, J.F. (1950), 'Indian Horses and Horsemanship'. *Southwest Review* 35, pp. 265–75.

Ewers, J.C. (1969), *The Horse in Blackfoot Indian Culture*. Smithsonian Institution Bureau of American Ethnology, Bulletin 159. Washington, DC, Smithsonian Institution Press.

Fronval, G. and D. Dubois (1985), *Indian Signals and Sign Language*. New York, Bonanza Books.

Gilmore, M.R. (1977), *Uses of Plants by the Indians of the Missouri River Region*. Lincoln, University of Nebraska Press.

Grinnell, G.B. (1923), *The Cheyenne Indians*, (2 volumes). New Haven, Yale University Press.

Kindscher, K. (1992), *Medicinal Wild Plants of the Prairie: An Ethnobotanical Guide*. Lawrence, KS, University Press of Kansas.

Kluckhohn, C. and D. Leighton (1962), *The Navaho*. Garden City, NY: Natural History Library.

Lawrence, E.A. (1985), *Hoofbeats and Society: Studies of Human–Horse Interactions*. Bloomington, Indiana University Press.

—— (1988), '"That by Means of which People Live": Indians and their Horses' Health'. *Journal of the West* 27, pp. 7–15.

Linderman, F.B. (1930), *American: The Life Story of A Great Indian*. New York, John Day.

Lowie, R.H. (1924), 'Minor Ceremonies of the Crow Indians'. *Anthropological Papers of the American Museum of Natural History* 2, pp. 325–65.

McCorkle, C.M. (1994), The Roles of Animals in Social, Cultural, and Agroeconomic Systems. Animal Agriculture and Natural Resources in Central America: Strategies for Sustainability. In *Proceedings of a Symposium in San José, Costa Rica*. San José, CATIE/UNIAAG/USAID-ROCAP, pp. 105–23.

Mandelbaum, D.G. (1979), *The Plains Cree*. Regina, Canadian Plains Research Center.

Murphey, E. Van Allen (1987), *Indian Uses of Native Plants*. Ukiah, CA, Mendocino County Historical Society.

Opler, M.E. (1965), *An Apache Life-Way*. New York: Cooper Square Publishers.

Powers, W.K. (1986), *Sacred Language: The Nature of Supernatural Discourse in Lakota*. Norman, University of Oklahoma Press.

Wallace, E. and E.A. Hoebel (1972), *The Comanches*. Norman, University of Oklahoma Press.

Wilson, G.L. (1924), 'The Horse and Dog in Hidatsa Culture'. *Anthropological Papers of the American Museum of Natural History* 15, pp. 125–311.

7. Tradition and modernity: French shepherds' use of medicinal bouquets

Blood, D.C., O.M. Radostits and J.A. Henderson (1983), *Veterinary Medicine: A Textbook of the Diseases of Cattle, Sheep, Pigs, Goats, and Horses (6th edition)*. London, Bailliere Tindall.

Bouteiller, M. (1966), *Médecine Populaire d'hier et d'aujourd'hui*. Paris, Maisonneuve et Larose.

Brie, J. de (1979), *Le Bon Berger. Le Vrai Règlement et Gouvernement des (1379) Bergers et des Bergères (transcription of the 1542 edition)*. Paris, Stock.

Brisebarre, A. (1978), *Bergers des Cévennes. Histoire et Ethnographie du Monde Pastoral et de la Transhumance en Cévennes*. Paris, Berger-Levrault.

—— (1984), 'À Propos de l'Usage Thérapeutique des Bouquets Suspendus dans les Bergeries Cévenoles'. *Bulletin d'Ethnomédecine* 32, pp. 129–63.

—— (1985), 'Les Bouquets Thérapeutiques en Médecine Vétérinaire et Humaine. Essai de Synthése'. *Bulletin d'Ethnomédecine* 35, pp. 3–38.

—— (1987), 'Pratique et Insertion Sociale d'un Berger-guérisseur Cévenol'. *Bulletin d'Ethnomédecine* 39, pp. 135–51.

—— (1989), Déprise, Maîtrise, Reprise, une Pratique Vétérinaire 'Traditionnelle' dans la Modernité. In *Anthropologie Sociale et Ethnologie de la France*. M. Segalen (ed.), pp. 395–404. Belgique, Bibliothèque des Cahiers de l'Institut de Linguistique de Louvain (BCILL), 44/2.

—— (1990), Ethnoveterinary Practices and Beliefs among French Shepherds: Traditional and Modern Practice of Phytotherapeutical Bouquets. Unpublished manuscript.

Collectif (1973), Thérapeutique. In *L'Aubrac*. Vol. 4, pp. 137–95. Paris, Centre National de Recherche Scientifique.

Corbin, A. (1982), *La Miasme et la Jonquille*. Paris, Aubier Montaigne.

Cornuau, C. (1989), 'Les Bouquets Suspendus . . . Magie? Sorcellerie? N'y-a-til rien d'autre . . . '? *Bulletin de l'Alliance Pastorale* Mar, p. 23.

Coste, H. (1901–06), *Flore Descriptive et Illustrée de la France, de la Corse et des Contrées Limitrophes*. Paris, Librairie des Sciences et des Arts.

Delpastre, M. (1982), *Sorcellerie et Magie Blanche*. Limoges, Lémouzi 83.

Descoeur, D. (1959), 'Les Traditions Populaires Médicales de la Haute-Auvergne'. *Revue de la Haute-Auvergne* 36, pp. 486–7.

Durand-Tullou, A. (1981), Religion Populaire en Cévennes. Le Culte à Saint Guiral. Annales du Milieu Rural 1. Béziers: Fédération Nationale des Foyers Ruraux.

Edeine, B. (1974), Les Techniques Thérapeutiques pour les Hommes et les Animaux: Pharmacopée Humaine et Pharmacopée Vétérinaire. In *La Sologne*, 1. pp. 539–69. Paris, Mouton.

Ensminger, M.E. (1970), *Sheep and Wool Science (4th edition)*. Danville, IL, Interstate.

Fournier, P. (1947–8), *Le Livre des Plantes Médicinales et Vénéneuses de France (3 vols.)*. Paris, P. Lechevalier.

Garnier, M. and V. Delamare (1974), *Dictionnaire des Termes Techniques de Médecine*. Paris, Maloine.

Lacrocq, L. (1921), *Saint Goussaud et son Culte. Mémoires de la Société de Sciences Naturelles et d'Archéologie de la Creuse XXI*. Gueret, SSAC.

Laplantine, F. (1981), 'Quelques Réflexions pour une Anthropologie des Systèmes de Représentation de la Maladie et de la Guérison à partir de l'Exemple du Culte de Saint Sabin (Loire)'. *Bulletin d'Ethnomédecine* 6, pp. 11–18.

Lévi-Strauss, C. (1962), *La Pensée Sauvage*. Paris, Plon.

Lieutaghi, P. (1983), *Les Simples entre Nature et Société. Catalogue d'Exposition*. Mane, Études Populaires et Initiatives.

Maupas, A. (1961), *Petit Lexique Botanique Français-Barnais-Gascon et Béarnais-Gascon-Français*. Pau, Guinarthe.

Mauss, M. and H. Hubert (1950), Esquisse d'une Théorie Générale de la Magie. In *Sociologie et Anthropologie*. M. Mauss (ed.), pp. 1–141. Paris, Presses Universitaires de France.

Nardonne, J. (1981), 'Le Verbe par Extension et ses Implications de Protection et de Guérison dans la Perspective de l'Ethnomédecine. Exemples des Cultes de Saint Sabin et de Saint Marcou'. *Bulletin d'Ethnomédecine* 6, pp. 23–31.

Rolland, E. (1896–1914), *Faune Populaire de la France (6 volumes)*. Paris, Maisonneuve et Larose.

Seguin, J. (1941), *L'Art de Soigner Gens et Bêtes en Basse-Normandie. 1980 reprinting*. Paris, Guénégaud.

Seignolle, C. (1969), *Le Berry Traditionnel*. Paris, Maisonneuve et Larose.

Van Gennep, A. (1937–58), *Manuel de Folklore Français Contemporain (9 volumes)*. Paris, Picard.

Vayssier, A. (1879), *Dictionnaire Patois-Français du Département de l'Aveyron. 1970 reprinting*. Geneva, Slatkine Reprints.

Villemin, M. (1982), *Les Vétérinaires Français au XIXe Siécle*. Paris, Le Point Vétérinaire.

—— (1984), *Dictionnaire des Termes Vétérinaires et Zootechniques*. Paris, Vigot.

8. The interpenetration of endogenous and exogenous in Saami reindeer raising

Aikio, P. (1987), Reindeer Herding in Norden. In *Norden—Man and Environment*. U. Varjo and W.Tietze (eds.), pp. 332–7. Berlin and Stuttgart, Gebrüder Borntraeger.

Anderson, M. (1978), Saami Ethnoecology: Resource Management in Norwegian Lapland. Thesis, Yale University, New Haven, CN.

—— (1981), *Vectors of Diversification and Specialization in Saami Society. In Contemporary Nomadic and Pastoral Peoples: Asia and the North*. P.C. Salzman (ed.), *Studies in Third World Societies* 18, pp. 97–124.

Anderson, M. (1984a), 'Dialectics of Intensivity and Extensivity in Saami Reindeer Management'. Review article. *Ethnos* 49, pp. 119–28.

—— (1984b), 'Proper Names, Naming, and Labeling in Saami'. *Anthropological Linguistics* 26, pp. 186–201.

———— (1986), 'From Predator to Pet: Social Relationships of the Saami Reindeer-herding Dog'. *Central Issues in Anthropology* 6, pp. 3–11.

Beach, H. (1981), 'Reindeer-herd Management in Transition: The Case of Tuorpon Saameby in Northern Sweden'. Acta Universitatis Upsaliensis/ Uppsala Studies in Cultural Anthropology No. 3. Stockholm, Almqvist and Wiksell.

———— (1990), 'Perceptions of Risk, Dilemmas of Policy: Nuclear Fallout in Swedish Lapland'. *Social Science and Medicine* 30, pp. 729–38.

Beach, H., M. Anderson and P. Aikio (1991), Dynamics of Saami Territoriality within the Nation-states of Norway, Sweden, and Finland. In *Pastoral and Nomadic Territoriality*. A. Rao and M.J. Casimir (eds.), pp. 55–90. Oxford, Berg Publishers.

Edelstein, M.R. (1988), *Contaminated Communities: The Social and Psychological Impacts of Residential Toxic Exposure*. Boulder, CO and London, Westview Press.

Haugerud, R.E. (1990), 'Moderne Reindrift og Parasittbehandling (Ivermectin del 3)'. *Boazodoallu-oddasat* 24, pp. 3–5.

Ingold, T. (1976), *The Skolt Lapps Today*. Cambridge, Cambridge University Press.

———— (1980), *Hunters, Pastoralists, and Ranchers*. Cambridge, Cambridge University Press.

Jones, B.-E.V. (1989), 'Effects of the Chernobyl Accident on Animal Husbandry and Production, from a Swedish Perspective'. *Journal of the American Veterinary Medical Association* 194, pp. 900–02.

Nesheim, A. (1966), Duol'lje—Coar've—Muorra: Samisk Sløydterminologi og dens Opprinnelse. In *Norrbottensläns Hembygdsförenings Årsbok 1967* [no editor given], pp. 23–30. Luleå, Norrbottensläns Hembygdsförening.

Nielsen, K. (1928), 'Litt om Nordiske Lånord i den Lappiske Ren- og Rendriftstermi-nologi'. *Tromsø Museum Skrifter* 2, pp. 179–83. (Reprinted in *Studia Septentrionalia* 1, Oslo, 1945.)

Paine, R. (1964), 'Herding and Husbandry: Two Basic Distinctions in the Analysis of Reindeer Management (Lapps of Kautokeino)'. *Folk* 6, pp. 83–8.

———— (1971), 'Animals as Capital: Comparisons among Northern Nomadic Herders and Hunters'. *Anthropological Quarterly* 44, pp. 157–72.

———— (1972), The Herd Management of Lapp Reindeer Pastoralists. In *Perspectives on Nomadism. International Studies in Sociology and Social Anthropology No. 13*. W.G. Irons and N. Dyson-Hudson (eds.), pp. 76–87. Leiden, E.J. Brill.

———— (1987), 'Accidents, Ideologies, and Routines: "Chernobyl" over Norway'. *Anthropology Today* 3, pp. 7–10.

———— (1988a), 'Reindeer and Caribou *Rangifer tarandus* in the Wild and under Pastoralism'. *Polar Record* 24, pp. 31–42.

———— (1988b), Coming to Terms: 'Chernobyl' and the Southern Saami of Snåsa. Paper presented at the 12th International Congress of Anthropological and Ethnological Sciences, Zagreb.

Ruong, I. (1968), 'Different Factors of Reindeer-breeding'. *Inter-Nord* 10, pp. 293–7.

Salthe, S.N. and M. Anderson (1989) Modeling Self-organization. In *Semiotics 1988*. T. Prewitt, J. Deely and K. Haworth (eds.), pp. 14–23. Lanham, MD, University Press of America.

Skjenneberg, S. (1965), *Rein og Reindrift*. Lesjaskog, A/S Fjell-Nytt.

Skjenneberg, S. and L. Slagsvold (1968), *Reindriften og dens Naturgrunnlag*. Oslo, Universitetsforlaget.

Turi, J. (1931), *Turi's Book of Lappland*. New York, Harper and Row.

———— (1965), *Mui'talus Samiid Birra*. Stockholm, Alimus Skuv'ladoimahat/Kungliga Skolöverstyrelsen.

Utsi, M. (1948), 'The Reindeer Breeding Methods of the Northern Lapps'. *Man* 48, pp. 97–101.

Vorren, Ø. (1973), Some Trends of the Transition from Hunting to Nomadic Economy in Finnmark. In *24 Circumpolar Problems: Habitat, Economy, and Social Relations in the Arctic*. G. Berg (ed.), pp. 185–94. Oxford, Pergamon Press.

Wiklund, K.B. (1916), 'Lapska Navn på Ren-oestriderna och deras Larver'. *Monde*

Orientale: Archives pour l'Histoire et le Technographie, les Langues et Litteratures, Religions et Traditions de l'Europe Orientale et de l'Asie 10, pp. 183–91.

Zeuner, F.E. (1963), The Reindeer. In *A History of Domesticated Animals*. F.E. Zeuner (ed.), pp. 79–128. London, Hutchinson.

9. Ethno-agroveterinary perspectives on poultry production in rural Nigeria

Abdu, P.A., A.A. Adesiyun and S.U. Abdullahi (1984), 'Serological Evidence of Brucellosis, Q-Fever, Salmonellosis and Mycoplasma in Chickens from Nomadic Herds Around Zaria'. *Nigerian Veterinary Journal* 13, pp. 61–2.

Abdu, P.A., S.U. Abdullahi and A.A. Adesiyun (1985a), 'Infectious Bursal Disease Virus Antibody in Chickens from Fulani Nomads Around Zaria'. *Nigerian Veterinary Journal* 14, pp. 61–2.

Abdu, P.A., J.B. George and J.U. Umoh (1985b), 'Study of Poultry Diseases Diagnosed at Zaria from 1981–1984'. *Nigerian Veterinary Journal* 14, pp. 63–5.

Abraham, R.C. (1958), *Dictionary of the Hausa Language*. London, Hodder and Stoughton.

Adesiyun, A.A. and P.A. Abdu (1985), 'Serological Survey of *Mycoplasma gallisepticum* Antibody in Four Domestic Poultry Species around Zaria, Nigeria'. *Bulletin of Animal Health and Production in Africa* 33, pp. 171–2.

AERLS (Agricultural Extension and Research Liaison Services) (1976), 'How to Improve the Performance of Local Chickens'. Extension Guide 79, *Poultry Series* 9:1–7. Zaria, Ahmadu Bello University.

Aire, T.A. and M.O. Ojo (1974), 'Response of White-leghorn and Nigerian Cockerels to Experimental Salmonella Infection'. *Tropical Animal Health and Production* 6, pp. 111–16.

Akinwumi, J.A., A.J. Adegeye, A.E. Ikpi and S.O. Olayide (1979), Economic Analysis of the Nigerian Poultry Industry. Lagos, Federal Livestock Department.

Ayeni, J.S.O. and J.O. Ayanda (1982), 'Studies of the Husbandry Practices and Social Acceptance of Guineafowl in Nigeria'. *Bulletin of Animal Health and Production in Africa* 30, pp. 139–48.

Ayorinde, K.L. (1988), 'Tips on Backyard Guineafowl Production in Nigeria'. *Nigerian Livestock Farmer* 8, pp. 10–12.

Ayorinde, K.L., J.A. Oluyemi and J.S.O. Ayeni (1988), 'Growth Performance of Four Indigenous Helmeted Guineafowl Varieties (*Numida, meleagris, galeata, pallas*) in Nigeria'. *Bulletin of Animal Health and Production in Africa* 36, pp. 356–60.

Bushman, D.M. (1974), 'Feeding for Egg Production in the Tropics and Subtropics'. *World Animal Review* 12, pp. 14–18.

Callaway, B.J. (1984), 'Ambiguous Consequences of the Socialisation and Seclusion of Hausa Women'. *Journal of Modern African Studies* 22, pp. 429–50.

CTA (Technical Centre for Agricultural and Rural Cooperation) (1987), 'City Chicks or Country Birds?' *Spore* 38, pp. 1–3.

Dalziel, J.M. (1937), *The Useful Plants of West Tropical Africa*. London, Crown Agents.

Ensminger, M.E. (1980), *Poultry Science (2nd edition)*. Danville, IL, Interstate.

Etkin, N.L. and P.J. Ross (1982), 'Food as Medicine and Medicine as Food'. *Social Science and Medicine* 16, pp. 1 559–73.

Ibrahim, M.A. (1986), Veterinary Traditional Practices in Nigeria. In *Livestock Systems Research in Nigeria's Subhumid Zone*. R. von Kaufmann, S. Chater and R. Blench (eds.), pp. 189–203. Addis Ababa, ILCA.

Ibrahim, M.A., N. Nwude, Y.O. Aliu and R.A. Ogunsusi (1983), 'Traditional Concepts of Animal Disease and Treatment among Fulani Herdsmen in Kaduna State of Nigeria'. Pastoral Development Network Paper No. 16C. London, Overseas Development Institute.

McArdle, A.A. (1972), 'Methods of Poultry Production in Developing Areas'. *World Animal Review* 2, pp. 28–32.

McClymont, G.L. and D.C. Duncan (1952), 'Studies on Nutrition of Poultry. III: Toxicology of *Sorghum* for Chickens'. *Australian Veterinary Journal* 28, pp. 229–33.

McCorkle, C.M. (1986), 'An Introduction to Ethnoveterinary Research and Development'. *Journal of Ethnobiology* 6, pp.129–49.

―――― (1989), 'Veterinary Anthropology'. *Human Organization* 48, pp. 156–62.

Merat, P. (1986), 'Potential Usefulness of the Naked Neck Gene in Poultry Production'. *World's Poultry Science Journal* 42, pp. 124–42.

Nawathe, D.R. and A.G. Lamorde (1982), 'Gumboro Disease: Problems of Control in Nigeria'. *Bulletin de l'Office International des Épizooties* 1, pp. 1163–8.

Nesheim, M.C., R.E. Austic and L.E. Card (1979), *Poultry Production (12th edition)*. Philadelphia, Lea and Febiger.

Nwosu, C.C. (1987), 'Is the Local Fowl Essential or Non-essential?' Paper presented to the Poultry Farmers Workshop, Agricultural Extension and Research Liaison Services, Zaria.

Nwude, N. and M.A. Ibrahim (1980), 'Plants Used in Traditional Veterinary Medical Practices in Nigeria'. *Journal of Veterinary Pharmacology and Therapeutics* 3, pp. 261–73.

Taran, M. (1974), 'The Development of the Poultry Industry in Israel and Poultry Improvement Schemes in Developing Countries'. *World Animal Review* 10, pp. 38–43.

Umoh, J.U., C.D. Ezeokoli, A.A. Adesiyun, P.A. Abdu and G. Bishu (1982), 'Surveillance of Infectious Bursal Disease by Precipitating Antibody Survey in the Zaria Area'. *Nigerian Journal of Animal Production Research* 2, pp. 153–62.

Waters-Bayer, A. (1988), *Dairying by Settled Fulani Agropastoralists in Central Nigeria*. Kiel, Wissenschaftsverlag Vauk Kiel.

Wilson R.T. (1979), 'Studies on the Livestock of Southern Dafur. Sudan VII: Production of Poultry under Simulated Traditional Conditions'. *Tropical Animal Health and Production* 11, pp. 143–50.

―――― (1986), 'Poultry Production in Sub-Saharan Africa'. *Outlook on Agriculture* 15, pp. 121–7.

Zeitlyn, D. (1991), 'Do Mambila Cockerels Lay Eggs? Reflection on Knowledge and Belief'. *Journal of the Anthropological Society of Oxford* 22, pp. 59–64.

10. *Madosha*: traditional castration of bulls in Ethiopia

Brumby, P.J. and R.G. Scholtens (1986), 'Management and Health Constraints for Small-scale Dairy Production in Africa'. *ILCA Bulletin* 25, pp. 9–12.

Elmi, A.A. (1984), Observations on the Browsing and Grazing Behaviour of the Camel. In *Camel Pastoralism in Somalia. Proceedings of a Workshop Held in Baydhabo, Somalia, April 8–13*. M.A. Hussein (ed.), Camel Forum Working Paper No. 7, pp. 115–36. Mogadishu, Somali Academy of Science and Arts.

Evans-Pritchard, E.E. (1940), *The Nuer: A Description of the Modes of Livelihood and Political Institutions of a Nilotic People*. London, Oxford University Press.

Ghirotti, M. (1988), Farming Systems, Household Economics and Child Malnutrition in Sidama. Report for the UNICEF/WHO Joint Nutritional Support Programme, Sidama. International Course for Primary Health Care Managers at District Level in Developing Countries. Rome, Istituto Superiore di Sanità.

Ghirotti, M. and M. Woudyalew (1990), Rapid Rural Appraisal (RRA) Techniques for Animal Production and Health in Agro-pastoral Societies: A Study on Ghibe Valley. Unpublished manuscript.

ILCA (International Livestock Centre for Africa) (1981), 'Animal Traction in Sub-Saharan Africa'. *ILCA Bulletin* 14, pp. 1–14.

Ligers, Z. (1958), 'Comment les Peuls de Koa Castrent leurs Taureaux'. *Bulletin de IFAN* 20B(1–2), pp. 191–204.

MacFarlane, J.S. (1966), 'Castration in Farm Animals'. *Veterinary Record* 78, pp. 436–41.

Mason, I.L. (1976), Factors Influencing the World Distribution of Beef Cattle. In *Beef Cattle Production in Developing Countries*. A.J. Smith (ed.), pp. 29–42. Edinburgh, Centre for Tropical Veterinary Medicine, University of Edinburgh.

Mathias-Mundy, E. and C.M. McCorkle (1989), *Ethnoveterinary Medicine: An Annotated Bibliography*. Bibliographies in Technology and Social Change No. 6. Center for Indigenous Knowledge and Agricultural and Rural Development (CIKARD). Ames, Iowa State University Research Foundation.

Pollera, A. (1926), *Lo Stato Etiopico e la sua Chiesa*. Rome, Edizioni SEAT.

Schwabe, C.W. and I.M. Kuojok (1981), 'Practices and Beliefs of the Traditional Dinka Healer in Relation to Provision of Modern Medical and Veterinary Services for the Southern Sudan'. *Human Organization* 40, pp. 231–8.

Sottochiesa, G. (1936), *La Religione in Etiopia*. Torino, Quaderni Nazionali.

Walker, C.H. (1933), *The Abyssinian at Home*. London, Sheldon Press.

11. Aspects of animal healthcare among Samburu pastoralists

Beaman, A. W. (1983), Women's Participation in Pastoral Economy: Income Maximization among the Rendille. Thesis, Boston University, Boston, MA.

Blood, D.C. and O.M. Radostits (1989), *Veterinary Medicine (7th edition)*. Philadelphia, Bailliere and Tindall.

Fumagalli, C. (1977), A Diachronic Study of Change and Socio-Cultural Processes among the Pastoral Nomadic Samburu of Kenya, 1900–1975. Thesis, State University of New York, Buffalo, NY.

Halderman, J.M. (1985), 'Problems of Pastoral Development in Eastern Africa'. *Agricultural Administration* 18, pp. 199–216.

Halpin, B. (1981), 'Vets—Barefoot and Otherwise'. Pastoral Network Paper No. 11c. London, Overseas Development Institute.

Heffernan, C. (1987), Traditional Veterinary Medicine among the Samburu Pastoralists of Northern Kenya. School of Veterinary Medicine, Tufts University, North Grafton, MA. Unpublished manuscript.

——— (1990), The Dynamics of Livestock Healthcare among the Samburu Pastoralists of Northern Kenya. Thesis, Tufts University, North Grafton, MA.

Hogg, R. (1986), 'The New Pastoralism: Poverty and Dependence in Northern Kenya'. *Africa* 56, pp. 319–33.

IPAL (Integrated Project on Arid Lands) (n.d.), Annotated Check List of Plants of Mount Kalal. Technical Report D-4. Maralel, Kenya, IPAL.

Jacobs, A.H. (1973), Pastoral Masai and Tropical Rural Development. Working paper for the Colloquium on Ecological–Cultural Analysis in Tropical Rural Development, University of California, Los Angeles.

Lamprey, H.F. and H. Yussef (1981), 'Pastoralism and Desert Encroachment in Northern Kenya'. AMBIO, pp. 130–34.

Losos, G. (1986), *Infectious Tropical Diseases of Domestic Animals*. New York, Churchill Livingston.

McCorkle, C.M. (1986), 'An Introduction to Ethnoveterinary Research and Development'. *Journal of Ethnobiology* 6, pp. 129–49.

Meck, M. (1971), *Problems and Prospects of Social Service in Kenya: A Study with Special Regard to Education and Health in Light of Regional Needs and Demographic Trends*. München, Welforam Verlag.

Ojang, F.F. and R.B. Ogendo (1973), *Kenya—A Study in Physical and Human Geography*. Nairobi, Longman Kenya.

Ominde, S.H. (1988), *Kenya's Population and Development to the Year 2000*. Nairobi and Athens, OH, Heineman Kenya and University of Ohio Press.

Raikes, P. (1981), *Livestock Development and Policy in East Africa*. Uppsala, Scandinavian Institute of African Studies.

Rigby, P. (1985), *Persistent Pastoralist—Nomadic Societies in Transition*. Totowa, NJ, Zed Books.

Schwabe, C.W. and I.M. Kuojok (1981), 'Practices and Beliefs of the Traditional Dinka Healer in Relation to Provision of Modern Medical and Veterinary Services for the Southern Sudan'. *Human Organization* 40, pp. 231–8.

Sollod, A.E. and C. Stem (1991), 'Appropriate Animal Health Information Systems for Nomadic and Transhumant Livestock Populations in Africa'. *Revue Scientifique Technique de l'Office Internationale des Épizooties* 10, pp. 89–101.

Sollod, A.E., K. Wolfgang and J.A. Knight (1984), Veterinary Anthropology: Interdisciplinary Methods in Pastoral Systems Research. In *Livestock Development in Africa: Constraints, Prospects, Policy*. J.R. Simpson and P. Evangelou (eds.), pp. 285–302. Boulder, CO, Westview Press.

Spencer, P. (1965), *The Samburu—Study of Gerontocracy in a Nomadic Tribe*. London, Routledge and Kegan Paul.

———— (1973), *Nomads in Alliance: Symbiosis and Growth among the Rendille and Samburu of Kenya*. London, University Press.

Sperling, L. (1984), 'Recruitment of Labor among the Samburu Herders'. Working Paper No. 414. Nairobi, University of Nairobi.

Stem, C. (1983), Vetscout: Animal Disease Monitoring through Veterinary Auxiliaries in Central Niger. Paper presented at the Workshop on Monitoring Change in Pastoral Livestock Systems, 4th International Symposium on Veterinary Epidemiology and Economics, Kuala Lampur and Singapore.

12. Traditional management of camel health and disease in North Africa and India

Abdalla, A.J. and F.O. Akasha (1988), Camel Pastoralists of Kordofan Region: Problems of Survival and Adaptation through Drought, 1983–1985. In *Camel Production as a Food System*. M. Salih and B. E. Musa (eds.), pp. 26–39. Camel Forum Working Paper No. 26. Mogadishu, Somali Academy of Sciences and Arts.

Acland, P.B.E. (1932), 'Notes on the Camel in Eastern Sudan'. *Sudan Notes and Records* 15, pp. 119–49.

Bernus, E. (1981), *Touaregs Nigériens: Unité Culturelle et Diversité Régionale d'un Peuple Pasteur*. Mémoires ORSTOM No. 94. Paris, ORSTOM.

Cauvet, Commandant (1925), *Le Chameau*. Paris, Librairie J.-B. Bailliere et Fils.

Cross, H.E. (1917), *The Camel and its Diseases*. London, Bailliere, Tindall & Cox.

Curasson, G. (1947), *Le Chameau et ses Maladies*. Paris, Vigot Frères.

Davis, R. (1957), *The Camel's Back*. London, John Murray.

Droandi, I. (1936), *Il Camello*. Florence, Istituto Agricolo Coloniale Italiano.

Froehner, R. (1936), 'Arabische Kamelheilkunde des Mittelalters'. *Archiv für Wissenschaftliche und Praktische Tierheilkunde* 70, pp. 358–61.

Higgins, A.J. (1983), 'Observations on the Diseases of the Arabian Camel (*Camelus dromedarius*) and their Control: A Review'. *Veterinary Bulletin* 53, pp. 1089–100.

Köhler-Rollefson, I., B.E. Musa and M.F. Achmed (1991), 'The Camel Pastoral System of the Rashaida in Eastern Sudan'. *Nomadic Peoples* 29, pp. 68–76.

Leese, A.S. (1927), *A Treatise on the One-humped Camel in Health and in Disease*. Stamford, CN, Haynes and Son.

Mahmoud, M.M. and M.O. Osman (1984), A Note of Trypanosomiasis in Sudanese Camels. In *The Camelid: An All-purpose Animal. Vol. 1*. R. Cockrill (ed.), pp. 502–08. Uppsala, Scandinavian Institute of African Studies.

Monteil, V. (1952), *Essaie sur le Chameau au Sahara Occidental*. Saint Louis du Sénégal, Centre IFAN- Mauritanie.

Nayel, M.N. and M.T. Abu-Samra (1986), 'Sarcoptic Mange in the One-humped Camel (*Camelus dromedarius*). A Clinico-pathological and Epizootiological Study of the Disease and its Treatments'. *Journal of Arid Environments* 10, pp. 199–211.

Nicolaisen, J. (1963), *Ecology and Culture of the Pastoral Twareg*. Nationalmuseets Skrifter Etnografisk Roekke 9. Copenhagen, The National Museum of Copenhagen.

Reid, J.A. (1930), 'Some Notes on the Tribes of the White Nile Province'. *Sudan Notes and Records* 13, pp. 149–209.
Schillinger, D. and J. Rottcher (1984), The Current State of Chemotherapy of *T. evansi* Infection in Camels. In *The Camelid: An All-purpose Animal. Vol. 1.* R. Cockrill (ed.) pp. 509–18. Uppsala, Scandinavian Institute of African Studies.
Schinkel, H.-G (1970), *Haltung, Zucht und Pflege des Viehs bei den Nomaden Ost- und Nordostafrikas.* Berlin, Akademie-Verlag.

13. Ethnoveterinary pharmacology in India: past, present and future

Ahmed, J. (1986), 'Use of Pestoban for Control of Lice in Poultry'. *Indian Journal of Indigenous Medicines* 5.
Ali, S.M. and R.K Mehta (1986), Taenicidal Activity of *Piper nigrum*. In *Proceedings of the 20th Indian Pharmaceutical Congress*, Ahmedabad, India.
Ambaye, R.V., M.A. Indap, M. Parchure and S.V. Ghokhale (1984), 'Plants and Novel Anti-Tumor Agents—A Review'. *Indian Drugs* Feb, pp. 173–91.
Angelo, S.J. and J.P. Lavania (1976), 'Therapeutic Management of Urethral Calculosis in a Bullock—A Case Report'. *Indian Veterinary Journal* 53, pp. 478–9.
Anjaria, J.V. (1969), 'Observations on Bovine Urethral Calculosis'. *Indian Veterinary Journal* 46, pp. 449–53.
———— (1981a), Recent Trends in the Use of Indigenous Drugs in Animal Production and Health Care: (i) Indian Herb our Legendary of Ancestral Vedic Heritage and National Health; (ii) *Leptadenia reticulata*—a Potential Lactogenic Herb in Aid of Animal Production; (iii) Indigenous Drugs as Cheap Effective Remedies in Routine Animal Health Care. Paper presented at the Summer Institute on Epidemiological Survey and Techno-economics of Diseases, Gujarat Veterinary College, Anand.
———— (1981b), Indigenous Drugs in Fertility and Contraception. Paper presented at University Grants Commission National Seminar on the Reproductive Biology Research Unit, Gujarat Agricultural University, Anand.
———— (1982), Clinical Pharmacology of the Bovine Digestive System with some Reference to Indigenous Drug Approach in Rural Clinics. Paper presented at the Indian Council of Agricultural Research's Summer Institute on Rural Clinical Services for Dairy Animals, Gujarat Veterinary College, Anand.
———— (1985), Treatment of Infected Wounds and Antimicrobial Activity of some Traditional Drugs. Paper presented at the National Workshop on Selected Medicinal Plants Used in Traditional/Indigenous System of Medicine, Chemexil, Bombay.
———— (1986a) Traditional (Indigenous) Veterinary Medicine Project. Final Report. Livestock Development Project, Sri Lanka Asian Development Bank. Gannoruwa, Peradeniya, Sri Lanka, Veterinary Research Institute.
———— (1986b), Recent Trends in the Use of Traditional (Indigenous) Drugs in Animal Health and Production. Traditional Veterinary Medicine—the Modern Trend. Indigenous Drug Research—A Brief Review. Paper presented at the Inservice Training Course of Veterinary Surgeons in Traditional Veterinary Medicine, Veterinary Research Institute, Gannoruwa, Peradeniya, Sri Lanka.
———— (1986c), Medicinal Plants in Health and Disease. Paper presented at a Research Colloquium at the Institute of Fundamental Studies, Hantana, Kandy, Sri Lanka.
———— (1986d), Traditional Drugs in Reproductive Disorders. Paper presented at the Faculty of Veterinary Medicine, Peradeniya, Sri Lanka.
———— (1986e), Herbs in Urinary, Respiratory and Cardiovascular Disorders. Paper presented at the Inservice Training Course of Veterinary Surgeons in Traditional Veterinary Medicine, Veterinary Research Institute, Gannoruwa, Peradeniya, Sri Lanka.
Anjaria, J.V. (1986f), Herbs in Digestive Disorders. Paper presented at the Inservice Training Course of Veterinary Surgeons in Traditional Veterinary Medicine, Veterinary Research Institute, Gannoruwa, Peradeniya, Sri Lanka.

—————— (1986g), Antimicrobial Activity of some Indigenous Drugs and its Therapeutic Applications. Paper presented at the Veterinary Research Institute, Gannoruwa, Sri Lanka.

—————— (1986h), Antimicrobial Activity of some Traditional Drugs and Practical Therapeutical Application. Paper presented at the International Workshop on Research Planning on Organic Fertilizers and Botanicals in Pest Control, Faculty of Agriculture, University of Peradeniya, Peradeniya, Sri Lanka.

Anjaria, J.V. and I. Gupta (1967), 'Studies on Lactogenic Property of *Leptadenia reticulata* (Jivanti) and Leptaden Tablets in Goats, Sheep, Cows and Buffaloes'. *Indian Veterinary Journal* 44, pp. 967–74.

—————— (1969a), 'Studies on Lactogenic Property of *Leptadenia reticulata* and Leptaden Tablets on some Clinical Cases'. *Gujvet* 3, p. 43.

—————— (1969b), 'The Pharmacognosy of *Leptadenia reticulata*'. *Gujvet* 3, pp. 10–12.

—————— (1970a), 'Preliminary Chemical Investigations and Extraction of *Leptadenia reticulata* (Jivanti)'. *Gujvet* 4, pp. 81–3.

—————— (1970b), Some Pharmacological Studies on *Leptadenia reticulata* and Leptaden Tablets. Paper presented at the 2nd Annual Conference of the Indian Pharmacological Society, Lucknow.

—————— (1972), 'Some Pharmacological Studies on *Leptadenia reticulata* (Jivanti) and Leptaden Tablets'. *Gujvet* 6, pp. 7–9.

Anjaria, J.V., K. Janakiraman, M.R. Varia and O.D. Gulati (1975a), Studies on *L. reticulata*; Effects on some Endocrine Glands and Reproductive Organs of Rats. Paper presented at the 7th Conference of the Indian Pharmacological Society, B.J. Medical College, Ahmedabad.

—————— (1975b), 'Studies on *L. reticulata*; Lactogenic Effects on Rats'. *Indian Journal of Experimental Biology* 13, p. 448.

Anjaria, J.V. and S.H. Kamboya (1970), 'A Preliminary Inquiry in the Efficacy of Cystone™ Tablets'. *Gujvet* 4, pp. 45–6.

Anjaria, J.V., S.H. Kamboya and J.F. Mithuji (1970), 'Preliminary Inquiry into the Effect of *Leptadenia reticulata* (Jivanti) on Egg Yield'. *Indian Poultry Gazette* 54, pp. 140–42.

Anjaria, J.V., S.H. Kamboya, V.N. Vaishnav and O.D. Gulati (1974), 'Studies on *Leptadenia reticulata* Effects on Gir Cow'. *Gujvet* 12, pp. 25–7.

Anjaria, J.V., M.S. Naphde, M.G. Tripathi and O.D. Gulati (1975c), 'Studies on *L. reticulata*—Effect on Egg Yields in Hens'. *Gujarat Agricultural University Research Journal* 1, pp. 59–63.

Annapurna, J., D.S. Iyenger, and U.T. Bhalerao (1989), 'Antimicrobial Activity of Leaf Extract of *Enterolobium saman*'. *Indian Drugs* 26, pp. 272–4.

Anonymous (1941a), Charaka Samhita (3rd edition). Vaid Jadavji Trikamji (ed.). Bombay: Narayan Sagar Press for Satyabhamabhai Pandurang Publisher.

—————— (1941b), Shusruta Samhita. Vaid Jadavji Trikamji (ed.). Bombay: Narayan Sagar Press for Pandurang Jivaji Publisher.

—————— (1954a), Agni Purana. Gorakhpur, Gorakhpur Press for Mahadev Ramchandra Jaguste Publisher.

—————— (1954b), Brahma Purana. Gorakhpur, Gorakhpur Press for Mahadev Ramchandra Jaguste Publisher.

—————— (1954c), Devi Purana. Gorakhpur, Gorakhpur Press for Mahadev Ramchandra Jaguste Publisher.

—————— (1954d), Garuda Purana. Gorakhpur, Gorakhpur Press for Mahadev Ramchandra Jaguste Publisher.

Anonymous (1954e), Linga Purana. Gorakhpur, Gorakhpur Press for Mahadev Ramchandra Jaguste Publisher.

—————— (1954f), Matsaya Purana. Gorakhpur, Gorakhpur Press for Mahadev Ramchandra Jaguste Publisher.

—————— (1954g), Skanda Purana. Gorakhpur, Gorakhpur Press for Mahadev Ramchandra Jaguste Publisher.

—— (1958a), Atharvaveda (3rd edition) [Sanskrit]. Bombay, Narayan Sagar Press for Vasant Shripad Satavlekar.

—— (1958b), Rugveda (3rd edition) [Sanskrit]. Bombay: Narayan Sagar Press for Vasant Shripad Satavlekar.

—— (1958c), Yajurveda (3rd edition) [Sanskrit}. Bombay, Narayan Sagar Press for Vasant Shripad Satavlekar.

—— (1958d), Mahabharata. Gorakhpur: Kalyan Karyalaya Gorakhpur Press, for Mahadev Ramchandra Jaguste Publisher.

Arora, R.B. (1965), Cardiovascular Pharmacotherapeutics of Six Medicinal Plants Indigenous to India. Report. New Delhi, Hamdard National Foundation.

Arora, S.P. and Mohini, M. (1984), 'A Note on Feeding Livol as a Feed Additive for Growth'. *Pashudhan* 9(76).

Aulakh, G.S. and G. Mahadevan (1989), Herbal Drugs for Asthma—a Review of Clinical Estimations of Antiasthmatic Drugs. *Indian Drugs* 26, pp. 593–9.

Azmi, M.N. (1970), Feeding Trials on Leptaden (Vet). Paper presented at the 19th Indian Veterinary Conference, Veterinary College, Ranchi, Bihar.

Bagayitkar, K. (1959), A Compilation of Jivanti. Jamnagar: Institute of Ayurvedic Research and Studies. Unpublished report.

Banerjee, A.K., K.K. Kaul and S.S. Nigam (1984), 'Chemical, Microbial and Anthelmintic Examination of *Aegle marmelos*'. *Indian Drugs* Feb, pp. 217–18.

Basak, B.R. (1986), 'Use of Himalayan Batisa in Broiler Mesh'. *Indian Journal of Indigenous Medicines* 5.

Basak, B.R. and A. Nandi (1982), 'Increased Feed Intake in Dairy Cattle with Himalayan Batisa'. *Pashudhan* 8, (67).

Bhutani, K.K., V. Kumar, R.W. Kaur and A.N. Sarin (1987), 'Potential Antidysenteric Candidates from Indian Plants: A Selective Screening Approach'. *Indian Drugs* 24, pp. 212–16.

Bhutani, K.K., Somraj, D.K. Gupta, S. Kumar, C.K. Atal and M.K. Kaul (1984), 'Profile of Kurchi in India'. *Indian Drugs* Feb, pp. 212–16.

Budavari, S., M.J. O'Neil, A. Smith and P.E. Heckelman (1989), *The Merck Index: An Encyclopedia of Chemicals, Drugs, and Biologicals (11th edition)*. Rahway, NJ, Merck & Co.

Chaddha, A.C., I.D. Mehta, R.D. Chugh, J.S. Bhullar, B.K. Nagpal and B.K. Juneja (1977), 'Field Trials of Galog as Galactagogue'. *Pashudhan* 3, (36–8).

Chaturvedi, S.K. and V.K. Saxena (1983), 'Antibacterial and Anthelmintic Activity of Essential Oil from *Senecio quinquelobus* leaves'. *Indian Drugs* Nov, pp. 50–51.

Chemexil (1986), Report of Conference on Chemical and Pharmaceuticals, Bombay, 19 February 1986. Bombay, Basic Chemical Pharmaceuticals and Cosmetic Export Council and London, Trade Agency for Developing Countries.

Chopra, K.K. (1970), Role of Varuna (*Crateva nurvala*), on Urinary Disorders. Thesis, Banaras Hindy University, Varanasi, India.

Dange, B.N. (1977), Clinical Trial with Aloes Compound and Myron in Cases of Bovine Infertility. Paper presented at the First Asian Congress on Fertility and Sterility, Bombay.

Das, R.C. (1956), 'Urethral Calculi in a Bullock and its Treatment with the Decoction of *Dolichos biflorus* (Horse Gram)'. *Indian Veterinary Journal* 32, pp. 369–70.

Dash, S.K., M.J. Owens and H.H. Voelker (1972), 'Effects of Feeding Leptaden to Dairy Cows'. *Journal of Dairy Science* 55, pp. 102–06.

Dave, M.R. (1969), Study of Galactopoietic Property of Leptaden in Cows. Thesis, Madras University, Madras, India.

Desai, P.U. (1985), Clinical Screening Trial with Seed of *Annona squamosa* in House Flies. Thesis, Royal Veterinary and Agricultural University, Copenhagen.

Deshpande, B. R. (1976), 'Functional Forms of Infertility with Reference to some Indigenous Herbal Remedies in Prolonged Post Partum Oestrus'. *Pashudhan* 24–5.

Devegowda, G. and B.S. Ramappa (1988), Supplementation of Livol in Diet on Broiler

Performance. Summary of paper submitted to Pashudhan. Bangalore, Department of Poultry Science, University of Agricultural Sciences.

Dubey, M.P. and I. Gupta (1969), 'Anthelmintic Activity of *Alangium lamarckii'*. *Indian Journal of Physiology and Pharmacology* 12, pp. 35–6.

Dutta, J.C., K.C. Deka and S. Rahman (1988), 'Treatment of Anoestrous Cattle with Aloes Compound'. *Indian Journal of Animal Health* 27, pp. 171–2.

Edwin, L. and J. I. Chungath (1988), 'Studies on *Swertia chirata'*. *Indian Drugs* 25, pp. 143–6.

Ehsham, M.D., D.K. Thakur, K.P. Sinha and R.P. Sinha (1977), 'Management of Tympany in Ruminants with Tympol'. *Pashudhan* 3, (40–41).

FAO (Food and Agriculture Organization) (1984a), Traditional (Indigenous) Systems of Veterinary Medicine for Small Farmers in India. Bangkok, Regional Office for Asia and the Pacific, Food and Agriculture Organization of the United Nations. (Based on the work of J.V. Anjaria.)

—— (1984b), Traditional (Indigenous) Systems of Veterinary Medicine for Small Farmers in Nepal. Bangkok, Regional Office for Asia and the Pacific, Food and Agriculture Organization of the United Nations. (Based on the work of D.D. Joshi.)

—— (1984c), Traditional (Indigenous) Systems of Veterinary Medicine for Small Farmers in Thailand. Bangkok, Regional Office for Asia and the Pacific, Food and Agriculture Organization of the United Nations. (Based on the work of P. Burana-manus.)

—— (1986), Traditional (Indigenous) Systems of Veterinary Medicine for Small Farmers in Pakistan. Bangkok, Regional Office for Asia and the Pacific, Food and Agriculture Organization of the United Nations. (Based on the work of M. Maqsood.)

—— (1991a), Traditional Veterinary Medicine in Indonesia. Bangkok, Regional Office for Asia and the Pacific, Food and Agriculture Organization of the United Nations. (Based on the work of S. Sukobagyo.)

—— (1991b), Traditional Veterinary Medicine in Sri Lanka. Bangkok, Regional Office for Asia and the Pacific, Food and Agriculture Organization of the United Nations. (Based on the work of S.B. Dhanapala.)

Foster, G.M. and B. Gallatin Anderson (1978), *Medical Anthropology.* New York, Alfred A. Knopf.

Gahlot, O.P. (1982), 'Usefulness of Galog for Increasing Milk Production'. *Pashudhan* 8, (68).

Galhotra, A.P., V.V. Bhaskar and O.P. Gautam (1970), 'Effect of Prajana on Inducing Heat in Cattle'. *Haryana Agricultural University Journal of Research* 1, pp. 66–73.

George, M., P.R. Venkatraman and K.M. Pandali (1946), 'Investigations on Plant Antibiotics. 2: A Search for Antibiotic Substances in some Indian Medicinal Plants'. *Journal of Scientific and Industrial Research* 6, pp. 42–46.

Ghokale, V.P. (1926), 'A Prescription for Increasing the Quantity of Milk in Cattle'. *Indian Veterinary Journal* 2: pp. 167–8.

Gowal, K.N. (1987), 'An Observation on the Effect of Himalayan Batisa and Livol in Overcoming Stress in Sheep'. *Pashudhan* 2(12).

GEC (Gujarat Export Corporation) (1987), Gujarat Export Bulletin, Statistical Number, Table 8. Ahmedabad, Gujarat Export Corporation.

Gupta, I. (1974), Antimycotic Drugs. Paper presented at the Summer Institute in Pharmacology, Haryana Agricultural University, Hissar, India.

Harkawat, D.S. and L.R. Singhvi (1977), 'Leptaden (Vet) to Enhance Lactation in Ewes'. *Livestock Adviser* 2, pp. 9–11.

Ishwar, A.K. (1980), Effect of Leptaden (Vet) on Growth, Age of Maturity and Egg Production in Poultry. Thesis, Govind Ballabh Pant Agricultural University, Patna-garh, India.

Ishwar, A.K. and M. Mohsin (1981a), 'Effect of Leptaden (Vet) on the Growth of Internal Organs in Broiler Chicks'. *Indian Journal of Poultry Science* 16, pp. 301–06.

—— (1981b), 'Leptaden (Vet), a Growth Promoting Agent in Broilers'. *Indian Veterinary Journal* 58, pp. 984–9.

———— (1981c), Leptaden (Vet) on Blood Calcium, Phosphorus and Total Cholesterol in Broiler Chicks. *Indian Poultry Gazette* 65, pp. 22–4.

———— (1981d), 'A Study on Leptaden (Vet) on Egg Production in Poultry Birds'. *Journal of Morphology and Physics Baroda PAVO* 10(1&2), pp. 14–20.

———— (1981e), A Study on Leptaden (Vet) on the Growth, Maturity and Blood Levels of Inorganic Calcium, Phosphorus and Total Cholesterol of White Leghorn Pullets. *Indian Journal of Poultry Science* 16, pp. 307–10.

Iyengar, M.A. (1976), *Bibliography of Investigated Indian Medicinal Plants (1950–1975)*. Manipal, College of Pharmacy, Kasturba Medical College.

Jain, M.P., V.N. Gupta and C.K. Atal (1984), 'Recent Advances in Vasika Alkaloids—A Review'. *Indian Drugs* May, pp. 313–22.

Jai, Singh (1977), Some Pharmacological Studies on Saxom. Thesis, Chandra Shekhar Azad University of Agriculture and Technology, Kanpur, India.

Jai, Singh and H.C. Joshi (1979), 'Effect of Saxom on Libido and Semen Quality of Rams'. *Pashudhan* 5(54–61).

———— (1981), 'Effect of Saxom on Mounting Behaviour of Buffalo Teaser Bulls'. *Pashudhan* 7(65).

Johari, M.P. and G.D. Singh (1970), Studies on Galactagogues in Buffaloes. Paper presented at the 19th Indian Veterinary Conference, Veterinary College, Ranchi, Bihar.

Kaikini, A.S., V.B. Hukeri and D.R. Pargaonkar (1968), Influences of Leptaden (Vet) in Milk Irregularities in Buffaloes. Paper presented at the 18th Indian Veterinary Conference, Hyderabad.

Kaikini, A.S. and D.R. Pargaonkar (1969), 'Studies on Leptaden (Vet) as a Galactagogue in Buffaloes'. *Food Farming and Agriculture* 1, pp. 16–19.

Kodagali, S.B., B.K. Bhavsar and F.S. Kavani (1973), 'Clinical Evaluation of "Prajana" for Anoestrous Conditions in Surti Buffaloes'. *Gujarat College of Veterinary Science and Animal Husbandry Magazine* 6, pp. 51–2.

Kulkarni, A.B. (1973), Oestrogenic Effect of some Indigenous Drugs. Thesis, Konkan Krishi Vidyapith (Konkan Agricultural University), Dapoli, India.

Kulkarni, M.J. (1976), 'Clinical Trials with Galog in Case of Hypogalactia'. *Pashudhan* 2(24–5).

Kulkarni, M.V. (1970), 'Lactogenic Property of Leptaden in Conditioned Hypogalactia'. *Indian Journal of Animal Health* 9, pp. 235–9.

Kumar, G.M., A.K. Sinha and B.N. Sahai (1973), 'Anthelmintic Efficacy of Wopell against Hook Worms in Dogs and Stomach Worms in Goats'. *Indian Journal of Animal Research* 7, pp. 78–80.

Lal, J., S. Chandra, V. Raviprakash and M. Sabir (1976), '*In Vitro* Anthelmintic Action of some Indigenous Medicinal Plants on *Ascaridia galli* Worms'. *Indian Journal of Physiology and Pharmacology* 20, pp. 64–8.

Lodrick, D.O. (1981), Sacred Cows, Sacred Places. Origins and Survivals of Animal Homes in India. Pp. 43–70. Berkeley, University of California Press.

Mahanta, P.N., D.L. Bijwsal, B. Prasad and P. Gupta (1983), 'Therapeutic Efficacy of Livol in Experimentally Induced Hepatitis in Buffalo Calves'. *Indian Journal of Veterinary Medicine* 3, pp. 73–8.

Mehta, R.K. and G.C. Parashar (1966), 'Effect of *Butea frondosa*, *Vernonia anthelmintica*, and *Carica papaya* against Oxyurids in Mice'. *Indian Veterinary Journal* 43, pp. 744–8.

Misra, S.C. (1983), 'A Note on the Efficacy of Wopell against *Toxocara canis* and *Dipylidium caninum* Infection in Pups'. *Indian Journal of Indigenous Medicines* 3.

Moulvi, M.V. (1963), 'Lactogenic Properties of "Leptaden"'. *Indian Veterinary Journal* 40, pp. 657–8.

Mukherjee, T., N. Bhalla, G.S. Auklah and S.C. Jain (1984), 'Herbal Drugs for Urinary Stones: Literature Appraisal'. *Indian Drugs* Mar, pp. 224–8.

Narang, J.R. (1981), 'Field Studies on Efficacy of Pestoban against Ectoparasites of Livestock'. *Pashudhan* 7.

Narasimhamurthy, G. (1969), 'A Preliminary Note on the Study of Lactogenic Properties of Leptaden (Alarsin Pharmaceuticals, Bombay)'. *Indian Veterinary Journal* 46, pp. 510–16.

Naresh Chand (1974), 'A Preliminary Report on the Effect of 'Prajana' on Reproductive Organs in Immature Mice'. *Indian Veterinary Journal* 51, pp. 167–9.

Natrajan, R.T. (1968), Leptaden (Vet) in Poultry and Effect of Leptaden in Culled Birds. Paper presented at the 18th Indian Veterinary Conference, Hyderabad.

Nooruddin, M. (1983), 'Clinical Trial of Himalayan Batisa in Loss of Appetite in Cattle'. *Pashudhan* 8(69).

Pachauri, S.P. (1965), Indigenous Drugs on Horn Cancer—Anticancer Drugs. Thesis, Agra University, Agra, India.

Pal, M. (1976), 'Clinical Trials of Tympol in Tympany'. *Pashudhan* 2(31–2).

Pal, M., I.D. Sharma and G.D. Dube (1979), 'Clinical Trial with Leptaden (Vet) in Cases of Hypogalactia in Buffaloes'. *Dairy Guide* 2, pp. 19–21.

Pande, P. N., and M. R. Rai (1982), 'Galog Drug of Choice for More Milk Production by Dairy Cows'. *Pashudhan* 8(69).

Pandey, G.P., P.N. Shrivastava and J.J. Sharma (1984), 'Livol(R)—a Drug for Liver Disorders'. *Livestock Adviser* 9, pp. 62–5.

Pandit, D. (1986), 'Tonic against Hepatic Disorders Caused by Liver Flukes in Ovines—Livol'. *Pashudhan* 1(4).

Patel, A.B. and U.K. Kanitkar (1969), '*Asparagus racemosus* Willd.-Form Bordi, as a Galactagogue, in Buffaloes'. *Indian Veterinary Journal* 46, pp. 718–21.

Patel, R.B., J.D. Raval, J.P. Gandhi and B.K. Chakhavarty (1988), 'Hepatoprotective Actions of Indian Medicinal Plants'. *Indian Drugs* 25, pp. 224–5.

Patil, J.S., N.S. Bugalia, A.K. Sinha, A.S. Khana and S.C. Chopra (1983), 'Clinical Efficacy of Prajana, Lugol's Paint and Utero-Ovarian Massage in Anoestrus Cows'. *Indian Veterinary Journal* 60, pp. 1019–20.

Pillai, S., C.R. Rajagopalan and K.P.D. Nair (1971), 'Clinical Trials with Neblon in Non-Specific Diarrhoea of Cattle and Goats'. *Kerala Journal of Veterinary Science* 2, pp. 109–12.

Pradhan, N.R. and S.K. Misra (1988), 'Effect of Feeding 'Livol' on the Egg Production of Layers'. *Indian Veterinary Journal* 65, pp. 714–18.

Prasad, A. (1970), Leptaden (Vet). Paper presented at the 19th Veterinary Conference, Veterinary College, Ranchi, Bihar, India.

Quimby, M.W. (1977), Foreword. In *Major Medicinal Plants*. J.F. Morton (ed.), pp. V-IX. Springfield, IL, Charles C. Thomas.

Raghavan, R.S., D. Kulkarni and M.M. Hussain (1976), 'Wopell in Treatment of Round Worms in Dogs'. *Pashudhan* 2(29–30).

Raghavan, R.S., D. Kulkarni and V.A. Sangvikar (1983), 'Clinical Trials of Teeburb and Himax in Treatment of Dermatological Conditions in Animals'. *Pashudhan* 9(71).

Raghavan Nambiar, M.O. (1980), 'Initiation of Lactation and Galactagogue Effect of Leptaden (Vet) on a Cross-Bred Jersey Heifer after Abortion'. *Indian Journal of Animal Research* 14, pp. 71–2.

Raghavan Nambiar, M.O. (1981), 'Leptaden (Vet) as a Galactagogue in an Elephant with Deficient Lactation'. *Indian Veterinary Journal* 58, pp. 667–8.

Rahman, A. and M. Nooruddin (1981), 'Clinical Trials with Neblon in Diarrhoea of Cattle'. *Pashudhan* 7, p. 66.

Rai, M.K. and S.K. Upadhyaya (1988), '*In Vitro* Efficacy of Different Extracts *Parthenium hysterophorus* against Human Pathogenic Fungi Using Different Techniques'. *Indian Drugs* 26, pp. 637–40.

Rajagopalan, M.K., M. Menachery and S.E. George (1972), 'Studies on the Lactogenic Properties of Leptaden'. *Indian Veterinary Journal* 49, pp. 196–203.

Raju, M.L. (1932), 'Use of *Euphorbia* in Increasing Milk'. *Indian Veterinary Journal* 9, p. 35.

Ramchandani, M. and J.I. Chugath (1987), 'Antibacterial and Antiviral Studies on *Phyllanthus fraternus* and *Jatropha glandulifera*'. *Indian Drugs* 25, pp. 134–5.

Rathore, H.S. and H. Rawat (1989), 'Liv-52 Protection against Cadmium Induced Histomorphological Changes in Mice Spleen, Duodenum and Small Intestine'. *Indian Drugs* 26, pp. 533–40.

Rathore, S.S. and S.R. Pattabhi Raman (1977), 'Clinical Trial of Myron in Post Partum Metritis in Buffaloes'. *The Haryana Veterinarian* 16, pp. 27–8.

Razak, M.A. (1982), Research Activities in Unani System of Medicine in India. Hamdard Nagar, Central Council of Research in Unani Medicine, Ministry of Health.

Samal, G.N. (1974), 'A Controlled Study of Leptaden (Vet) Therapy on Growth, Laying Performance and Disease Control of Poultry'. *Indian Poultry Review* 6 (Dec).

Satyavati, G.V. (1982), 'Some Traditional Medical Systems and Practices of Global Importance'. *Indian Journal of Medical Research* 76(Supplement Dec), pp. 1–26.

Sharma, H.N., K.N. Deka and S.C. Pathak (1981), 'Clinical Trial of Himax in the Treatment of Wounds in Animals'. *Pashudhan* 7, (64).

Sharma, M.C., O.P. Gupta and A.S. Pandey (1982), 'Clinical Trial of Himax against Mange in Buffaloes'. *Agricultural Science Digest* 2, p. 124.

Sharma, R. (1978), 'Massage in Gingivitis and other Painful Oral Conditions in Veterinary Practice'. *Livestock Adviser* 3, pp. 23–5.

Sharma, S.C. (1969), 'Effect of Oral Administration of "Fortege" on Bovine Semen'. *Indian Journal of Animal Health* 8, pp. 219–22.

Shirlaw, L.H. (1940), 'A Short History of Ayurvedic Veterinary Literature'. *Indian Journal of Veterinary Science* 10, pp. 1–39.

Shrivastava, P.N., D.B. Shrivastava and A. Ahmed (1970), 'Pharmacological Studies on Leptaden'. *Indian Journal of Pharmacology* 3, p. 68.

Shrivastava, P.N., D.N. Shrivastava and A. Ahmed (1974), 'Pharmacological Studies on Indigenous Drugs, *Leptadenia reticulata* and *Breynia patens*'. *Indian Veterinary Journal* 51, pp. 7–8.

Shrivastava, P.S., V.K. Sinha and S.P. Sinha (1988), 'Control of Canine Ectoparasites through Application of Herbal Preparation Blaze'. *Pashudhan* 3(1).

Shrivastava, S.C. and C.S. Sissodia (1970), 'Analgesic Studies on *Vitex negundo* and *Valeriana wallichii*'. *Indian Veterinary Journal* 47, pp. 170–75.

Singh, M., S.L. Garg, J.P. Puri and O.P. Nangia (1980), 'Effect of Himalayan Batisa on Performance of Buffalo Calves'. *Indian Veterinary Medical Journal* 4, pp. 28–32.

Singh, N. (1969), 'Anthelmintic Studies of *Zanthoxylum alatum* Roxb. against Ascarids'. *Indian Journal of Animal Sciences* 39, pp. 332–44.

Singh, S., N.A. Ansari, M.C. Shrivastava, M.K. Sharma and S.N. Singh (1985), 'Anthelmintic Activity of *Vernonia anthelmintica*'. *Indian Drugs* 22, pp. 508–511.

Singh, S.P., N. Misra, K.S. Dixit, N. Singh, and R.P. Kohli (1984), 'An Experimental Study of Analgesic Activity of *Cissus quadrangularis*'. *Indian Journal of Pharmacology* 16, pp. 162–3.

Singh, U.B. (1980), 'Treatment of Demodectic Mange in Dogs with Teeburb and Neem Oil'. *Pashudhan* 6(62).

Sinha, R.P., R.S. Prasad, S. Roy and M. Zahinuddin (1987), 'Effect of Pestoban against Ectoparasites of Livestock and Poultry'. *Livestock Adviser* 12, pp. 26–30.

Soni, J.L., R.N. Gupta and B.K. Dave (1980), 'Neblon in Non-Specific Diarrhoea in Large White Yorkshire Pigs'. *Indian Veterinary Journal* 57, p. 521.

Supekar, P.G. and H.K. Mehta (1986), 'Blaze: An Efficacious Ectoparasiticide and Hair Conditioner in Dogs'. *Indian Journal of Indigenous Medicines* 5.

Thaker, A.M. and J.V. Anjaria (1986), 'Antimicrobial and Infected Wound Healing Response of some Traditional Drugs'. *Indian Journal of Pharmacology* 18, pp. 171–4.

Thakur, D.K. (1975), 'Wound Healing by Himax'. *Pashudhan* 1(4).

Tripathy, S.B., P.K. Das and S.N. Tripathy (1987), 'Study of the Utility of Herbal Ectoparasite Shampoo (Blaze), on Dogs'. *Pashudhan* 2(11).

Tripathy, S.B. and Pradhan, R. (1977), 'Some Observations on First Aid Therapy of Tympany in Ruminants'. *Pashudhan* 3(34–5).

Tripathy, S.B., S.N. Tripathy and P.K. Das (1986), 'Studies on the Therapeutic Efficacy of Himax on Sarcoptic Mange of Goats and Dogs'. *Indian Journal of Indigenous Medicines* 5.

Tyler, V.E., L.R. Brady and J.E. Robbers (1988), *Pharmacognosy (9th edition)*. Philadelphia, Lea & Febiger.

UNCTAD/GATT (1982), *Markets for Selected Medicinal Plants and Their Derivatives*. Geneva, International Trade Centre UNCTAD/GATT.

Vaishnav, V.N. and H.B. Buch (1965), 'A Preliminary Note on the Study of Lactogenic Properties of "Leptaden"'. *Indian Veterinary Journal* 42, pp. 796–800.

Vashishtha, M.S. and R.P. Singh (1975), 'Effect of Caflon in Camels Suffering from Coryza'. *Pashudhan* 2(19).

Vinayagamoorthy (1982), Bacterial Activity of some Medicinal Plants of Sri Lanka. *Journal of Biological Sciences* 15, pp. 50–59.

Vohora, S.B. (1989), 'Research on Medicinal Plants in India—A Review on Reviews'. *Indian Drugs* 26, pp. 526–32.

WHO (World Health Organization) (1976), *WHO Handbook on Basic Health Policy: Alternative Approaches to Meeting the Basic Health Needs of Developing Countries*. Fifth Meeting, September 1976, SEA/RC.29/Min.5.

Zysk Keni (1979), 'In Wilder Fields'. *Hemisphere* 23, pp. 200–205.

14. Ethnoveterinary medicine in western India

Agarwal, D.C., S. Khurana, A.K. Shrivastava, K.K. Shrivastava and A.W. Bhagwat (1987), 'Preliminary Studies on the *In Vitro* Antimicrobial Activity of *Tephrosea purpurea*'. *Indian Journal of Physiology and Pharmacology* 31, pp. 284–6.

Agarwal, J.S., R.P. Rastogi and O.P. Srivastava (1976), 'In Vitro Toxicity of Constituents of *Rumex maritimus* Linn. to Ringworm Fungi'. *Current Science* 45, pp. 619–20.

Agshikar, N.V., V.R. Naik, G.J.S. Abraham, C.V.G. Reddy, S.W.A. Naqvi and P.K. Mittal (1979), 'Analgesic, Anti-inflammatory Activity of *Acanthus illicifolius* Linn'. *Indian Journal of Experimental Biology* 17, pp. 1257–8.

Anand, K.K., M.L. Sharma, B. Singh and B.J. Ray Ghatak (1978), 'Anti-inflammatory, Antipyretic and Analgesic Properties of Bavachinin—A Flavanone Isolated from Seeds of *Psoralea corylifolia* Linn. (Babchi)'. *Indian Journal of Experimental Biology* 16, pp. 1216–17.

Anjaria, J.V., M.R. Varia, K. Janakiraman and O.D. Gulati (1975), 'Studies on *Leptadenia reticulata*: Lactogenic Effect on Rats'. *Indian Journal of Experimental Biology* 13, pp. 448–9.

Banerjee, A. and S.S. Nigam (1976), 'Antifungal Activity of Essential Oil of *Curcuma caesia* Roxb'. *Indian Journal of Medical Research* 64, pp. 1318–21.

——— (1977), 'Antifungal Activity of the Essential Oil of *Curcuma angustifolia* Roxb'. *Indian Journal of Pharmacy* 39, pp. 143–5.

Bhargava, A.K., J. Lal, P.R. Vanamayya and P.N. Kumar (1989), 'Experimental Evaluation of a Few Indigenous Drugs as Promoters of Wound Healing'. *Indian Journal of Animal Sciences* 59, pp. 66–8.

Bhargava, M.K., H. Singh and A. Kumar (1988), 'Evaluation of *Adhatoda vasica* as a Wound Healing Agent in Buffaloes: Clinical, Mechanical and Biochemical Studies'. *Indian Veterinary Journal* 65, pp. 33–8.

Chandel, R.S. and R.P. Rastogi (1978), 'Schwallin, the Antidermatophytic Constituent from *Schima wallichii*'. *Indian Journal of Pharmaceutical Sciences* 40, p. 228.

Deshpande, P.J., M. Sahu and P. Kumar (1982), '*Crataeva nurvala* Hook and Forst (Varuna)—the Ayurvedic Drug of Choice in Urinary Disorders'. *Indian Journal of Medical Research* 76 (supplement), pp. 46–53.

Garg, G.M., S.V. Vadnere and V.D. Sharma (1983), 'Efficacy of Garlic (*Allium sativum*) Treatment against Non-specific Uterine Infections in Repeat-breeding Cows'. *Indian Journal of Animal Reproduction* 3, pp. 9–11.

Gehlot, N.K., V.N. Sharma and D.S. Vyas (1976), 'Some Pharmacological Studies on

310 *Ethnoveterinary Research and Development*

Ethanolic Extract of Roots of *Bergenia ligulata'. Indian Journal of Pharmacology* 8, p. 92.

Ghosh, S.B., S. Gupta and A.K. Chandra (1980), 'Antifungal Activity in Rhizomes of *Curcuma amada* Roxb'. *Indian Journal of Experimental Biology* 18, pp. 174–6.

Gopalakrishnan, C., D. Shankaranarayanan, S.K. Nazimudeen, S. Viswanathan and L. Kameswaran (1980), 'Anti-inflammatory and CNS Depressant Activities of Xanthones from *Calophyllum inophyllum* and *Mesua ferrea'. Indian Journal of Pharmacology* 12, pp. 181.

Gupt, R.P. (1961), *Pashuon Ka Ilaj (Treatment of Animals).* New Delhi, Sasta Sahitya Mandal.

Gupta, O.P., M. Ali, B.J. Ray Ghatak and C.K. Atal (1977), 'Some Pharmacological Investigations of Embelin and its Semisynthetic Derivatives'. *Indian Journal of Physiology and Pharmacology* 21, pp. 31–9.

Kar, K., S. Singh and N.M. Khanna (1976), 'A Diuretic Flavone Glycoside from *Millingtonia hortensis* Linn'. *Indian Journal of Pharmacy* 38, pp. 26–7.

Katti, S.B., Y.N. Shukla and J.S. Tandon (1979), 'Arnebin Derivatives for Anticancer Activity'. *Indian Journal of Chemistry* 18B, pp. 440–42.

Khan, N.H., M. Rahman and M.S.A. Nur-e-Kamal (1988), 'Antibacterial Activity of *Euphorbia thymifolia* Linn'. *Indian Journal of Medical Research* 87, pp. 395–7.

Kumar, A. and R.S. Gupta (1984), 'A Note on the Sensitivity of Enterotoxigenic *Staphylococcus aureus* for Garlic Extract (*Allium sativum* Linn.)'. *Indian Veterinary Journal* 61, pp. 718–19.

Lal, J., S. Chandra, V. Raviprakash and M. Sabir (1976), '*In Vitro* Anthelmintic Action of some Indigenous Medicinal Plants on *Ascaridia galli* Worms'. *Indian Journal of Physiology and Pharmacology* 20, pp. 64–8.

Malik, J.K., A.M. Thaker and J.G. Sarvaiya (1988), Pharmacological Investigations on some Indigenous Medicinal Plants. Annual Progress Report, 18th Meeting of Research Subcommittee on Animal Health 1988–9, Gujarat Agricultural University, Sardar Krushinagar. [No page numbers available.]

Malik, J.K., J.G. Sarvaiya and M. Pal (1991a), Activity of some Indigenous Plants against Systemic Fungal Pathogens. Paper presented at the 24th Annual Conference of the Indian Pharmacological Society, Ahmedabad.

Malik, J.K., J.G. Sarvaiya and K.S. Prajapati (1991b), Studies on the Local Anaesthetic Action of *Lycopersicum esculentum.* Abstracts of the 8th All Gujarat Annual Meeting of the Indian Pharmacological Society, Jamnagar. [No page or abstract number available.]

Mathew, M.D. (1990), 'Red Hot Iron as a Styptic'. *Pashudhan* 5(7).

Mehta, S.C., H. Vardhan and S.P. Saxena (1986), 'Some Pharmacological Actions of the Essential Oil of *Blumea membranacea'. Indian Journal of Physiology and Pharmacology* 30, pp. 149–54.

Mishra, S.K. and K.C. Sahu (1977), 'Screening of some Indigenous Plants for Antifungal Activity against Dermatophytes'. *Indian Journal of Pharmacology* 9, pp. 269–72.

Pandey, B.L. and P.K. Das (1989), 'Immunopharmacological Studies on *Picrorhiza kurroa* Royle-Ex-Benth. Part IV: Cellular Mechanism of Anti-inflammatory Action'. *Indian Journal of Physiology and Pharmacology* 33, pp. 28–30.

Patel, R.G. (1967), Pashuon ki Siddh Vanaushadhi Chikitsa (Siddh Herbal Treatment of Animals). Indore, Gandhi Smarak Nidhi, Mishra Kheti Yojna.

Pendse, V.K., A.P. Dadhich, P.N. Mathur, M.S. Bal and B.R. Madan (1977), 'Anti-inflammatory, Immunosuppressive and some Related Pharmacological Actions of the Water Extract of Neem Giloe (*Tinospora cordifolia*): A Preliminary Report'. *Indian Journal of Pharmacology* 9, pp. 221–4.

Rao, J. T. (1976), 'Antifungal Activity of the Essential Oil of *Curcuma aromatica'. Indian Journal of Pharmacy* 38, pp. 53–4.

Rastogi, R.P. and B.N. Dhawan (1982), 'Research on Medicinal Plants at the Central Drug Research Institute, Lucknow (India)'. *Indian Journal of Medical Research* 76(supplement), pp. 27–45.

Ray, P.G. and S.K. Majumdar (1976), 'Antifungal Flavonoid from *Alpinia officinarum* Hance'. *Indian Journal of Experimental Biology* 14, p. 712.

—— (1977), 'Antifungal Activity of *Saussurea lappa* Clarke'. *Indian Journal of Experimental Biology* 15, pp. 334.

Rusia, K. and S.K. Srivastava (1988), 'Antimicrobial Activity of some Indian Medicinal Plants'. *Indian Journal of Pharmaceutical Sciences* 50, pp. 57–8.

Sarvaiya, J.G., M.P. Verma, A.M. Thaker, S.K. Bhavsar and J.K. Malik (1990), Studies on the Antimicrobial Activity of *Prosopis juliflora*. Paper presented at the 7th Gujarat State Conference of Pharmacologists, Baroda.

Satyavati, G.V., M.K. Raina, and M. Sharma (1976), *Medicinal Plants of India. Vol. 1.* New Delhi, Indian Council of Medical Research.

Sharma, M.C. and S.K. Dwivedi (1990), 'Efficacy of a Herbal Drug Preparation against Dermatomycosis in Cattle and Dog'. *Indian Veterinary Journal* 67, pp. 269–71.

Sharma, V.D., M.S. Sethi, A. Kumar and J. R. Rarotra (1977), 'Antibacterial Property of *Allium sativum* Linn: In Vivo and In Vitro Studies'. *Indian Journal of Experimental Biology* 15, pp. 466.

Singh, R.C.P., J.K. Malik, K.S. Roy and B.S. Paul (1978), 'Investigations into the Local Anaesthetic Activity of the Ether Extract of the Leaves of Tomato in the Case of Buffalo Calves'. *Journal of Research of Punjab Agricultural University* 15, pp. 120–26.

Sinha, A.K., M.S. Mehra, R.C. Pathak and G.K. Sinha (1977), 'Antibacterial Activity of Volatile Oils from some Indigenous Plants'. *Indian Journal of Experimental Biology* 15, pp. 339–40.

Thaker, A.M. and J.V. Anjaria (1986), 'Antimicrobial and Infected Wound Healing Response of some Traditional Drugs'. *Indian Journal of Pharmacology* 18, pp. 171–4.

Tirkey, K., R.P. Yadava, T.K. Mandal and N.C. Banerjee(1988), 'Pharmacological Study of *Ipomoea carnea*'. *Indian Veterinary Journal* 65, pp. 206–10.

Tripathi, V.D., S.K. Agarwal and R.P. Rastogi (1977), 'Atylosol, an Antibacterial Constituent from *Atylosia trinervia*'. *Indian Journal of Pharmacy* 39, p. 165.

Tripathi, V.D., S.K. Agarwal and R.P. Rastogi (1978a), 'An Antibacterial Biphenyl Derivative and other Constituents of *Atylosia trinervia*'. *Phytochemistry* 17, pp. 2 001–3.

Tripathi, V.D., S.K. Agarwal, O.P. Srivastava and R.P. Rastogi (1978b), 'Antidermatophytic Constituents from *Inula racemosa* Hook'. *Indian Journal of Pharmaceutical Sciences* 40, pp. 129–31.

Udupihille, M. and M.T.M. Jiffry (1986), 'Diuretic Effect of *Aerna lanata* with Water, Normal Saline and Coriander as Controls'. *Indian Journal of Physiology and Pharmacology* 30, pp. 91–7.

Varshney, A.C., A. Kumar and N.S. Jadon (1989), 'Treatment of Deep Seated Abscess Cavities with Granulated Sugar Paste: Clinical Case Reports in Cattle, Buffaloes and Dogs'. *Indian Veterinary Journal* 66, pp. 656–9.

Wahab, S., R.N. Tandon, Z. Jacob, B. Chandra and O.P. Srivastava (1982), 'Comparative In Vitro and In Vivo Effect of Lactones and Arnebins on *Trichophyton mentagrophytes* and *Candida albicans*'. *Indian Journal of Medical Research* 76 (supplement), pp. 77–82.

Zutshi, S.K., S.K. Joshi and M.M. Bokadia (1976), 'The In Vitro Antimicrobial Efficiency of some Essential Oils'. *Indian Journal of Medical Research* 64, pp. 854–7.

15. Banjarese management of duck health and nutrition

Chávez, E.R. and A. Lasmini (1978), 'Comparative Performance of Native Indonesian Egg Laying Ducks'. Center Report No.6. Bogor, Center for Animal Research and Development.

Clayton, G.A. (1972), 'Effects of Selection on Reproduction in Avian Species'. *Journal of Reproductive Fertility* 15 (supplement), pp. 1–21.

Cumming, R.B. (1980), Infectious Poultry Diseases in Tropical Areas. Paper presented to the South Pacific Poultry Science Convention, Auckland, New Zealand.

DJP (Direktorat Jenderal Peternakan), (1979), Laporan Inventarisasi Masalah Tehnik Peternakan Itik. Proyek Pengembangan Produksi Pusat. Jakarta, DJP.

———— (1982), Petjunjuk Tehnis Peternakan Itik. Proyek Bimas Ayam Pusat. Jakarta: DJP.

Gunawan, B. (1989), Importance of Animal Agriculture in Asian Production Systems. In *Summary Report of the Animal Agriculture Symposium: Development Priorities toward the Year 2000.* [No editor given.] pp. 39–52. Washington, DC, USAID.

Hetzel, J. and I. Sutikno dan Soeripto (1981), Beberapa Pengaruh Aflatoksin Terhadap Pertumbuhan Itik-itik Muda. In *Proceedings Seminar Penelitian Peternakan,* Pusat Penelitian dan Pengembangan Ternak (ed.), pp. 400–04. Ciawi, Balai Penelitian Ternak.

IEMVT (Institut d'Élevage et de Médecine Vétérinaire des Pays Tropicaux), (1987), *Manual of Poultry Production in the Tropics.* Wallingford, UK, Commonwealth Agricultural Bureaux International.

Kingston, D.J. and R. Dharsana (1977), 'Isolation of a Mesogenic Newcastle Disease from an Acute Outbreak of Mortality in Indonesian Ducks'. *Seminar Pertama Ilmu dan Industri Perunggasan* 1, pp. 1–21. Bogor, Center for Animal Research and Development.

Kingston, D.J., D. Kosasih and Iberani Ardi (1979), 'The Rearing of Alabio Ducklings and Management of the Laying Duck Flocks in the Swamps of South Kalimantan'. Center Report No. 9. Bogor, Center for Animal Research and Development.

McCorkle, C.M. (1989), Veterinary Anthropology. *Human Organization* 48, pp. 156–62.

McDowell, R.E. (1989), Technical Issues in Animal Agricultural Development. In *Summary Report of the Animal Agriculture Symposium: Development Priorities toward the Year 2000.* [No editor given.] pp. 105–21. Washington, DC, USAID.

Nari J., S. Hardjoutomo, Soetedjo, P. Ronohardjo, S. Hastiono and N. Ginting (1979), 'Situasi Penyakit Unggas di Indonesia: Pencegahan dan Pemberantasannya'. *Proceedings Seminar Ilmu dan Industri Perunggasan II.* Pp. 142–60. Ciawi, Balai Penelitian Ternak.

Prodjoharjono, S. (1977), 'Sindrom Sinusitis Kontagiosa Pada Anak Itik'. *Seminar Pertama Industrierunggasan* 1(1–8). Ciawi, Balai Penelitian Ternak.

Rahardi, F. and F.W. Kastyanto (1982), *Itik Alabio.* Jakarta, P.T. Penebar Swadaya.

Robinson, D.W., A. Usman, E. Dartojo and E.R. Cáhvez (1977), 'The Husbandry of Alabio Ducks in South Kalimantan Swamplands'. Center Report No. 3. Bogor, Center for Animal Research and Development.

Siregar, A.P. (1982), 'Sejarah Itik di Indonesia'. *Poultry Indonesia* 26, pp. 35–8.

Soedjai, H.R.A. (1974), *Beternak Itik.* Bandung, N.V. Masa Baru.

USDA (United States Department of Agriculture) (1973), 'Raising Ducks'. *Farmers' Bulletin No. 2215.* Washington, DC, USDA.

Vondal, P.J. (1984), Entrepreneurship in an Indonesian Duck Egg Industry: A Case of Successful Rural Development. Thesis, Rutgers University, New Brunswick, NJ.

———— (1987), 'Intensification through Diversified Resource Use: The Human Ecology of a Successful Agricultural Industry in Indonesian Borneo'. *Human Ecology* 15, pp. 27–51.

———— (1989), The Ecology of Farm Management in a Swamplands Region of Indonesia. In *Human Systems Ecology: Studies in the Integration of Political Economy, Adaptation and Socionatural Regions.* E. Reeves and S. Smith (eds.), pp. 107–23. Boulder, CO, Westview Press.

Witono, S., I.G. Sudana, Hartaningsih and M. Malole (1981), Studi Pasteurella multocida Sebagai Penyebab Fowl Cholera Pada Itik. In *Proceedings of a Seminar Penelitian Peternakan.* pp. 440–47. Ciawi, Balai Penelitian Ternak.

16. Sheep husbandry and healthcare among Tzotzil Maya shepherdesses

Foster, G.M. (1962), *Traditional Cultures and the Impact of Technological Change (1st edition)*. New York, Harper & Brothers.

Fraser, C.M. (ed.) (1986), *The Merck Veterinary Manual: A Handbook of Diagnosis, Therapy, Disease Prevention and Control, for the Veterinarian (6th edition)*. Rahway, NJ, Merck and Co.

Holland, W.R. (1978), *Medicina Maya en Los Altos de Chiapas*. México, DF, Instituto Nacional Indigenista.

King, L. (1966), *Weeds of the World: Biology and Control (1st edition)*. New York, Interscience.

Klein, J. (1920), *The Mesta: A Study in Spanish Economic History 1273–1836*. Cambridge, Harvard University Press.

Laughlin, R.M. (1975), *The Great Tzotzil Dictionary of San Lorenzo Zinacantan*. Smithsonian Contributions to Anthropology No. 19. Washington, DC, Smithsonian Institution Press.

Ley, G., P. Pedraza, R. Perezgrovas, I. Pimentel and G. Skromne-K. (1986), *Estacionalidad Reproductiva del Borrego Chiapas*. Cuadernos de Investigación No. 3. Tuxtla Gutiérrez, Universidad Autónoma de Chiapas.

Lucero, R. (1990), Etnozoología y Epizootiología de la Fascioliasis Ovina en el Municipio de San Juan Chamula, Chiapas. Thesis, Facultad de Estudios Superiores Cuautitlán, Universidad Nacional Autónoma de México.

McCorkle, C.M. (1986), 'An Introduction to Ethnoveterinary Research and Development'. *Journal of Ethnobiology* 6, pp. 129–49.

―――― (1989), 'Veterinary Anthropology'. *Human Organization* 48, pp. 156–62.

Manrique, G. (1968), Tradiciones Pastoriles. In *El Folklore Español*. J. Gómez-Tabanera (ed.), pp. 368–86. Madrid, Instituto de Antropología Aplicada.

Mathias-Mundy, E. and C.M. McCorkle (1989), Ethnoveterinary Medicine: An Annotated Bibliography. Bibliographies in Technology and Social Change No. 6. Center for Indigenous Knowledge and Agricultural and Rural Development (CIKARD). Ames, Iowa State University Research Foundation.

Ochiai, K. (1985), *Cuando los Santos Vienen Marchando*. Serie Monografías No. 3. San Cristóbal de las Casas, Chiapas, Centro de Estudios Indígenas.

Pérez Inclan, M.A. (1981), Situación Actual de la Ovinocultura en México. In *Memorias del Curso sobre Producción Ovina*. [No editor given.] pp. 1–12. México, DF, Facultad de Medicina Veterinaria y Zootecnia, Universidad Nacional Autónoma de México.

Perezgrovas, R. (ed.) (1990), *Los Carneros de San Juan: Ovinocultura Indígena en los Altos de Chiapas*. Serie Monografías No. 5. San Cristóbal de las Casas, Chiapas, Centro de Estudios Indígenas.

Perezgrovas, R. and P. Pedraza (1984), *Ovinocultura Indígena I: Desarrollo Corporal del Borrego Chiapas*. Cuadernos de Investigación No. 1. Tuxtla Gutiérrez, Universidad Autónoma de Chiapas.

―――― (1985), *Ovinocultura Indígena II: Infestación Parasitaria Natural en el Borrego Chiapas*. Cuadernos de Investigación No. 2. Tuxtla Gutiérrez, Universidad Autónoma de Chiapas.

Perezgrovas, R., A. Villalobos and P. Pedraza (1989), Milk Production in Mexican Breeds of Sheep. In *Proceedings of the North American Dairy Sheep Symposium*. W. Boylan (ed.), pp. 21–32. St. Paul, University of Minnesota.

Pozas, R. (1977), *Chamula: Un Pueblo Indio de los Altos de Chiapas*. México, DF, Instituto Nacional Indigenista.

Razgado, F. (1989), Características de la Producción Lanar en el Borrego Criollo de Chiapas y en sus Cruzas con Ovejas Romney Marsh. Thesis, Universidad Autónoma de Chiapas, Tuxtla Gutiérrez, México.

Sarmiento, J. (1989), Estudio Zoométrico de los Diferentes Fenotipos de la Oveja Criolla de los Altos de Chiapas. Thesis, Universidad Autónoma de Chiapas, Tuxtla Gutiérrez, México.

Villalobos, A. and R. Perezgrovas (1989), *Producción de Leche de la Borrega Criolla de Los Altos de Chiapas.* Cuadernos de Investigación No. 4. Tuxtla Gutiérrez, Universidad Autónoma de Chiapas.

Wasserstrom, R. (1980), *Ingreso y Trabajo Rural en Los Altos de Chiapas.* Serie Documentos No. 6. San Cristóbal de Las Casas Chiapas, Centro de Investigaciones Ecológicas del Sureste.

17. Care of cattle versus sheep in Ireland: south-west Donegal in the early 1970s

AFT (An Foras Taluntais) (1969), *West Donegal Resource Survey (4 parts).* Dublin, AFT.

ARTAI (An Roinn Talmhaiochta Agus Iascaigh), (1965), 'Fence Off Liver Fluke'. Leaflet No. 138. Dublin, Department of Agriculture and Fisheries.

Attwood, E.A. and J.F. Heavey (1964–5), 'Determination of Grazing Livestock Units'. *Irish Journal of Agricultural Research* 3, pp. 249–51.

McCorkle, C.M. (1994), The Roles of Animals in Social, Cultural, and Agroeconomic Systems. In *Animal Agriculture and Natural Resources in Central America: Strategies for Sustainability Proceedings of a Symposium/Workshop held in San José, Costa Rica.* San José, CATIE/ UGAAG/USAID-ROCAP, pp. 105–23.

Nuallain, T.O. (1973), Helminth Infestation in Cattle, Sheep and Horses in Eire. In *Helminth Disease of Cattle, Sheep and Horses in Europe.* G.M. Urquhart and J. Armour (eds.), pp. 144–7. Glasgow, Robert MacLahose.

Ogg, J.S. (1977), 'Eradication of *Hypoderma* species in Northern Ireland'. *Veterinary Parasitology* 3, pp. 229–37.

Orme, A.R. (1970), *Ireland.* Chicago, Aldine.

Primov, G. (1992), The Role of Goats in Agropastoral Production Systems of the Brazilian Sertao. In *Plants, Animals and People.* C.M. McCorkle (ed.), pp. 51–8. Boulder, CO, Westview Press.

Shanklin, E. (1985), *Donegal's Changing Traditions: An Ethnographic Study.* New York, Gordon and Breach.

———— (1988), 'Sure and What Did We Ever Do But Knit? Women's Lives in Early 20th Century Donegal'. *Donegal Annual* 40, pp. 40–54.

———— (1994), Life Underneath the Market: Herders and Gombeenmen in 19th Century Donegal. In *Herders and Markets.* C. Chang and H.A. Koster (eds.), pp. 103–21. Tucson, University of Arizona Press.

18. Ethnoveterinary R&D in production systems

Akerejola, O.O., T.W. Schillhorn van Veen and C.O. Njoku (1979), 'Ovine and Caprine Diseases in Nigeria: A Review of Economic Losses'. *Bulletin of Animal Health and Production in Africa* 27, pp. 65–70.

Bembello, H. (1970), 'Note se Rapportant aux Effets de la Sécheresse sur le Bétail'. *Bulletin of Epizootic Diseases in Africa* 18, pp. 35–9.

Bernus, E. (1969), 'Maladies Humaines et Animales chez les Touaregs Sahéliens'. *Journal de la Société des Africanistes* 34, pp. 111–37.

———— (1975) *Les Tactiques des Éleveurs Face à la Sécheresse: Le Cas du Sud-Ouest de l'Air, Niger.* Paris, ORSTOM.

———— (1981), 'Touaregs Nigériens: Unité Culturelle et Diversité Régionale d'un Peuple Pasteur'. Mémoires ORSTOM No. 94. Paris, ORSTOM.

Bernus, E., S. Bernus, C. Desjeux and B. Desjeux (1983), *Touaregs.* Paris, l'Harmattan.

Bohnel, H. (1971), 'Recherche sur des Causes de Mortalité des Veaux dans la Savane Sous-Soudanienne dans le Nord de la Côte-d'Ivoire'. *Bulletin of Epizootic Disease in Africa* 1, pp. 145–57.

Campbell, D.J. (1984), 'Response to Drought among Farmers and Herders in Southern Kajiado District, Kenya'. *Human Ecology* 12, pp. 35–64.
Casley, D.J. and K. Kumar (1988), *The Collection, Analysis and Use of Monitoring and Evaluation Data*. Baltimore, Johns Hopkins University Press.
Cord, L.J., C. Stem and N. El Inguini (1986), *Successful Drought Strategies among Twaregs of the Eduk-Kao Region*. Tahoua, Niger Integrated Livestock Production Project/Tufts University/ USAID.
Day, J. (1989), 'Hope for the Sahel?' *Agricultural Outlook* Jul, pp. 24–8.
Devereux, S. and J. Hoddinott (eds.) (1993), *Fieldwork in Developing Countries*. Boulder, CO, Lynne Rienner Publishers.
Dupire, M. (1972), 'Les Facteurs Humains de l'Économie Pastorale'. *Études Nigériennes* No. 4.
Fabiyi, J. P. (1970), 'An Investigation into the Incidence of Goat Helminth Parasites in the Zaria Area of Nigeria'. *Bulletin of Epizootic Disease in Africa* 18, pp. 29–34.
Fine, K., C. Prouty and C. Stem (1990), Traditional Concepts of Disease and Animal Health Care in Sheep among Members of the Beni Guil Tribe of Eastern Morocco. Report from the Eastern Pastoral Livestock Development Project, Morocco. North Grafton, MA, Tufts University.
Graber, M. (1966), 'Étude dans Certaines Conditions Africaines de l'Action Antiparasi- taire du Thiabendazole sur Divers Helminthes—II. Dromadaire'. *Revue d'Élevage et Médecine Vétérinaire des Pays Tropicaux* 19, pp. 527–43.
—— (1967), 'Enquête sur les Helminthes du Dromadaire Tchadien'. *Revue d'Élevage et Médecine Vétérinaire des Pays Tropicaux* 20, pp. 213–25.
—— (1972), 'À Propos de l'Action du Tartrate de Pyrantel sur Certains Nématodes Gastro-intestinaux du Zébu et du Mouton d'Afrique Centrale'. *Bulletin of Epizootic Disease in Africa* 20, pp. 121–6
Gretillat, S. (1976), 'De la Variation de la Formule Sanguine de la Chèvre Rousse de Maradi en Function de son Parasitisme Gastro-intestinal'. *Acta Tropica* 33, pp. 240–45.
Grigg, D.B. (1985), *The World Food Problem: 1950–1980*. Oxford, Basil Blackwell.
Haan, C. de and N.J. Nissen (1985), 'Animal Health Services in Sub-Saharan Africa'. World Bank Technical Paper No. 44. Washington, DC, World Bank.
Halderman, J.M. (1985), 'Problems Facing Pastoral Development in Eastern Africa'. *Agricultural Administration* 18, pp. 199–216.
Halpin, B. (1981), 'Vets—Barefoot and Otherwise'. Pastoral Development Network Paper No. 11c. London, Overseas Development Institute.
Hart, J. A. (1964), 'Observations on the Dry Season Strongyle Infestations of Zebu Cattle in Northern Nigeria'. *British Veterinary Journal* 120, pp. 87–95.
Hogg, R. (1983), 'Restocking the Isiolo Boran: An Approach to Destitution among Pastoralists'. *Nomadic Peoples* 14, pp. 35–9.
—— (1986), 'The New Pastoralism: Poverty and Dependence in Northern Kenya'. *Africa* 56, pp. 319–33.
Horowitz, M.M. (1980), Ideology, Policy and Praxis in Pastoral Livestock Development. In *Anthropology and Rural Development in West Africa*. M.M. Horowitz and T.M. Painter (eds.), pp. 249–72. Boulder, CO, Westview Press.
—— (1981), Research Priorities in Pastoral Studies: An Agenda for the 1980s. In *The Future of Pastoral Peoples*. J.G. Galaty, D. Aronson and P.C. Salzman (eds.), pp. 61–88. Ottawa, International Development Research Center.
—— (1983), On Listening to Herders: An Essay on Pastoral Demystification. In *Third International Symposium on Veterinary Epidemiology and Economics*. pp. 416–25. Edwardsville, KS, Veterinary Medical Publishing Co.
Horowitz, M.M. and F. Jowkar (1992), 'Pastoral Women and Change in Africa, the Middle East, and Central Asia'. IDA Working Paper No. 91. Binghamton, NY, Institute for Development Anthropology for UNIFEM and UNDP.
Howes, M. (1980), The Uses of Indigenous Technical Knowledge in Development. In *Indigenous Knowledge Systems and Development*. D. Brokensha, D.M. Warren and O. Werner (eds.), pp. 335–51. Lanham, MD, University Press of America.

Jowkar, F. and M.M. Horowitz (1991), *Gender Relations of Pastoral and Agropastoral Production: A Bibliography with Annotations*. Binghamton, NY, Institute for Development Anthropology for UNIFEM and UNDP.

Lamb, P.J. (1986), 'On the Development of Regional Climatic Scenarios for Policy-oriented Climatic-impact Assessment'. *Bulletin of the American Meteorological Society* 68, pp. 1116–23.

Lindenmayer, J.S., E. Stem, D. Marshall and S. Sama (1988), Field Trials with Exhelm (Morantel tartrate) and Vitamin A in Sheep in Niger. In *Proceedings of the 5th International Symposium on Veterinary Epidemiology and Economics*, Copenhagen, Denmark. R. Willeberg, J.F. Aggar and H.P. Rieman (eds.), *Acta Veterinaria Scandinavica* 84 (supplement), pp. 151–4.

Little, P.D. (1985a), 'Absentee Owners and Part-time Pastoralists: The Political Economy of Resource Use in Northern Kenya'. *Human Ecology* 13, pp. 131–51.

——— (1985b), 'Social Differentiation and Pastoralist Sedentarization in Northern Kenya'. *Africa* 55, pp. 243–61.

McCorkle, C.M. (1989a), 'Toward a Knowledge of Local Knowledge and its Importance for Agricultural RD&E'. *Agriculture and Human Values* 6, pp. 4–12.

——— (1989b), 'Veterinary Anthropology'. *Human Organization* 48, pp. 156–62.

McCorkle, C.M., M.F. Nolan, K. Jamtgaard and J.L. Gilles (1989), 'Social Research in International Agricultural R&D: Lessons from the Small Ruminant CRSP'. *Agriculture and Human Values* 6, pp. 42–51.

Malo, R. and S.E. Nicholson (1990), 'A Study of Rainfall and Vegetation Dynamics in the African Sahel Using Normalized Difference Vegetation Index'. *Journal of Arid Environments* 19, pp. 1–24.

Mishra, G.S., E. Camus, J. Berlot and A.E. N'Depo (1979), 'Enquête sur le Parasitisme et la Mortalité des Veaux dans le Nord de la Côte-d'Ivoire: Observations Préliminaires'. *Revue d'Élevage et Médecine Vétérinaire des Pays Tropicaux* 32, pp. 353–9.

Morel, P.C. (1959), 'Les Helminthes des Animaux Domestiques de l'Afrique Occidentale'. *Revue d'Élevage et Médecine Vétérinaire des Pays Tropicaux* 12, p. 153.

Nichols, P. (1991), 'Social Survey Methods: A Fieldguide for Development Workers'. Development Guidelines No. 6. Oxford, Oxfam.

Packard-Winkler, M. (1989), 'Putting the Culture Back into Development'. *The Fletcher Forum of World Affairs* 13, pp. 251–270.

Penning de Vries, F.W.T. (1983), 'The Productivity of Sahelian Rangelands—A Summary Report'. Pastoral Development Network Paper No. 15b. London, Overseas Development Institute.

Remillard, R.L., C. Stem, K.E. Michel, L. Engleking and A.E. Sollod (1990), 'Oral Vitamin A Supplementation to Debilitated Cattle during Sahelian Dry Seasons'. *Preventive Veterinary Medicine* 9, pp. 173–83.

Rhoades, R.E. (1986), Breaking New Ground: Agricultural Anthropology. In *Practicing Development Anthropology*. E.C. Green (ed.), pp. 22–67. Boulder, CO, Westview Press.

Salzman, P.C. (1983), 'The Psychology of Nomads'. *Nomadic Peoples* 12, pp. 48–55.

Schillhorn van Veen, T.W. (1980), 'Fascioliasis (*Fasciola gigantica*), in West Africa: A Review'. *Veterinary Bulletin* 50, pp. 529–33.

Schillhorn van Veen, T.W., R.A.O. Shonekan and J.P. Fabiyi (1975), 'A Host Parasite Checklist of Helminth Parasites of Domestic Animals in Northern Nigeria'. *Bulletin of Animal Health and Production in Africa* 23, pp. 269–88.

Schwabe C.W. and I.M. Kuojok (1981), 'Practices and Beliefs of the Traditional Dinka Healer in Relation to the Provision of Modern Medical and Veterinary Services for the Southern Sudan'. *Human Organization* 40, pp. 231–38.

Scott, M.F. and B. Gormley (1980), The Animal of Friendship (*Habbanaae*): An Indigenous Model of Sahelian Pastoral Development in Niger. In *Indigenous Knowledge Systems and Development*. D. Brokensha, D.M. Warren and O. Werner (eds.), pp. 92–110. Lanham, MD, University Press of America.

Skinner, E.P. (1989), 'Development in Africa: A Cultural Perspective'. *The Fletcher Forum of World Affairs* 13, pp. 205–16.
Sollod, A.E. (1990), 'Rainfall, Biomass and the Pastoral Economy of Niger'. *Journal of Arid Environments* 18, pp. 97–107.
Sollod, A.E. and C. Stem (1991), 'Appropriate Animal Health Information Systems for Nomadic and Transhumant Livestock Populations in Africa'. *Revue Scientifique Technique de l'Office Internationale des Épizooties* 10, pp. 89–101.
Sollod, A.E., K. Wolfgang and J.E. Knight (1984), Veterinary Anthropology: Interdisciplinary Methods in Pastoral Systems Research. In *Livestock Development in Subsaharan Africa: Constraints, Prospects, Policy*. J.R. Simpson and P. Evangelou (eds.), pp. 285–302. Boulder, CO, Westview Press.
Sprent, J.F.A. (1946), 'Studies on the Life History of *Bunostomum phlebotomum* (Railliet, 1900), a Hookworm Parasite of Cattle'. *Parasitology* 37, p. 192.
Stem, C. (1985), Vetscout: Animal Disease Monitoring through Veterinary Auxiliaries in Central Niger. Paper presented at the Workshop on Monitoring Change in Pastoral Livestock Systems, 4th International Symposium on Veterinary Epidemiology and Economics, Kuala Lumpur and Singapore.
—— (1986a), *Clinical Field Trials. Evaluation of Interventions: Salmonellosis in Camels, Coccidiosis in Sheep, Louse in Drought Stricken Animals, Bacterial Pneumonia in Sheep*. Tahoua, Niger Integrated Livestock Production Project/Tufts University/USAID.
—— (1986b), *Vitamin A Studies*. Tahoua, Niger Integrated Livestock Production Project/Tufts University/USAID.
—— (1986c), *Final Report of the Epidemiology and Reproduction Advisor*. Tahoua, Niger Integrated Livestock Production Project/Tufts University/USAID.
Stryker, J.D. (1984), Land Use Development in the Pastoral Zone of West Africa. In *Livestock Development in Subsaharan Africa: Constraints, Prospects, Policy*. J.R. Simpson and P. Evangelou (eds.), pp. 175–85. Boulder, CO, Westview Press.
Swift, J. and A. Maliki (1984), 'A Cooperative Development Experiment among Nomadic Herders in Niger'. Pastoral Development Network Paper No. 18c. London, Overseas Development Institute.
Tager-Kagan, P. (1984), 'Résultats d'Enquêtes sur les Helminthiases du Dromadaire dans le Département de Zinder (République du Niger), leur Évolution dans l'Année—moyens de Lutte'. *Revue d' Élevage et Médecine Vétérinaire des Pays Tropicaux* 37, pp. 19–25.
USDA (United States Department of Agriculture) (1981), 'Food Problems and Prospects in Sub-Saharan Africa: The Decade of the 1980s'. USDA Economic Research Service Foreign Agricultural Research Report No. 166. Washington, DC, USDA.
Vassiliades, G. (1981), 'Parasitisme Gastro-intestinal chez le Mouton au Sénégal'. *Revue d'Élevage et Médecine Vétérinaire des Pays Tropicaux* 34, pp. 169–77.
—— (1984), 'Essais de Traitement Anthelminthique par le Fenbendazole chez les Ovins en Zone Sahélienne au Sénégal'. *Revue d'Élevage et Médecine Vétérinaire des Pays Tropicaux* 37, pp. 293–8.
Vassiliades, G. and S.M. Toure (1975), 'Essais de Traitement des Strongyloses Digestives du Mouton en Zone Tropicale par le Tartrate de Morantel'. *Revue d'Élevage et Médecine Vétérinaire des Pays Tropicaux* 28, pp. 481–9.
Werner, O. and G.M. Schoepfle (1987), *Systematic Fieldwork: Foundations of Ethnography and Interviewing (Vol. 1)*, and *Systematic Fieldwork: Ethnographic Analysis and Data Management (Vol. 2)*. Newbury Park, CA, SAGE Publications.
White, C. (1986), 'Food Shortages and Seasonality in Wodaaɓe Communities in Niger'. *Institute for Development Studies Bulletin* 17, pp. 19–25
—— (1987), Changing Animal Ownership and Access to Land among the Wodaaɓe (Fulani), of Central Niger. Paper presented at the Workshop on Changing Rights in Property and Pastoral Development, University of Manchester, Manchester, UK.
Wolfgang, K. (1983), An Ethnoveterinary Study of Cattle Health Care by the Fulbe Herders of South Central Upper Volta. Thesis, Hampshire College, Amherst, MA.

19. Collection and use of ethnoveterinary data in community-based animal health programmes

Grandin, B.E. (1984a), Livestock Transactions Data Collection. In *Proceedings of the ILCA/IDRC Workshop on Pastoral Systems Research in Sub-Saharan Africa, March 1983*. Addis Ababa, International Livestock Centre for Africa.

———— (1984b), Towards a Maasai Ethnoveterinary. Nairobi, ILCA. Unpublished manuscript.

———— (1988), *Wealth Ranking in Smallholder Communities: A Field Manual*. London, IT Publications Ltd.

———— (n.d.), Restocking of Long-term Destitute Pastoralists: Some Lessons from Kenya Boran in Isiolo District. Draft manuscript.

Grandin, B.E., R. Thampy and J. Young (eds.), (1991), *Village Animal Health Care: A Community-based Approach to Livestock Development in Kenya*. London, IT Publications Ltd.

Iles, K. (1991), *The Oxfam/ITDG Livestock Project Samburu: A Report of a Base-line Study and Implications for Project Design*. Rugby, UK, ITDG.

McCorkle, C.M. (1994) *Ethnoveterinary R&D and Gender in the ITDG/Kenya Rural Agricultural and Pastoral Development Programme*. Nairobi, ITDG.

Njeru, F. (1991), *Some Features of Smallholder Livestock Production in Lowland Areas of Machakos District and Their Implications for a Livestock Programme with the Utooni Development Group*. Rugby, UK, ITDG.

Sperling, L. (1987), The Labor Organization of Samburu Pastoralism. Thesis, McGill University, Montreal.

Wanyama, J. (in progress–a), ITDG/OXFAM Ethnoveterinary Treatment Study among the Samburu and Turkan Communities in Baragoi. Nairobi, ITDG.

———— (in progress–b), Ranking of Confidently Treated Diseases among Samburu and Turkana. Nairobi, ITDG.

Young, J. (1987), *Livestock Production in Lower Meru and Implications for a Livestock Programme at Kamujine Farmers' Centre*. Rugby, UK, ITDG.

———— (1988), *Some Aspects of Livestock Ownership, Use, Constraints to Production, and Traditional Ethnoveterinary Knowledge among the Pokot of Nginyang Division, Baringo District*. Rugby, UK, ITDG.

20. Methods and results from a study of local knowledge of cattle diseases in coastal Kenya

Barnett, S.F. (1968), Theileriosis. In *Infectious Blood Diseases of Man and Animals*. D. Weinman and M. Ristic (eds.), pp. 269–328. New York, Academic Press.

Buruchara, R. (1988), Agriculture and Animal Production. In *District Socio-Cultural Profiles: Kilifi District*. pp. 50–67. Nairobi, Kenya Ministry of Planning and National Development and University of Nairobi Institute of African Studies.

Delehanty, J. (1990), Local Knowledge of Cattle Diseases in Kaloleni Division, Kilifi District, Kenya. Nairobi, ILRAD (unpublished report).

Grandin, B. (1985), Towards a Maasai Ethnoveterinary. Nairobi, ILCA (unpublished paper).

ILCA (International Livestock Centre for Africa) (1989), Cattle Census, Kaloleni Division, Kilifi District, Kenya. Mtwapa, Kenya, ILCA. Unpublished report.

ITDG (Intermediate Technology Development Group) (1989), Pokot Knowledge of Livestock Diseases. EPAP/KFFHC Livestock Project Survey. Appendix 2, Ethnoveterinary Data. Rugby, UK, ITDG. Unpublished report.

Irvin, A.D. and D.M. Mwamachi (1983), 'Clinical and Diagnostic Features of East Coast Fever (*Theileria parva*) Infection of Cattle'. *Veterinary Record* 113, pp. 192–8.

Jaetzold, R. and H. Schmidt (1982), *Farm Management Handbook of Kenya. Vol. IIc: East Kenya*. Nairobi, Kenya Ministry of Agriculture.

KMALD (Kenya Ministry of Agriculture and Livestock Development) (1986), Background information on Farmer Circumstances in Chonyi Location, Kaloleni Division, Kilifi District. Mtwapa, Kenya, KMALD. Unpublished report.

McCorkle, C.M. (1986), 'An Introduction to Ethnoveterinary Research and Development'. *Journal of Ethnobiology* 6, pp. 129–49.

—— (1989), Veterinary Anthropology. *Human Organization* 48, pp. 156–62.

McCorkle, C.M. and E. Mathias-Mundy (1990), Ethnoveterinary Medicine in Africa. In *Proceedings of the Eighth Small ruminants CRSP Scientific Workshop, 7–8 March, ILRAD, Nairobi.* pp. 45–67.

Maloo, S. (1990), Serological Results. Mtwapa, Kenya, ILCA. Unpublished report.

Mathu, G. (1988), History. In *District Socio-Cultural Profiles: Kilifi District.* pp. 4–20. Kenya Ministry of Planning and National Development, and University of Nairobi Institute of African Studies.

Mochoge, B. (1987), Agriculture. In *Kwale District Socio-Cultural Profile.* pp. 61–77. Kenya Ministry of Planning and National Development, and University of Nairobi Institute of African Studies.

Mukhebi, A. (1991), The Economic Impact of Theileriosis and its Control in Africa. In *The Epidemiology of Theileriosis in Africa.* R.A.I. Norval, B.D. Perry and A.S. Young (eds.) London and San Diego, Academic Press.

Ohta, I. (1984), 'Symptoms are Classified into Diagnostic Categories: Turkana's View of Livestock Diseases'. *African Studies Monographs* 3 (Supplement), pp. 71–93.

Wolfgang, K. and A. Sollod (1986), Traditional Veterinary Medical Practice by Twareg Herders in Central Niger. Niamey, Niger and North Grafton, MA, Integrated Livestock Development Project, Niger Ministry of Animal Resources, and Tufts University, School of Veterinary Medicine. Unpublished report.

21. Veterinary science and savvy among the Ferlo Fulße

Bonfiglioli, A. Maliki (1990), West African Pastoralists' Knowledge of the Environment and Animal Behavior. Paper presented at the First International Symposium on Sustainable Agriculture, New Delhi.

Bonfiglioli, A. Maliki and Y.D. Diallo, with the collaboration of S. Fagerberg-Diallo (1988), *Kisal: Production et Survie au Ferlo.* Dakar, Oxfam.

Diallo, Y.D. (1989a), *Nguurndam Ferlaŋkooɓe: Renndo, Ngaynaakam e Demal (Life of the People in the Ferlo: Society, Herding Practices and Agricultural Techniques).* Dakar, Goomu Winndiyaŋkooɓe Demɗe Ngenndiije (Group for the Promotion of Publishing in National Languages).

—— (1989b) *Nguurndam Ferlaŋkooɓe: Nabbuuji Na'i (Life of the People in the Ferlo: Cattle Diseases).* Dakar, Goomu Winndiyankooße Demɗe Ngenndiije.

22. Traditional and re-applied veterinary medicine in East Africa

Beaman-Mbaya, V. and S.I. Muhammed (1976), 'Antibiotic Action of *Solanum incanum* L'. *Antimicrobial Agents and Chemotherapy* 9, pp. 920–24.

Budavari, S., M.J. O'Neil, A. Smith and P.E. Heckelman (1989), *The Merck Index: An Encyclopedia of Chemicals, Drugs, and Biologicals (11th edition).* Rahway, NJ, Merck & Co.

Chhabra, S.C., J.F. Shao and E.N. Mshiu (1982), 'Antifungal Activity among Traditionally Used Herbs in Tanzania'. *The Dar es Salaam Medical Journal* 9, pp. 68–73.

Chhabra, S.C., J. F. Shao, E.N. Mshiu and F.C. Uisu (1981), 'Screening of Tanzanian Medicinal Plants for Antimicrobial Activity'. *Journal of African Medicinal Plants* 4, pp. 93–8.

Chhabra, S.C., F.C. Uisu and E.N. Mshiu (1983), Unpublished data. Traditional Medicine Research Unit, Muhimbili Medical Centre, Dar es Salaam.

—— (1984), 'Phytochemical Screening of Medicinal Plants I'. *Journal of Ethnopharmacology* 11, pp. 157–79.

Goutarel, R., X. Monseur and J. LeMen (1962), 'On the Alkaloids of *Diplorrhynchus mossambicensis*'. *Chemical Abstracts* 56, p. 7373c.

Gupta, S.S., A.W. Bhagwat and A.K. Ram (1972), 'Cardiac Stimulant Activity of the Saponin of *Achyranthes aspera*'. *Indian Journal of Medical Research* 60, pp. 462–71.

Haerdi, F. (1964), Die Eingeborenen-Heilpflanzen des Ulanga-Distriktes Tanganjikas (Ostafrika). Afrikanische Heilpflanzen/Plantes Médicinales Africaines. *Acta Tropica (Supplementum)* 8, pp. 1–278.

Hedberg, I., O. Hedberg, P.J. Madati, K.E. Mshigeni, E.N. Mshiu and G. Samuelsson (1982), 'Inventory of Plants Used in Traditional Medicine in Tanzania. I: Plants of the Families Acanthaceae-Cucurbitaceae'. *Journal of Ethnopharmacology* 6, pp. 29–60.

Hegnauer, R. (1963), *Chemotaxonomie der Pflanzen: Eine Übersicht über die Verbreitung und die systematische Bedeutung der Pflanzenstoffe. Vol. 2: Monocotyledonae.* Basel, Birkhäuser Verlag.

——— (1973), *Chemotaxonomie der Pflanzen: Eine Übersicht über die Verbreitung und die systematische Bedeutung der Pflanzenstoffe. Vol. 4: Rafflesiaceae-Zygophyllaceae.* Basel, Birkhäuser Verlag.

Hudson, J.B. (1990), *Antiviral Compounds from Plants.* Boca Raton, FL, CRC Press.

ICRAF (International Council for Research in Agroforestry) (1986), *Entries of Database on Woody Plants with Pesticidal Properties.* Nairobi, International Council for Research in Agroforestry.

Kapoor, V.K. and H. Singh (1967), Investigation of *Achyranthes aspera*. Indian Journal of Pharmacy 29, pp. 285–8.

Kokwaro, J.O. (1976), *Medicinal Plants of East Africa.* Kampala, East African Literature Bureau.

Mathias-Mundy, E. and C.M. McCorkle (1989), *Ethnoveterinary Medicine: An Annotated Bibliography.* Bibliographies in Technology and Social Change No. 6. Center for Indigenous Knowledge and Agricultural and Rural Development (CIKARD). Ames, Iowa State University Research Foundation.

Milks, H.J. (1917), *Practical Veterinary Pharmacology and Therapeutics.* New York, Macmillan.

Perry, L.M. (1980), *Medicinal Plants of East and Southeast Asia: Attributed Properties and Uses.* Cambridge, MA, MIT Press.

Raymond-Hamet (1969), 'Total Extract of *Diplorrhynchus mossambicensis* Useful as Sympatolytic'. *Chemical Abstracts* 71, p. 53587u.

Riley, B.W. and D. Brokensha (1988), *The Mbeere in Kenya. II: Botanical Identities and Uses.* Lanham, MD, University Press of America.

Stauffacher, D. (1961), 'Alkaloide aus *Diplorrhyncus condylocarpon mossambicensis*'. *Helvitica Chimica Acta* 44, pp. 2006–15.

Sur, R.N. and S.N. Pradham (1964), 'Cissampelos Alkaloids. I: Action of Hayatine Derivatives on the Central Nervous System of Cats and Dogs'. *Archives Internationales de Pharmacodynamie et de Thérapie* 152, pp. 106–114.

Trease, G.E. and W.C. Evans (1983), *Pharmacognosy (12th edition).* London, Baillèire Tindall.

Tyler, V.E., L.R. Brady and J.E. Robbers (1988), *Pharmacognosy (9th edition).* Philadelphia, Lea & Febiger.

Watt, J.M. and M.G. Breyer-Brandwijk (1962), *Medicinal and Poisonous Plants of Southern and Eastern Africa (2nd edition).* Edinburgh, E.&S. Livingstone.

23. Field trials in ethnoveterinary R&D: Lessons from the Andes

Agrawal, A. (1995), 'Dismantling the Divide Between Indigenous and Scientific Knowledge'. *Development and Change* 26, pp. 413–39.

Arévalo, F. and H. Bazalar (1989a), Eficacia Antihelmíntica de la Semilla de Zapallo. In *Estudios Etnoveterinarios en Comunidades Alto-Andinas del Perú.* H. Bazalar and C.M. McCorkle (eds.), pp. 111–18. SR–CRSP Technical Publication No. 99—Community Studies Series. Lima, Lluvia Editores for the SR–CRSP.

———— (1989b), Eficacia de la Alcachofa y Jaya-Shipita contra Alicuya (*Fasciola hepatica*). In *Estudios Etnoveterinarios en Comunidades Alto-Andinas del Perú*. H. Bazalar and C.M. McCorkle (eds.), pp. 99–108. SR–CRSP Technical Publication No. 99—Community Studies Series. Lima, Lluvia Editores for the SR–CRSP.

Bazalar, H. and C.M. McCorkle (eds.) (1989), *Estudios Etnoveterinarios en Comunidades Alto-Andinas del Perú*. SR–CRSP Technical Publication No. 99—Community Studies Series. Lima, Lluvia Editores for the SR–CRSP.

Bazalar, H. and F. Arévalo (1989), Eficacia del Utashayli contra la Falsa Garrapata (*Melophagus ovinus*). In *Estudios Etnoveterinarios en Comunidades Alto-Andinas del Perú*. H. Bazalar and C.M. McCorkle (eds.), pp. 87–95. SR–CRSP Technical Publication No. 99—Community Studies Series. Lima, Lluvia Editores for the SR–CRSP.

Blond, R.D. (ed.) (n.d.), *Partners in Research*. Davis, CA, SR–CRSP Management Entity.

Carlier, A.B. de (1981), Así Curamos en el Canipaco: Manual de Medicina del Pueblo—Medicina Tradicional del Valle del Canipaco. Huancayo: no publishing house indicated.

Chambers, R., A. Pacey and L.A. Thrupp (eds.) (1989), *Farmer First: Farmer Innovation and Agricultural Research*. London, Intermediate Technology Publications.

Córdova, P. (1981), 'Así Curamos el Ganado en el Canipaco'. *Revista Minka* 5, p. 11.

Davis, D.K. (1995), 'Gender-based Differences in the Ethnoveterinary Knowledge of Afghan Nomadic Pastoralists'. *Indigenous Knowledge and Development Monitor* 3, pp. 3–5.

Dennis, W.R., W.H. Stone and L.E. Swansen (1954), 'A New Laboratory and Field Diagnostic Test for Fluke Ova in Faeces'. *Journal of the American Veterinary Association* 124, pp. 47–50.

Fals-Borda, O. and M.A. Rahman (eds.) (1991), *Action and Knowledge: Breaking the Monopoly with Participatory Action-Research*. New York and London, Apex Press and Intermediate Technology Publications.

Farrington, J. and A. Martin (1990), 'Farmer Participation in Agricultural Research: A Review of Concepts and Practices'. Agricultural Administration Unit Occasional Paper 9. London, Overseas Development Institute. [Originally published 1988.]

Fernández, M.E. (1986), 'Particpatory-Action-Research and the Farming Systems Approach with Highland Peasants'. SR–CRSP Technical Publication No. 72. Columbia, MO, University of Missouri Department of Rural Sociology. [Also available in Spanish.]

———— (1989), 'Consideraciones para la Investigación Participativa en Comunidades Campesinas Alto-Andinas'. SR–CRSP Technical Publication No. 98—Community Studies Series. Lima, Lluvia Edtores for the SR–CRSP.

———— (1991), Participatory Research with Community-Based Farmers. In *Joining Farmers' Experiments: Experiences in Participatory Technology Development*. B. Haverkort, J. van der Kamp, and A. Waters-Bayer (eds.), pp. 77–92. London, Intermediate Technology Publications.

———— (1992), The Social Organization of Production in Community-based Agropastoralism in the Andes. In *Plants, Animals & People: Agropastoral Systems Research*. C.M. McCorkle (ed.), pp. 99–108. Boulder, CO, Westview Press.

Fernández, M.E. and A.A. Huaylinos S. (1986), *Sistemas de Producción Agropecuarios y Zonas Agroecológicas del Valle del Mantaro*. Lima, Ediciones Betaprint for the SR–CRSP.

———— (1989), Participatory Technology Validation in Highland Communities of Peru. In *Farmer First: Farmer Innovation and Agricultural Research*. R. Chambers, A. Pacey and L.A. Thrupp (eds.), pp. 146–50. London, Intermediate Technology Publications.

Grupo Yanapai (1989), *Taller Interinstitucional sobre la Investigación Acción Participativa en la Produccióm Agropecuaria de Comunidades*. Lima, Lluvia Editores.

Haverkort, B., J. van der Kamp and A. Waters-Bayer (eds.) (1991), Joining Farmers'

Experiments: Experiences in Participatory Technology Development. London, Intermediate Technology Publications.

Hiemstra, W., C. Reijntjes and E. van der Werf (eds.) (1992), *Let Farmers Judge: Experiences in Assessing the Sustainability of Agriculture.* London, Intermediate Technology Publications for ILEIA.

IIED (International Institute for Environment and Development) (1995), 'Critical Reflections From [sic] Practice'. PLA Notes—Notes on Participatory Learning and Action (Formerly RRA Notes) No. 24. London, IIED Sustainable Agriculture Programme.

McCorkle, C.M. (1982), 'Management of Animal Health and Disease in an Indigenous Andean Community'. SR–CRSP Technical Publication No. 5. Columbia, MO, University of Missouri Department of Rural Sociology.

——— (1987), Punas, Pastures, and Fields: Grazing Strategies and the Agropastoral Dialectic in an Indigenous Andean Community. In *Arid Land Use Strategies and Risk Management in the Andes: A Regional Anthropological Perspective.* D. Browman (ed.), pp. 57–79. Boulder, CO, Westview Press.

——— (1994), Farmer Innovation in Niger. Studies in Technology & Social Change No. 21. Ames, IA, Iowa State University Research Foundation in collaboration with the Center for Indigenous Knowledge for Agriculture and Rural Development (CIKARD) and the Leiden Ethnosystems and Development Programme (LEAD) of the Institute of Cultural and Social Studies, University of Leiden, The Netherlands.

——— (1995), 'Back to the Future: Lessons from Ethnoveterinary RD&E for Studying and Applying Local Knowledge'. *Agriculture and Human Values* 12, pp. 52–80.

McCorkle, C.M. (ed.) (1990), *Improving Andean Sheep and Alpaca Production: Recommendations from a Decade of Research in Peru.* Columbia, MO, University of Missouri Printing Services.

McCorkle, C.M. (ed.) (1992), *Plants, Animals & People: Agropastoral Systems Research.* Boulder, CO, Westview Press.

Mathias-Mundy, E. and C.M. McCorkle (1989), *Ethnoveterinary Medicine: An Annotated Bibliography. Bibliographies in Technology and Social Change No. 6.* Center for Indigenous Knowledge and Agricultural and Rural Development (CIKARD). Ames, Iowa State University Research Foundation.

Okali, C., J. Sumberg and J. Farrington (1994), *Farmer Participatory Research: Rhetoric and Reality.* London, Intermediate Technology Publications on behalf of the Overseas Development Institute.

Abbreviations and acronyms

AD	Anno Domini
AERLS	Agriculture Extension and Research Liason Service
AFT	An Foras Taluntais (Irish)
ARTAI	An Roinn Talmhaichta Agus lascaigh (Irish)
ATP	Adenosine Triphosphate
BC	Before Christ
bq	Bequerels
CAR	Central African Republic
CATIE	Centro Agronómico Tropical de Investigación y Enseñanza
CBAHP	Community-based Animal Health Program
CBPP	Contagious Bovine Pleuropneumonia
CCPP	Contagious Caprine Pleuropneumonia
CIKARD	Center for Indigenous Knowledge for Agriculture and Rural Development
CTA	Technical Centre for Agricultural and Rural Cooperation
DDT	Dichloro-diphenyl-trichloroethane (Dicophan)
ECF	East Coast Fever
EEC	European Economic Community (now European Union)
EIG	Ethnoveterinary Interview Guide
ENDA	Environment and Development in the Third World
EPI	Expanded Programme of Immunization
ER&D	Ethnoveterinary Research and Devlopment
ESEP	Epidemiology and Socioeconomics Program
FAO	Food and Agriculture Organization
FMD	Foot and Mouth Disease
g	Grams
GATT	General Agreement on Tariffs and Trade
GIPLLN	Groupe d'Initiative pour le Promotion du Livre en Langues Nationales
GIS	Geographic Information System
GTZ	German Agency for Technical Cooperation
ha	Hectares
HPI	Heifer Project International
ICRAF	International Centre for Research in Agroforestry
IDRC	International Development Research Centre (of Canada)
IEMVT	Institut d'Élevage et de Médécine Vétérinaire des Pays Tropicaux
IFAD	International Fund for Agricultural Development
IFAN	Institute Francophone d'Afrique Noire
IIRR	International Institute for Rural Reconstruction
ILCA	International Livestock Centre for Africa
ILRAD	International Laboratory for Research on Animal Disease
INR	Indian Rupees
IPAL	Integrated Project on Arid Lands
ISS	Instituo Superiore di Sanità
ITDG	Intermediate Technology Development Group
IVITA	Instituto Veterinario de Investigaciones Tropicales y de Altura

KARI	Kenya Agricultural Research Institute
kg	Kilograms
KLP	Kenya Livestock Programme
km	Kilometres
KMALD	Kenya Ministry of Agriculture and Livestock Development
l	Litres
L.	Linnean System
LR	*Leptadenia reticulata*
m	Meters
ml	Millilitres
mm	Millimetres
NAHA	Nomadic Animal Health Auxiliary
NAPRI	Nigerian Animal Production Research Institute
NDDP	National Dairy Development Programme (Kenya)
NFA	National Farmers Association (Kenya)
NGO	Non-governmental Organization
NILPP	Niger Integrated Livestock Production Project
ODI	Overseas Development Institute (UK)
ORSTOM	L'Ofice de la Recherche Scientifique et Technique Outre-Mer
OXFAM	Oxford Committee for Famine Relief
PVTC	Project for the Validation of Technologies in Communities
R&D	Research and Development
RD&E	Research Development and Extension
RRA	Rapid Rural Appraisal
SD	Standard Deviation
SR-CRSP	Small Ruminant Collaborative Research Support Program
TM	Trademark
UK	United Kingdom
UN	United Nations
UNCTAD	United Nations Council for Trade and Development
UNESCO	United Nations Educational, Scientific and Cultural Organization
UNICEF	United Nations International Children's Emergency Fund
US	United States
(US) AID	(United States) Agency for International Development
USDA	United States Department of Agriculture
USSR	Union of Soviet Socialist Republics
UV	Ultra-violet
VRI	Veterinary Research Institute (Sri Lanka)
WAPC	Women's Agricultural Production Committee
WHO	World Health Organization

Index

forage 54–6, 65, 95, 98, 182, 248, 249
see also feed; fodder
Fouta Jalon 27
fowl cholera 160
France 10, 76–90
Fraxinus excelsoir 81
fruits 48, 130, 131, 143, 144, 152–3, 199, 257
Fulani 9, 26–8, 31, 54–9, 104, 107–9, 111, 113, 116
see also Fulɓe; Peul
Fulɓe 246–53
fumigation 30, 77, 251, 252
fungi/mushrooms 94, 98, 99, 188, 258
see also antifungal/fungicides

Gaelic 179, 181, 184, 185, 187, 188
galactagogue 139–40, 263
Gardenia gummifera 142
garlic 56, 112, 151, 152, 174, 176, 259, 260
gastrointestinal problems 58, 123, 150, 195, 197, 201, 272–3
gelatin 261, 262
gelding/castration 56, 63, 65–6, 96, 97, 116–20
geldings 93, 96–7, 98
gender 194, 196–7, 211, 224, 269, 277
see also men; women
Geranium robertianum 81, 88
Geranium spp 262
ghee 150, 151
Ghibe 117, 118
gid 184, 214
Giriama 230, 231, 232, 233
Glycyrrhiza glabra 142
Gnidia kraussiana 55
goats 56, 196, 225, 231, 259, 266
gout 152
government(s) 41–4, 51, 62, 73–4, 91, 100, 183–4, 197
see also regulations
grains 109, 180, 246
grass 29, 65, 84, 169, 185, 195, 249
grazing 29, 30, 54, 169–70, 183, 211, 248
Grewia bicolor 251
rewia hirsuta 516
Guiera senegalensis 246
Guinea 27
guineafowl 103, 104, 107, 108, 109–10, 112
Gujurat 145, 152, 153
gum arabica 262
Gumboro disease 112

haemonchosis 171, 199
Hagenia abyssinica 259
Halogeton spp 56
Harrisonia abyssinica 258
Hausa 54–9, 103–13, 131
hawk 112

hay 181, 182, 200
healers/herbalists/practitioners/specialists 33, 37–43, 51–2, 78, 86–7, 125, 138, 148, 250–1
horse doctors 62, 64, 67, 69
priests 37–40, 77, 167, 187, 189, 191
shaman 60, 62–3, 68, 70, 71, 93
heartwater disease 25, 29, 31, 212, 216, 241
Hedera helix 81
Hedychinum spicatum 156
Heeria insignis 251
Heliotropum indicum 57
hellebore 71, 80, 81
Helleborus foetidus 81
helminthosis/worms 112, 172, 220–1, 224, 234, 236, 262, 272–4
see also anthelmintic; hookworms; lung-worms; roundworms
henbane 76, 82
henna 133, 150, 151, 152
hepatic distomatosis see fasciolosis/liverfluke disease
herbs 67, 70, 125, 138–9, 141–2, 144–5, 148, 152, 252
herd/flock composition 48, 95, 107, 158, 162
herd/flock size 48, 93, 95, 107, 158, 169, 197, 238–9
herding 9, 29, 34, 94–5
Heuchera spp 70
Hidatsa 60, 61, 65–6, 71, 72
hides 62, 72, 95, 96, 97, 184, 252, 269, 270
hieroglyphs 39, 40
Holarrhena antidysenterica 142, 143, 144
holistic approaches 1, 2, 5, 72, 139, 202, 277
honey 149
hookworms 143
hooves/feet 57, 67, 71–2, 84, 98, 149, 252
see also footrot
horns/antlers 91, 96, 97, 144, 149, 151
Horse Dance 62, 63, 64, 66, 73
horseracing/racehorses 67, 68, 69
horses 30, 48, 60–74, 138
horsetail 98
HPI (Heifer Project International) 19, 256
human–animal relationships 14, 31, 44, 60–1, 63, 72–3, 91–2, 94
human health 31, 38–9, 49–54, 58–9, 72, 99–100, 187, 189
human medicine 13, 37, 39–41, 46–53, 63, 139, 256–8, 262–3, 272–4
see also comparative medicine; reciprocity
hunting 55, 91, 93
Hydnocarpus wightiana 256
Hydrilla verticillata 163
hydrogen peroxide 150
hygiene/sanitation 160, 161, 163–4, 216

Index

www.ingramcontent.com/pod-product-compliance
Lightning Source LLC
Jackson TN
JSHW011350130125
77033JS00015B/546